Frans P.G.M. van der Linden

Problems and Procedures in Dentofacial Orthopedics

Problems and Procedures in Dentofacial Orthopedics

Frans P.G.M. van der Linden, D.D.S., Ph.D.
Diplomate of the American Board of Orthodontics
Professor and Chairman
Department of Orthodontics
University of Nymegen, The Netherlands
Visiting Scientist
Center for Human Growth and Development
The University of Michigan, Ann Arbor, Michigan

John F. Jefferys, M.D., B.D.S.
Translator

quintessence books

Quintessence Publishing Co., Ltd.
Chicago, London, Berlin, Tokyo, São Paulo, Hong Kong

Library of Congress Cataloging-in-Publication Data

Linden, Frans, P.G.M. van der, 1932-
Problems and procedures in dentofacial orthopedics / Frans P.G.M. van der Linden.

p. cm. — (The Van der Linden series; 4)
Includes bibliographical references.
ISBN 0-86715-212-5
1. Orthodontics. I. Title. II. Series: Linden, Frans P.G.M. van der, 1932- Van der Linden series; 4.
[DNLM: 1. Orthodontics. WU 400 L744p]
RK521.L574 1990
617.6'43--dc20
DNLM/DLC 89-24119
for Library of Congress CIP

Typesetting, printing, and binding: Samsom-Sijthoff grafische bedrijven bv, Alphen aan den Rijn, Holland

Preface

Problems and Procedures in Dentofacial Orthopedics builds upon the three works earlier published in this series: *Development of the Dentition, Facial Growth and Facial Orthopedics*, and *Diagnosis and Treatment Planning in Dentofacial Orthopedics.* In the latter volume, orthodontic anomalies were considered principally as single entities, as deviations in different parts of the face. In outlining standard therapies little was said about the presence of a combination of anomalies in function, in development of the dentition, and in facial growth.

In *Problems and Procedures in Dentofacial Orthopedics* the emphasis is on complex situations where discrepancies in tooth position, occlusion, and jaw relationships are involved with or without combination with yet other disturbances. The approach has been directed at clinical situations as they are found in practice. The integration of knowledge of distinct anomalies has been employed as a tool to penetrate the obscurities of complex situations.

The content and arrangement of the 20 chapters are based, on the one hand, on development from birth to maturity and, on the other hand, on a selection of the problems and procedures that present most often. Further, the variation in dental development—particularly concerning the changing of the dentition in the anterior and posterior regions—as it affects the recognition of problems is thoroughly illuminated. This part (Chapters 2 to 7) is derived from the previous book *Transition of the Human Dentition* by the author together with P.J.M.R. Bakker and H.J.W. Wassenberg.

Problems and Procedures in Dentofacial Orthopedics is written primarily for dental students and dentists. Nevertheless, the book contains sensible and useful information for orthodontists (and oral surgeons). The nature of the text assumes that a general practitioner should be able to perform simple orthodontic treatment and be able to recognise complicated cases and refer them to an orthodontist or oral surgeon. Generally, no hard and fast borderlines have been drawn as to the areas of competence or fields of operation for anyone; the variation in knowledge and technical skills of general practitioners precludes this.

Relatively little consideration is given to the technical performance of orthodontic therapy. Only occasionally is detailed reference made. The accent lies on theoretical bases that change less and change less rapidly than do treatment techniques. Above all, most faulty decisions and errors in clinical orthodontics are due to inadequate theoretical knowledge, not lack of practical ability.

It is hoped that the contents of this book will lead to an enhancement of the insight that is essential for the recognition of complex orthodontic situations, and result, when treatment is undertaken, in its application in the correct manner, in the most appropriate phase of development, as simply as is possible, and with the best results.

The author wishes to acknowledge the expertise of Henry C.M. Reckers and Jos L.M. van de Kamp in preparing the illustrations that appear in this book.

A number of colleagues have been willing to comment on the manuscript and offer suggestions for improvements. Most advice for changes has been followed, through which the content of the book has improved. For this the author is most indebted to the following:

Drs. P.G.F.C.M. Battistuzzi, H. Boersma, C. Booy, R.C.W. Burgersdijk, C. Carels, H.S. Duterloo, H.P.M. Freihofer, J.F. Jefferys, A.M. Kuijpers-Jagtman, N.E.A. Myrberg, B. Prahl-Andersen, and H.H. Renggli.
These remarks do not imply that the persons mentioned support every opinion presented in this work. Indeed, only the author is responsible for the content.

Contents

Introduction

Usually, the development of the dentition is described in terms of the normal sequence of events from birth to maturity. Little is said about the many variations, including those that lead to a good end result. In practice one is often confronted by conditions of the dentition that do not correspond with the normal picture. It is then not easy to tell if one is dealing with divergent development and if so, if this will deteriorate further or indeed will improve. A complex of factors is involved in the situation. In order to know if it is or is not desirable to intervene, a good comprehension of the normal and abnormal development of the dentition is essential. For this reason Chapters 2 to 7 are devoted to this theme. Only in subsequent chapters are commonly presenting problems and procedures appropriate to them taken into account.

The transition of the incisors and posterior teeth, including the canines, is particularly critical. Much orthodontic treatment is begun during the second transitional period. Furthermore, there is a tendency to begin treatment at a younger age, something that in most situations is not to the patient's advantage. One would be less inclined to go in that direction if one had a good understanding of the processes that occur in the first transitional period and knew which factors involved in the development were favourable and which ones would have an unfavourable influence.

Particularly during the periods of incisor transition, it is difficult to distinguish between normal and problematic situations. Gauging whether a normal or a distorted picture will develop is not simple. It is important to be able to do this at the right time because sometimes interceptive measures without the use of orthodontic appliances can achieve the necessary objective.

The more the development of the dentition and facial growth has progressed, the easier it is to estimate what end result can be expected. To the extent that development has advanced, the uncertainty in prediction decreases; the possibilities for guiding the development reduce to a comparable degree. The best results can be obtained by making use of the possibilities of influencing the development of the dentition and facial growth and by calling upon the mechanism nature has provided for that purpose. Orthodontic guidance and therapy on that biologic basis is the most justifiable intervention.

In a number of chapters the comprehensive approach to prevention of aberrations in the dentition, facial morphology, and function is dealt with in detail. Division of problems into parts has considerable didactic value, particularly when the necessary insight has yet to be acquired. In clinical situations one seldom encounters a simple problem on its own. Usually one is confronted by a combination of anomalies. In discussing problems, therefore, an integrated approach is used as the basis and takes the situation in practice as its model.

In writing this book it was assumed that the reader would be familiar with the contents of the previous works in this series. This applies in particular to *Diagnosis and Treatment Planning in Dentofacial Orthopedics*, which deals with many fundamental principles and also clinical aspects such as interceptive treatment.
Orthodontics is not a simple professional area. To practise it well demands a strong theoretical background, the gift of observation, ability to make deductions and combine and integrate details, and to think on a long-term basis. It is necessary to have a good feeling for timing, insight as to whether or not to intervene and when to do so, and the technical skill to execute simple and complex treatment. As well, experience and breadth and vigour of intellect play a role in professional performance.
As important as any other attribute of an orthodontist is the capacity to develop empathy with mostly young patients and their parents under often demanding and sometimes difficult circumstances.
Possession of the above qualities, potential, and skills is not the destiny of every dentist. It is unrealistic not to recognise the great individual variations that exist in that respect and not to accept the inherent consequences. It is of course the responsibility of the practising dentist to know himself or herself and to be objective enough to assess personal abilities and draw sensible conclusions about what he or she can achieve in a terrain where not every dentist can (learn to) practise adequately.

Chapter 1

Problems from Birth to the Transition of the Incisors

1.1 Introduction

In the first year after birth orofacial structures show marked growth and development. The relatively small lower part of the face increases greatly in size. Jaw growth in the first 6 months after birth provides sufficient space for the originally overlapping and rotated deciduous incisors and canines to arrive in good alignment alongside each other.

Development of the dentition and eruption of the deciduous teeth occur in conjunction with a considerable increase in height of the jaws and with increase in size of the alveolar processes. The tongue, which in the infant lies across the maxillary and mandibular alveolar processes, becomes contained within the arches.

The problems described in this chapter are sometimes noticed by the child and his or her parent(s), sometimes by the family doctor or dentist. They are dealt with in the following order: deciduous teeth present at birth, troublesome emergence of deciduous teeth, thumb-sucking and finger-sucking, use of dummies, injuries and loss of deciduous teeth, lateral forced bites, reversed overbites, and serious congenital anomalies.

1.2 Deciduous teeth present at birth

Children are rarely born with teeth already emerged (natal teeth, approximately 1:1,000). Teeth emerging in the first month seem to occur even less frequently (neonatal teeth). However, this impression is probably incorrect, because deciduous teeth present at birth would usually be recorded, whereas subsequent early emergence is less likely to be noticed. Both situations principally involve the mandibular central and lateral incisors; only very occasionally will a maxillary incisor be involved. It is very rare indeed for deciduous molars and canines to be found in the mouth at birth or soon afterwards.[25,32,98,127,130]

Such early teeth usually have little or no root formation. The crowns often are badly formed, small, conical, yellowish in colour, and hypoplastic in their enamel and dentine. The teeth are not firmly fixed, which is understandable because they cannot yet form an attachment between bone and tooth: there is, of course, no root yet.

It is likely that the presence of deciduous teeth in the mouth at birth is due to a genetically determined laying down of the germs of the relevant teeth close to the occlusal aspect of the jaw. They can be associated with gingivitis and tongue damage and can cause distress during breast-feeding, both for the child and the mother (nipple trauma). They often exfoliate as the result of forces applied during feeding or otherwise, with some danger of inhalation. Possibly the danger of inhalation is more imaginary than real; there is in fact no case on record where inhalation has occurred.[98,202] If advice and help are asked for, it depends mainly on the quality of the tooth and its mobility as to whether or not it should be ground down or removed. In this connection the root formation and attachment to the alveolar bone are deciding factors. The later they have emerged the more reasonable it is to retain them. Where teeth are reasonably firm and look clinically acceptable, sharp corners can be rounded, thus largely eliminating the problems. If they are very mobile and there is a likelihood that they will exfoliate or that the discomfort will interfere with feeding, then removal is indicated. Removal is technically simple but for the first 10 days after birth there is a possibility of excessive bleeding. During the first weeks there exists a physiological hypoprothrombinaemia that becomes eliminated when the intestinal flora of the infant begin to produce vitamin K. Excessive bleeding in these circumstances can be dealt with by administering vitamin K.[73,130]
Parents should be informed of the implications of extraction. Fortunately the consequences usually are unimportant. After very early loss of deciduous central incisors it appears that at the age of 5 to 5.5 years the space in the involved part of the dental arch is not demonstrably smaller than in normal cases.[66] When there is a very early loss of deciduous canines and molars, and also lateral incisors, the development of the dentition can be unfavourably influenced.[123]

1.3 Troublesome emergence of deciduous teeth

Before teeth emerge a fusion takes place between the dental and oral epithelium, which enables the tooth to perforate the gingiva without ulceration. For some children emergence of their deciduous teeth occurs without difficulty. But for the majority, local symptoms of differing degrees of severity develop. A few days before emergence the tissues overlying the tooth swell and redden. The child shows signs of local irritation, wants to rub the offending gum with fingers or anything handy, and drools frequently. The gingivae over the place where the tooth will appear are blanched. This corresponds with the keratinization of the fused dental and oral epithelium. After emergence, the gingivae retract, the crown comes into view, and the irritation disappears. Many remedies have been tried to counteract local and supposed general symptoms related to emerging deciduous teeth. In general, there are more disadvantages than advantages to such ministrations. For example, a high concentration of aspirin in a salve can even produce burning and ulceration of the gingivae.[30] A rubber ring is the best thing that can be used, because it is easy to clean, is too large to swallow, and will not damage the gingivae. This conclusion is based on the obvious relief provided by just rubbing the painful place.[127]

1.4 Thumb-sucking and finger-sucking

Thumb-sucking and finger-sucking should be considered normal in the first years of childhood. The desire to suck is inborn; sucking provides comfort, promotes sleep, and quiets the infant.[100]
Although thumb-sucking and finger-sucking can lead to an open bite and can alter the form of the alveolar process locally, these effects are temporary if the habit ceases before the transition of the incisors.
When sucking is indulged in frequently, intensively, and for long periods, the morphology of the facial skeleton can be negatively influenced in Angle Class II/1 anomalies. Moreover, the lower lip can come to lie behind the maxillary incisors and so provide an unfavourable local environment. But the situation is seldom so serious that giving up the habit is of great importance in early childhood.
Should it be desirable to give up the habit, one must set to work conservatively and gain the willing and active cooperation of the child. The different approaches to this problem are discussed in Volume 3 of this series.[226]

1.5 Use of dummies

Giving a dummy to a baby can prevent development of a thumb-sucking or finger-sucking habit. Sucking the dummy has comparable benefits of comforting and helping the infant to sleep without introducing significant external forces into the oral environment. However, if the child has already found his or her thumb or fingers, it will not be easy to employ the dummy. Because not all babies suck their thumbs, one should only introduce a baby to a dummy if by his or her actions shortly after birth it is clear that he or she does wish to suck a thumb or fingers.
Use of a dummy involves fewer disadvantages than thumb-sucking. The influence on the dentition is more limited and that on the facial skeleton is nil. This is principally because use of a dummy falls off rapidly with age. Almost half of the children who use a dummy have permanently given it up by the age of 4 years.[116]
Dummies should be given to children who show a desire to suck something and have a hereditary predisposition to a Class II/1 anomaly. Whenever one of the parents, and certainly if both, has or did have a Class II/1 anomaly, it is sensible before their child is born to advocate the use of a dummy and explain why.
Dipping a dummy in sugary things will lead to widespread caries. Fortunately, practices such as dipping dummies in brandy and sugar seem to have become unfashionable; still, misinformed yet well-meaning parents do not recognise the dangers of fruit syrups. For that reason parents should specifically be warned of the consequences of offering infants continual access to a feeding bottle containing sugary drinks or milk, something that is done for no other reason than to offer comfort.

1.6 Injury and loss of deciduous teeth

Particularly between the ages of 1.5 to 2.5 years, when children learn to walk and investigate the environment, they often fall, and injuries mount up. Most damage to

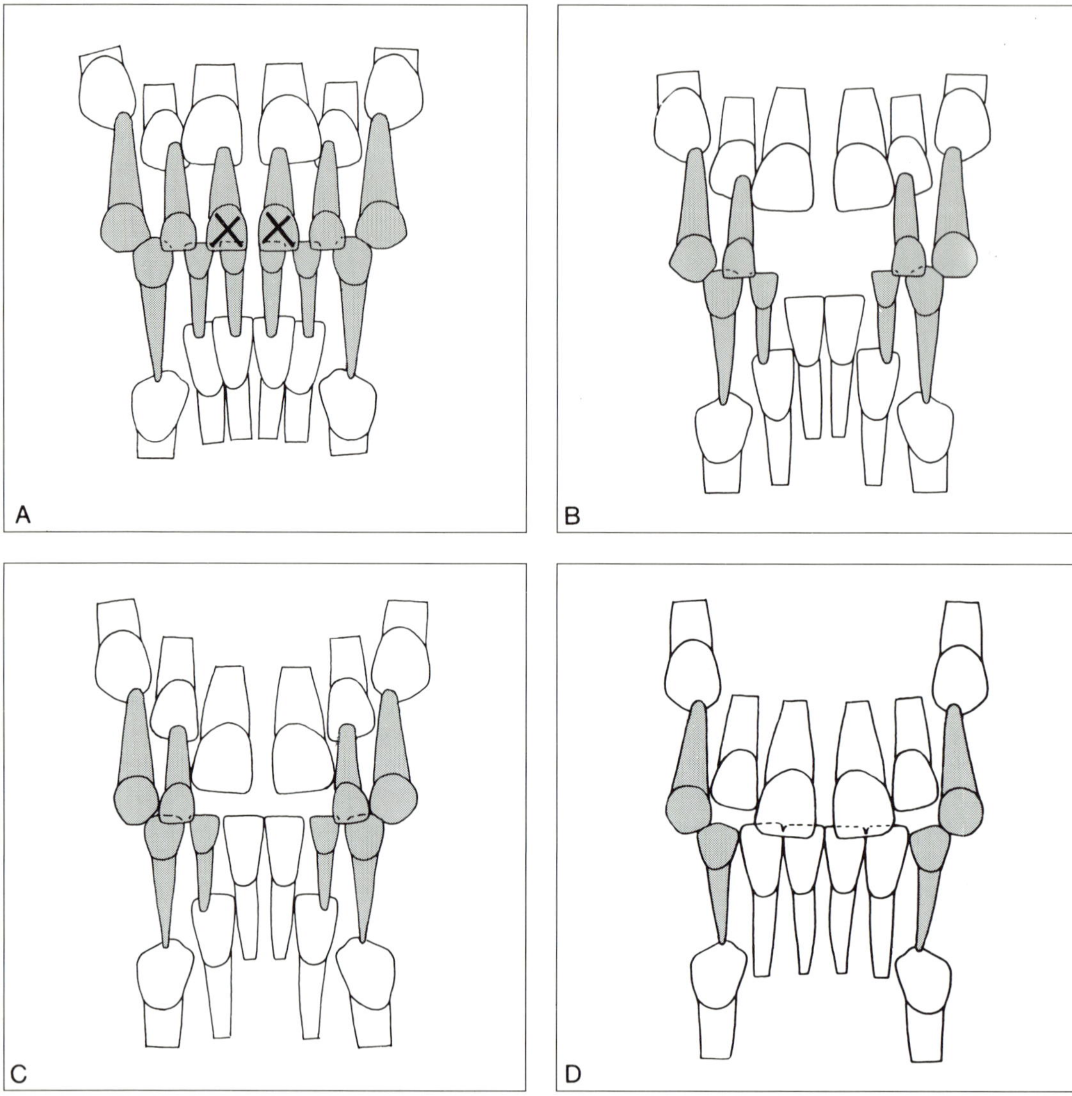

Fig. 1-1 Loss of two maxillary central deciduous incisors at an early age, without damage or displacement of their successors. Loss without further complications will usually not affect the development of the dentition. The central deciduous incisors are not instrumental in the increase of the distances between the deciduous canines associated with the transition of the incisors.

A *In general, the eruption of the maxillary central permanent incisors does not start before 5 years of age. Their distoincisal corners contact the roots of the adjacent deciduous lateral incisors.*

B *Even after premature loss of the maxillary central deciduous incisors the erupting central permanent incisors will displace the lateral deciduous incisors distally.*

C, D *Subsequent development of the dentition proceeds normally (Fig. 2-4, page 34). Further eruption of the central incisors leads to reduction and closure of the diastemata mesial of the deciduous canines.*

Premature loss of deciduous incisors is usually associated with delayed eruption and late emergence of successors, as is particularly evident in cases of unilateral premature loss. The displacement of the deciduous lateral incisor and canine in lateral and distal directions occurs when the critical contact relations are established. In cases of delayed eruption of only one central permanent incisor, the associated displacement will take place later also on that side.

deciduous teeth occurs in this period.[94] The damage that results depends on the severity of the accident and the age of the child. If there is a significant injury before the age of 2 years, then the prognosis for the permanent incisors is dubious. The formation of the crowns can be disturbed (hypoplasia and hypocalcification) and the position of the already formed part of the crown can be changed. With children of 2 years of age or older there is usually no direct mechanical damage; instead, there is the danger of subsequent infection that can disturb enamel and dentine formation. Also, displacement of the tooth germ can lead to dilaceration. Where the resulting kink in the root occurs and how marked it will be depend on the stage of tooth formation at the time of the trauma and on the extent of the displacement.[196]
In a minor injury, a small part of the crown of a deciduous tooth may be broken off. An irritating sharp corner can be ground smooth. If subsequently the colour of the tooth changes, it should be observed closely. If a periapical lesion appears, it should be dealt with (see 8.5.1). When a major fracture of the crown occurs with pulp exposure, prompt endodontic treatment or extraction is indicated.
Root fractures in the cervical third of the root necessitate removing the whole deciduous tooth. Simple fractures in the apical third need no treatment. Fractures between these points can be stabilised with a simple splint of composite resin over the incisors for a maximum of 3 weeks in order to encourage formation of a "cement callus." Complex fractures require extraction.[117] Intrusion of deciduous incisors is the most common consequence of traumata. Usually these teeth resume eruption without intervention. Meanwhile, it is best to institute careful periodic observation (see 8.5.5). If eruption is not resumed, the retained deciduous tooth must be removed.[3]
When a deciduous tooth is lost by injury no direct therapeutic action is usually required. Replantation is not indicated. Possible damage to the permanent dentition can be evaluated more adequately later (see 8.5.2, 8.5.3, and 8.5.4). Drifting of adjacent teeth is usually limited and loss of arch length that might result can be regained later if necessary (Fig. 1-1).

1.7 Lateral forced bites

There is insufficient information to suggest that a lateral forced bite in the deciduous dentition will unfavourably influence the subsequent development of the dentition and facial growth or that orthodontic intervention is justifiable. Nonetheless, selective occlusal grinding can in some cases correct the displacement with minimal effort. Whether or not this should be attempted will depend on the attitude and opinions of the child and parents.

1.8 Reversed overbites

Reversed overbites in the deciduous dentition are seen less frequently than in the permanent dentition. This difference can be attributed to the progressive development of some Class III anomalies. In the deciduous dentition a reversed overbite involving all the incisors is twice as common as those involving a small number of teeth.[57]
Reversed overbites in the deciduous dentition can be subdivided into ventral forced bites (which often are associated with lateral forced bites), into true Class III anomalies, and into combinations of both. The most important diagnostic criterion is the extent to which the bite can be displaced dorsally from the position of habitual occlusion.
In ventral forced bites in the deciduous dentition, occlusal displacement usually originates at the incisors and sometimes the canines. Normally selective grinding there is sufficient if it is desired to correct the forced bite.
Patients with true Class III anomalies should start treatment at the deciduous dentition stage. A simple chin cap pulling from the back of the head should be considered. Where the midface is retruded, ventral traction to the maxilla is recommended (using a facial mask according to Delaire).

1.9 Serious congenital anomalies

If no teeth at all are laid down (anodontia) or if many are lacking (oligodontia), prosthetic replacement should be considered. Regular adjustment of the appliance should be provided to allow for growth of the face and jaws.
Clefts of lip and/or jaw and/or palate are found in one in 700 to 1,000 children. Sometimes these clefts are a part of a more comprehensive syndrome. The treatment of such anomalies calls for a multidisciplinary regimen depending on a team of experts. Such treatment can best be given in centres developed for that purpose, whether or not the centre is associated with orthodontists established outside the centre. In such centres the most appropriate treatment can be provided from birth on. With team planning, optimal goals for immediate and long-term results can be chosen and instituted at the appropriate point in development.

1.10 Supplementary remarks

Orthodontic aberrations are relatively rare in the deciduous dentition. Usually a normal lip relationship exists with a closed mouth. Supernumerary teeth, anomalous crown formation, and crowding are much less often seen than in the permanent dentition. The same applies to agenesis. Very rarely is a deciduous lateral incisor missing, which usually is associated with lack of the corresponding lateral permanent incisor. In exceptional cases there is one tooth less than normal (hypodontia) because two tooth germs have fused to make one tooth (synodontia). In similarly exceptional cases one tooth is supernumerary (hyperdontia) because there has been a division of the tooth germ (schizodontia).

Treatment of orthodontic anomalies in the deciduous dentition as a rule is unwise. This is especially so in regard to use of appliances. An exception to this might be extreme deviations in sagittal jaw relationships. This would apply not only for the Class III anomalies already mentioned but also for pronounced Class II/1 anomalies. For both, facial orthopedic therapy is warranted in the deciduous dentition.

Finally, it should be pointed out that no relationship has been shown in humans between the development of the dentition and either the course of pregnancy, nutritional status, or psychomotor development. It is highly improbable that there is any connection between these variables and the time at which deciduous teeth emerge. Nor can any statements connecting the presence or absence in the mouth of deciduous teeth at a particular age with any other aspects of development be justified.

Chapter 2

Variations in Transition of Mandibular Incisors*

2.1 Introduction

The mandible precedes the maxilla in the transition of the incisors. The first deciduous tooth to be lost — the mandibular central incisor — is exfoliated about 1 year earlier than the corresponding maxillary incisor.

The tooth-containing parts of the mandible differ markedly from those in the maxilla in size, shape, and structure. Consequently, the transition of the mandibular incisors differs from that of the maxillary incisors. In the mandible less space is available for the crowns of the not-yet-erupting permanent teeth and the roots of the deciduous and permanent ones than in the maxilla. Further, the mandible does not have an interstitial growth site in the form of a midsagittal suture that can contribute to an increased transverse jaw dimension in the median plane. The aforementioned differences partly explain why the transition of incisors in the mandible varies less than that in the maxilla.

The combination of four features allows the alignment of the larger permanent incisors in the region where previously the smaller deciduous ones were located: *(1)* the presence of diastemata between the deciduous teeth, *(2)* the increase in intercanine distance associated with the transition of the incisors, *(3)* the more labial inclination of the permanent incisors, and *(4)* the fact that the permanent incisors are more labially positioned than their predecessors. In general, all four features exert a larger effect on the maxilla than the mandible.[13, 141, 143, 145, 223]

The transition of the mandibular incisors is discussed in relation to the size and shape of the anterior section of the apical area. The variation in location of the permanent incisors and canines prior to emergence and their relation to the adjacent deciduous predecessors are indicated. The eruption is divided into preemergence and postemergence phases. Common features in the transition of the mandibular incisors are explained. Three eruption patterns are presented by means of longitudinal records of dental casts and schematic drawings.

* Reproduced from: "Transition of the lower incisors" by Paul J.M.R. Bakker, Hein J.W. Wassenberg and Frans P.G.M. van der Linden. In: *Transition of the human dentition.* Monograph No. 13. Craniofacial Growth Series., Pg 19-38. Ed. Frans P.G.M. van der Linden. Center for Human Growth and Development. The University of Michigan, Ann Arbor, U.S.A., 1982.

2.2 The anterior section of the apical area* and arrangement of anterior teeth before emergence

The size, shape, and structure of the mandible determine the space available for the teeth. Considerable individual variation exists in the form of the anterior part of the mandible, as is expressed by the course of the lower border, the prominence of the chin, and the arrangement of the teeth in the dental arch. Critical in this respect is the location of the permanent canine crowns as determined by the sites where their formation started. The same holds for the location of the apices of the mandibular permanent canines after eruption is completed.

The anterior section of the apical area is bounded laterally by the location of the permanent canines and in the sagittal direction by the lingual and labial cortical walls. In the developing dentition, a considerable amount of tooth material is stacked in the anterior region of the mandible. Prior to the transition, the roots of the deciduous incisors and the forming permanent teeth fill the space available in a typical manner. The crowns of the permanent incisors with their large mesiodistal dimensions at the incisal edge and their large labiolingual dimensions at the cementoenamel junction are arranged in a way that utilises the available space efficiently.

The mandibular permanent incisors are formed parallel to each other behind the roots of their predecessors in a more or less perpendicular angulation. Invariably the crowns of mandibular central permanent incisors do not cross the midline and are placed labially to those of the lateral incisors. The central incisors are slightly labially inclined; the lateral incisors are slightly lingually inclined. The amount of overlap of the lateral incisors by the central incisors shows little variation; it ranges, when these teeth are not rotated, between one quarter to one third the width of the incisal edge of the lateral incisors. The amount of overlap of the lateral incisors by the canine crowns shows marked variation, can be completely absent, and is directly related to the size of the anterior section of the apical area.

Rotation of anterior permanent teeth prior to emergence is not necessarily a sign of crowding. In a number of cases the morphogenesis of the mandibular permanent incisors starts in a rotated orientation that is maintained in their subsequent formation and their initial eruption.

Some asymmetry may exist in the positioning of corresponding left and right mandibular permanent incisors and canine crowns. This applies not only to the

* The concept of *apical area* was introduced by the author in 1978 and is described as follows: the apical area in an infant is comprised of the region that contains the forming parts of the deciduous and permanent teeth. In the deciduous dentition the apical area is constituted of the region in which the apices of the deciduous teeth can be located and the forming parts of the permanent teeth are situated. In the mixed dentition the apical area consists of the region where the roots of the deciduous and permanent teeth can be located and the forming parts of the nonerupted teeth are situated. In the adult state the apical area is the region where the apices of the fully formed teeth can normally be located. The apical area in both jaws can be divided in three sections: anterior, middle, and posterior. The anterior section is formed by the region between the mesial surfaces of the forming parts of the permanent canines and those of the apices after eruption is completed. The middle section lies between the anterior section and the mesial surface of the forming part of the first permanent molar and following complete eruption slightly mesial to its apex. The posterior section is situated dorsally to the middle section and includes the maxillary tuberosity and lingual tuberosity in the mandible.

anteroposterior location and rotation but also to the amount of overlap of adjacent teeth.
The arrangement of the tooth material within the anterior region of the mandible, before the emergence of the permanent incisors, differs, depending on the relation between the space available and the space needed (Figs. 2-1 to 2-3).
The anterior section of the apical area is large when the distance between the crowns of the mandibular permanent canines is large in relation to the mesiodistal crown dimensions of the permanent incisors. Favourable conditions are then present for the transition of the incisors. Frequently, a large anterior section of the apical area is associated with many and wide diastemata between the mandibular anterior deciduous teeth and a small anterior section of the apical area with few and small diastemata or even no diastemata. However, the correlation between the sum of the mesiodistal crown dimensions of the mandibular incisors of the two dentitions is rather low.[144] So, large mesiodistal crown dimensions of deciduous incisors are not always associated with corresponding large permanent teeth, as well as vice versa. This has consequences when it is necessary to estimate the spatial requirements of the permanent anterior teeth.

2.3 Eruption before emergence*

The mandibular central permanent incisors are the first anterior teeth to commence eruption. They move in the direction of the occlusal plane according to their orientation within the jaw. The overlapping of the crowns of the adjacent lateral incisors reduces. After about 1 year, when the central incisors have reached the level of the occlusal plane, the lateral incisors are free to start to erupt. Normally the overlapping is fully eliminated and the lateral incisors move in the direction of the occlusal plane. Before the onset of eruption and in the preemergence eruption phase, the lateral incisors are more lingually inclined than the central incisors, as indicated above. Correspondingly, the lateral incisors usually follow a more lingually inclined path of eruption than that of the central incisors, and their incisal edges emerge more lingually. Figure 2-4 shows the transition of the mandibular and maxillary incisors. Figure 2-5 shows six specimens of prepared skulls to illustrate the process of transition of the mandibular incisors and some variations in the size of the anterior section of the apical area.
Teeth erupting normally do not change their course of eruption before emergence. In a large anterior section of the apical area eruption is usually not impeded and only a limited amount of displacement of neighbouring deciduous teeth is required, if any. In a medium anterior section of the apical area the mechanism of displacement of deciduous teeth can lead to a considerable increase in available space within the dental arch and to an enlarged distance between the left and right deciduous canine crowns.[223] In a small section of the anterior apical area the maximum possible displacement of adjacent deciduous teeth may not be sufficient and one or more deciduous teeth may become resorbed and be exfoliated prematurely (Fig. 2-6).

* The term *eruption* is used for the movement in an occlusal direction; *emergence* is used for the perforation of the gum tissue and the appearance of the crown in the mouth. The eruption process can be subdivided into a preemergence phase, the emergence itself, and the postemergence phase.

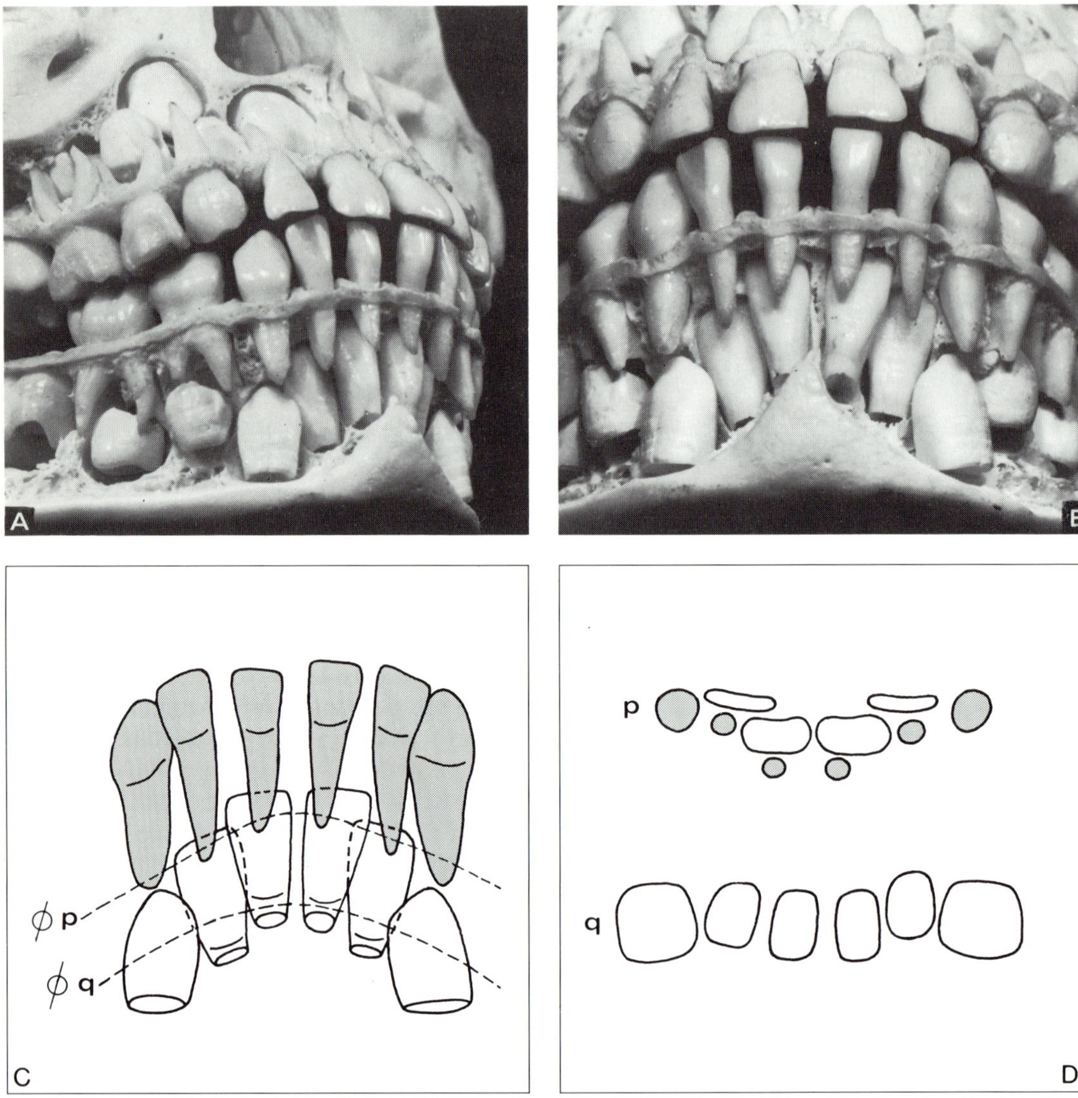

Fig. 2-1 Large anterior section of the apical area in the mandible.

A, B Many and large diastemata between the anterior deciduous teeth usually indicate the presence of a large section of the apical area. The mandibular permanent canines are only slightly lingually inclined and mesially angulated. The central permanent incisors are separated and overlap the neighbouring lateral incisors for about one quarter of their mesiodistal crown width. The cusp tips of the mandibular canines are located slightly distal to the apices of their predecessors.

C *Schematic drawing with dotted lines indicating the sections presented in D. The central permanent incisor crowns do not contact the adjacent lateral deciduous incisor roots. The same holds true for the crowns of the permanent lateral incisors and the roots of the deciduous canines. Some asymmetry exists in the arrangement of the permanent incisors. The left central incisor is more lingually inclined and more distally angulated than the right one.*

D *In the region of the incisal borders of the permanent incisors (p) the lateral incisors are located lingual to the central incisors. Note the relations indicated under C. No overlapping exists of the permanent incisors (q) in the region of the cementoenamel junctions, where the central incisors are only slightly labial to the lateral incisors.*

(Legend 2-2 continued)

D *In the region of the incisal borders of the permanent incisors (p), the crowns of the permanent teeth and the roots of the adjacent deciduous teeth are in close proximity. In the region of the cementoenamel junctions of the permanent incisors (q), the available space does not markedly exceed the space required. Note the asymmetry in the relationship between the lateral permanent incisors and canines.*

(Legend 2-3 continued)

D *In the region of the incisal borders of the permanent incisors (p), the crowns of the permanent teeth and the roots of the deciduous ones are close together. In the region of the cementoenamel junctions (q), crowding exists where the lateral incisors are lingual to the central incisors and canines and are overlapped by the latter.*

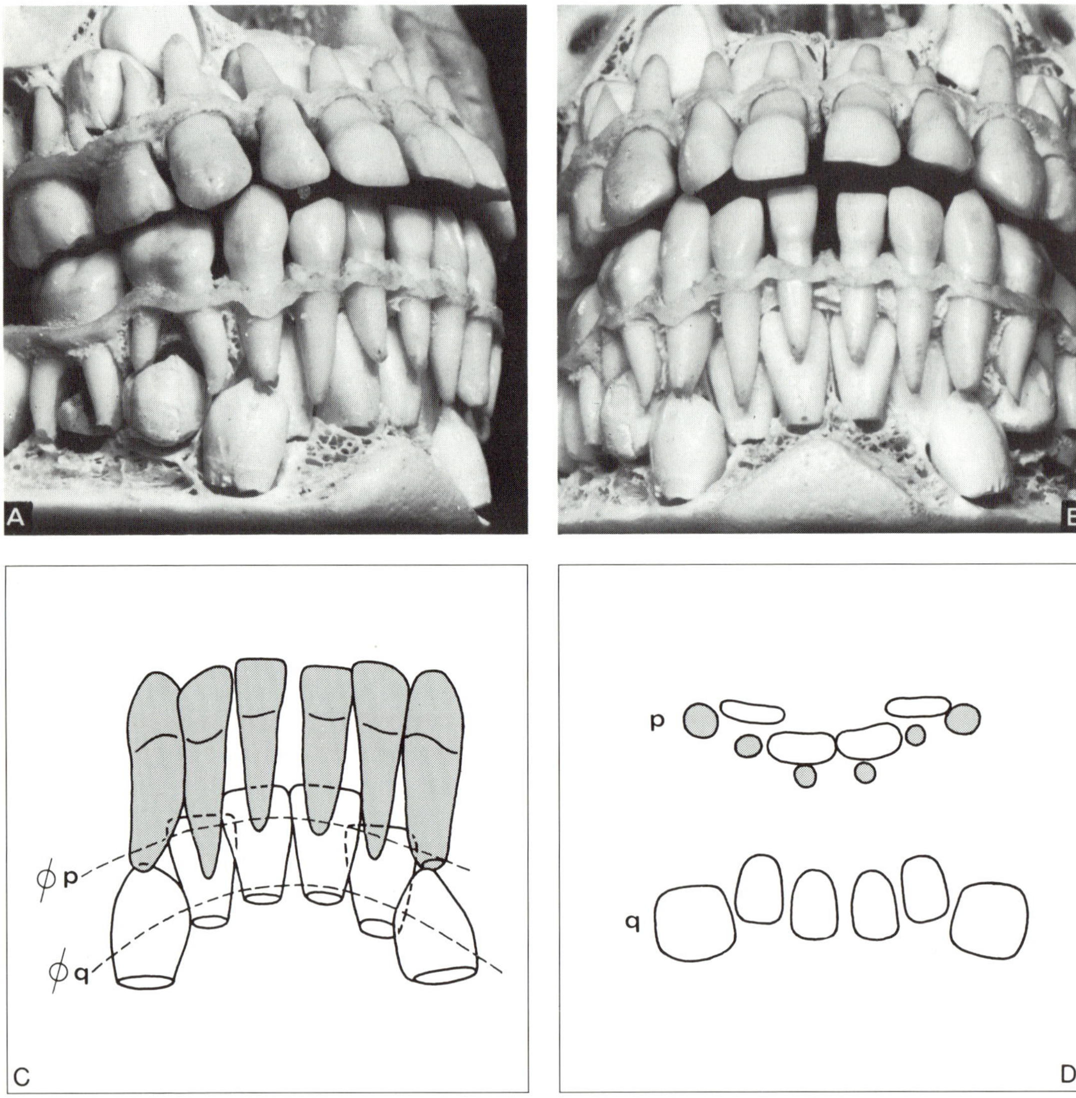

Fig. 2-2 Medium anterior section of the apical area in the mandible.

A, B *Limited spacing between the anterior deciduous teeth. The mandibular permanent canines are lingually inclined and mesially angulated. The crowns of the lateral permanent incisors are partly overlapped by those of the central incisors and also by those of the permanent canines. The cusp tips of the permanent canines are close to the apices of their predecessors.*

C *The distal corners of the crowns of the lateral permanent incisors are in close proximity to the roots of the adjacent deciduous canines. The left permanent canine is more mesially angulated than the right one; the left lateral incisor is overlapped more than the right one.*
(Legend continues on page 31)

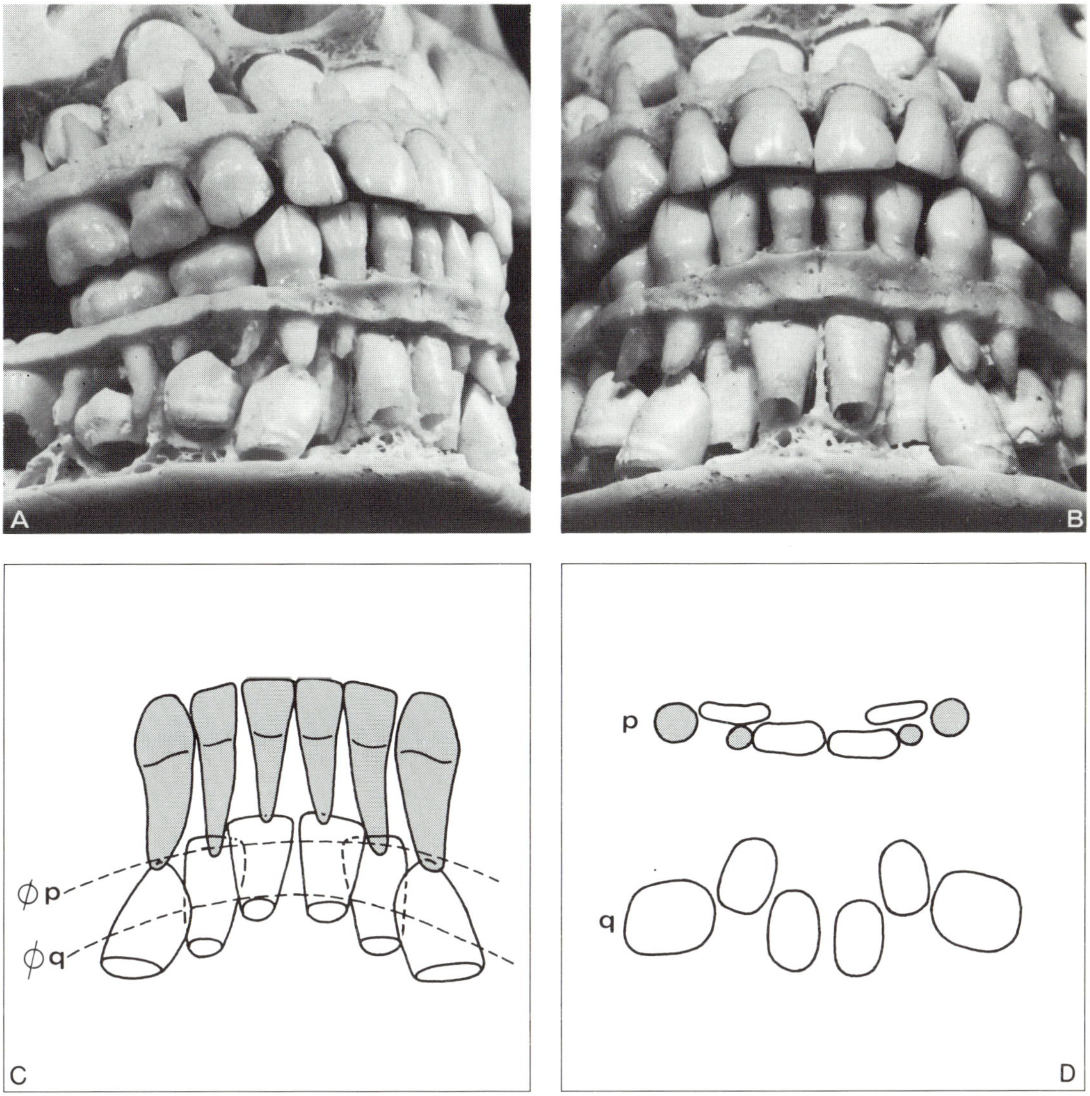

Fig. 2-3 Small anterior section of the apical area in the mandible.

A, B *Few and only small diastemata between the anterior deciduous teeth. The mandibular permanent canines are markedly lingually inclined and mesially angulated. Their crowns overlap those of the lateral incisors. The cusp tips of the permanent canines are in close proximity to the apices of their predecessors.*

C *The central permanent incisor crowns are close together and their distal corners are in contact with the roots of the adjacent lateral deciduous incisors. The distal corners of the crowns of the lateral permanent incisors are slightly lingual to the roots of the adjacent deciduous canines.*

(Legend continues on page 31)

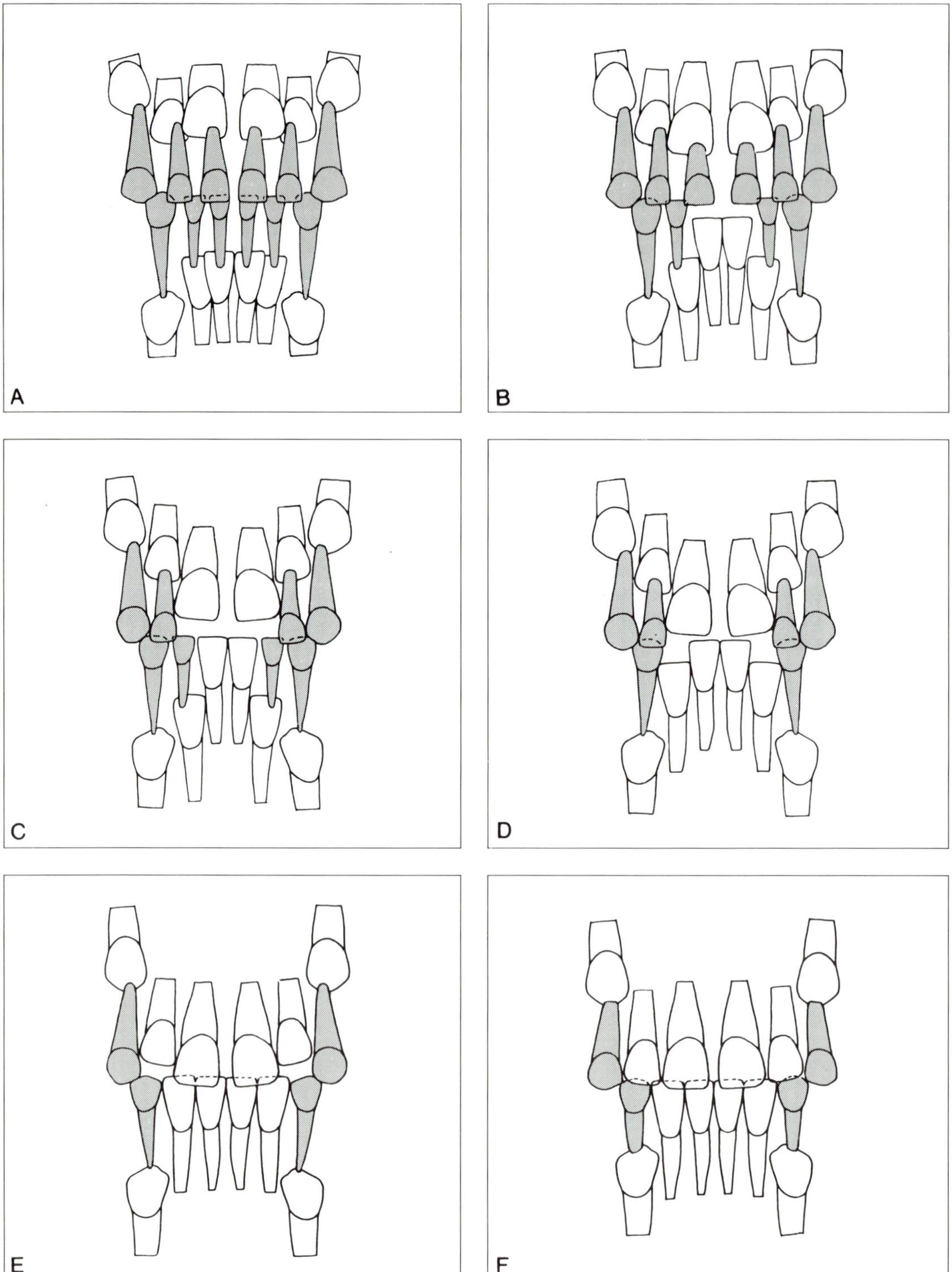

Figure 2-4

Fig. 2-4 Schematic presentation of the transition of the mandibular and maxillary incisors. (From Van der Linden.[223])

A Situation at approximately 5 years of age, prior to the start of eruption. All permanent crowns are placed lingually to the apices of their predecessors.
The mandibular central permanent incisors are located slightly nearer to the occlusal plane than the adjacent lateral incisors. The crowns of the latter are lingual to those of the central incisors.
In the maxilla the incisal edges of the lateral permanent incisors are located nearer to the occlusal plane than those of the central incisors. The distoincisal corners of the central permanent incisors are in contact with the mesial surfaces of the roots of the adjacent lateral deciduous incisors.

B After loss of the mandibular central deciduous incisors the successors emerge, frequently in close proximity to each other. The overlapping of the mandibular lateral permanent incisors disappears before eruption of the central incisors is completed.
In the maxilla the erupting central permanent incisors pass the lateral incisors. The contacts between the distoincisal corners of the central permanent crowns and the mesial surface of the roots of the lateral deciduous incisor lead to a distal movement of the latter. The diastemata mesial to the deciduous canines reduce in width, and more space becomes available for the central permanent incisors to emerge.

C The mandibular central permanent incisors have reached the level of the occlusal plane before the lateral incisors start to erupt. In a medium anterior section of the apical area, the distoincisal corners of the mandibular central permanent incisors may contact the mesial surfaces of the roots of the lateral deciduous incisors, resulting in a distal displacement of the latter and a reduction of the diastemata mesial to the deciduous canines. In the maxilla, the central deciduous incisors are lost and their successors have erupted further. The concomitant distal displacement of the lateral deciduous incisors has continued. The overlapping of the lateral permanent incisors disappeared with the continuing eruption of the central incisors.

D The erupting mandibular lateral permanent incisors reach the deciduous canines, and their distoincisal corners make contact with the mesial surfaces of the latter. Subsequently, the mandibular intercanine distance increases.
In the maxilla, the emerging central permanent incisors continue to move the lateral deciduous incisors distally. This in turn causes distal movement of the canines, resulting in an increase in intercanine distance in the maxilla also.

E The mandibular lateral permanent incisors have completed their eruption.
In the maxilla the lateral permanent incisors start their eruption after the central incisors have reached the level of the occlusal plane. It is then possible for the lateral incisors to erupt in the direction of their orientation within the jaws. They move labially from their initially more palatal location. When the erupting lateral incisors establish contact with the central incisors, the central diastema may become reduced in width. This reduction, however, can also take place when this contact is not established. After emergence of the lateral incisors, more room becomes available within the jaw to allow the roots of the central incisors to move distally, leading to a change in mesiodistal angulation of these teeth.

F The maxillary lateral permanent incisors are the last incisors to reach the level of the occlusal plane. The roots of these teeth are close to the crowns of the permanent canines. The relation will not change until the latter start to erupt.

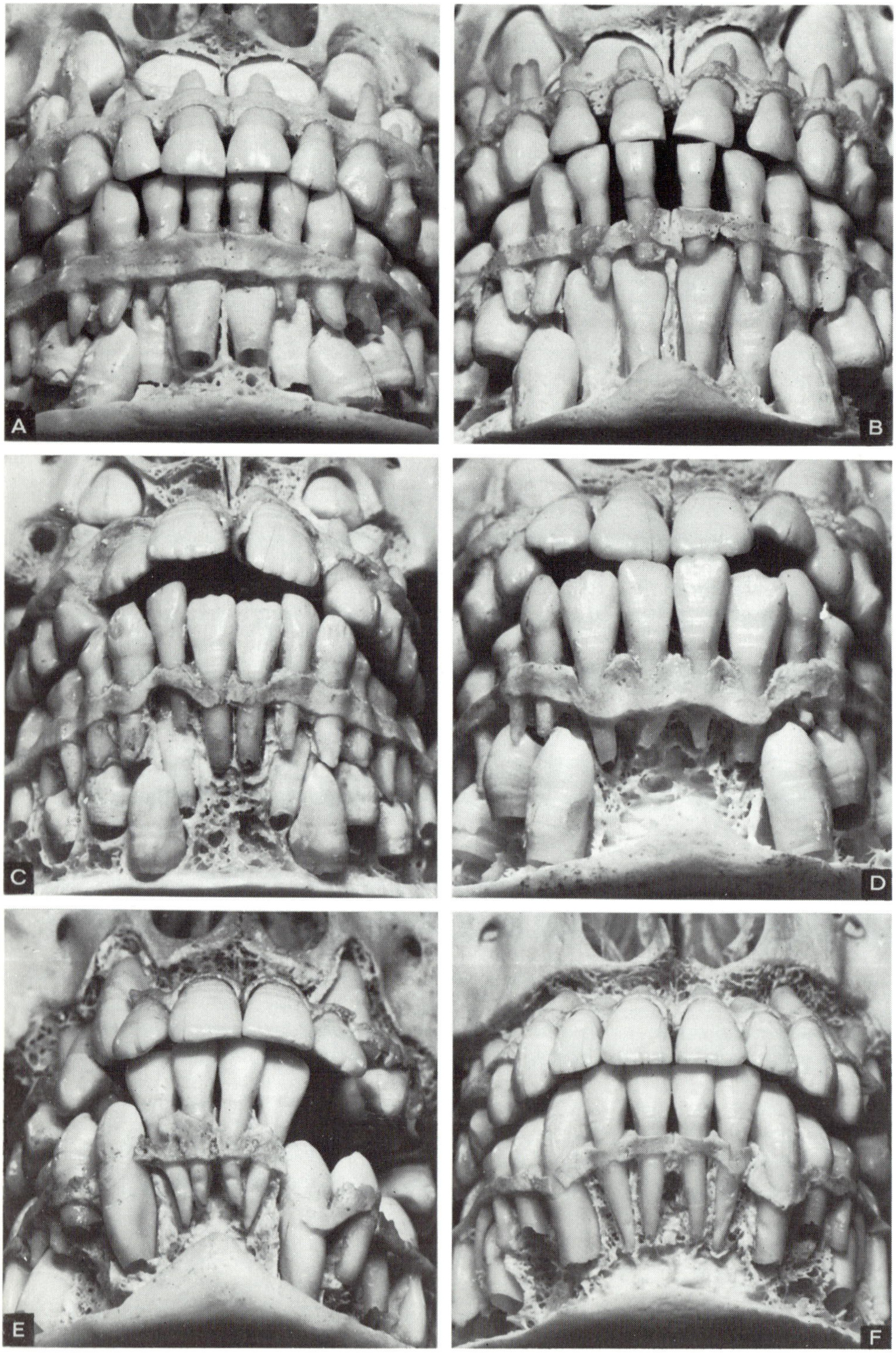

Figure 2-5

Fig. 2-5 Six preparations of human skulls with small and medium anterior sections of the apical areas in the mandible, showing different stages and aspects of the transition of the mandibular incisors and canines.

A Small anterior section of the apical area. No diastemata between the mandibular deciduous incisors and a small distance between the mandibular permanent canine crowns. Note the overlapping of the lateral permanent incisors by the adjacent permanent canine crowns and the marked mesial angulation and lingual inclination of the latter.

B Medium anterior section of the apical area. In the mandible diastemata are present between the deciduous incisors. The distance between the mandibular permanent canine crowns is large. The lateral permanent incisors are only slightly overlapped by the central incisors and only just by the canines. The distoincisal corners of the mandibular central permanent incisors contact the mesial surfaces of the roots of the adjacent lateral deciduous incisors. The distal corners of the crowns of the lateral permanent incisors are in close proximity to the roots of the deciduous canines. No diastemata are present between the lateral deciduous incisors and canines.

C Small anterior section of the apical area. The distance between permanent canine crowns is small. The central permanent incisors have emerged but have not yet completely erupted. The distal corners of the lateral permanent incisor crowns are positioned lingual to the roots of the adjacent deciduous canines.

D Medium anterior section of the apical area. The mandibular lateral permanent incisors have almost completed their eruption. The canines have not commenced eruption. The left lateral permanent incisor overlaps the crown of the deciduous canine buccally.

E Small anterior section of the apical area. The apices of the four mandibular incisors are close together. The mandibular right permanent canine is erupted further than the left one.

F Medium anterior section of the apical area. The permanent canines are almost fully erupted. Their root formation is not yet completed. The apices of the lateral incisors are subsequently able to move distally.

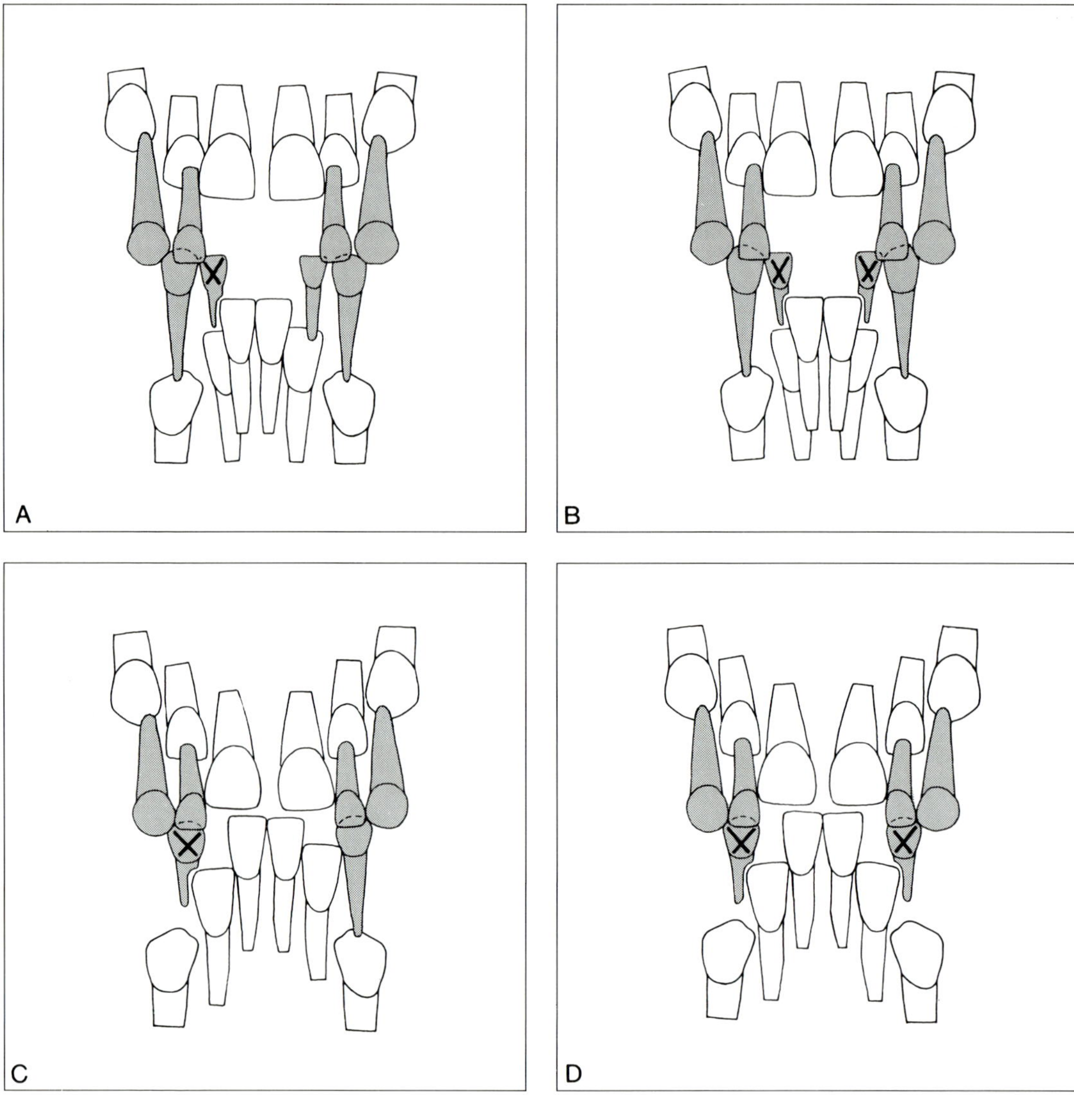

Fig. 2-6 Premature loss of lateral deciduous incisors and canines in the mandible associated with the eruption of adjacent permanent teeth in small anterior sections of the apical area. (From Van der Linden.[223])

A Unilateral loss of a lateral deciduous incisor as may occur with an asymmetrical location and eruption of the central permanent incisors.
B Same as A, bilaterally; the mandibular intercanine distance will not increase with the eruption of the mandibular central permanent incisors.
C Unilateral loss of a mandibular deciduous canine that will be followed by migration of the mandibular incisors and a deviation between the midlines of the two dental arches.
D Same as C, bilaterally; usually without the occurrence of a midline deviation.

Permanent incisors and canines emerge a few weeks or months after the loss of their predecessors. The wound left in the gingival tissue after the loss of the deciduous tooth is soon healed. The successor must later pierce the mucosa. This process is preceded by a stretching and protuberance of the gingival tissue. After penetration, the gingival tissue retracts and a large part of the crown becomes exposed in a relatively short period of time compared to the subsequent increase in clinical crown height.

2.4 Eruption after emergence and subsequent change in orientation

The position of mandibular permanent incisors becomes affected after emergence by forces exerted by the tongue and the lips, particularly the lower lip. Other factors, such as abnormal habits as exemplified by thumb-sucking, will influence the eruption path and final location of the teeth.

In a normal course of events the mandibular permanent incisors emerge more lingually than where their predecessors were located. Under influence of the tongue they subsequently move labially and the eruption path alters in that direction. Their final position depends on the distribution of forces exerted on these teeth by the tongue, lips, and other possible factors. The spatial conditions within the dental arch partly determine the extent of the displacement of the teeth resulting from the forces exerted upon them. If crowding exists, teeth may be unable to move to positions they would normally occupy. Excessive tongue pressure may move the mandibular incisors labially. On the other hand, extreme forces of the lower lip or an abnormal habit with a comparable influence may tip the mandibular incisors lingually.

Mandibular incisors, like all other permanent teeth, will continue to erupt until something slows down their vertical movement. Normally this is caused by the contact established with the maxillary teeth. In a deviating sagittal relationship between the dental arches, the mandibular incisors may not contact the maxillary ones and will continue to erupt until they contact the palate. Abnormal functional behaviour, such as improper tongue positioning, thumb-sucking, and lip biting may interfere with the continued eruption of the mandibular incisors and result in a lack of contact between the mandibular anterior teeth and their antagonists or the palatal structures in habitual occlusion.

The mandibular lateral permanent incisors emerge more lingually in the dental arch than the central permanent incisors. In addition, the central incisors have moved more labially in the time between their emergence and completion of their eruption. The combination of these two aspects results in a clearly more lingual position of the mandibular lateral incisors upon emergence than where their adjacent central incisors are then located. When sufficient space is available within the dental arch, the lateral incisors will gradually become aligned with the central incisors. Frequently, however, insufficient space is available initially and the improvement in orientation of the lingually positioned lateral incisors must wait until the transition of the posterior teeth provides the extra space needed. However, that is not always the case, and when no room or insufficient room becomes available, later on the improvement in location of the mandibular lateral incisors may take place only partly or not at all.

Central and lateral incisors that emerge in a rotated position will normally become aligned when sufficient space is available. A rotational component is exerted by the forces of the tongue and lips on the more or less flat lingual and labial surfaces of the mandibular incisors.

2.5 Patterns in transition of mandibular incisors

The transition of the mandibular incisors frequently does not occur symmetrically and synchronously. Differences between the left and the right sides often occur.
Three main patterns can be distinguished in the transition of the mandibular incisors. The degree of rotation around the long axis of the mandibular incisors during emergence serves as the guideline for the differentiation into groups. The different patterns will be presented by means of photographs of longitudinal series of dental casts and by schematic drawings that show the typical changes involved.

2.5.1 Mandibular Incisor Transition Pattern A

Emergence of the central and lateral permanent incisors in nonrotated or only slightly rotated positions (Figs. 2-7 and 2-8). The central and lateral incisors emerge

Fig. 2-7 Frontal and occlusal views of a mainly longitudinal series of dental casts of a medium anterior section of the apical area, demonstrating bilaterally the Mandibular Incisor Transition Pattern A, characterized by emergence of the central and lateral permanent incisors in nonrotated or slightly rotated positions.

A, B *Some small diastemata are present in the anterior region between the deciduous teeth.*
C, D *The central permanent incisors have emerged lingually and are slightly rotated. Sufficient space is available. The lateral deciduous incisors have been displaced distally and are now in contact with the adjacent deciduous canines.*
E, F *The central incisors have erupted to the level of the occlusal plane. Their incisal edges are located more labially than those of their predecessors. The slight rotations initially present at emergence have been corrected. The left lateral incisor precedes the right one in emergence, eruption, and correction of the slight rotation. The intercanine distance increased substantially with the eruption of the lateral permanent incisors.*
G, H *Situation after emergence of the mandibular permanent canines. The angulation of the central and lateral incisors changed as more room became available in the anterior section of the apical area. The narrower canine root takes up less space than its crown had done previously.*

Note: The age at which the dental casts were obtained is indicated in the photographs, in years and in months (9.5 = 9 years, 5 months). The ages frequently deviate from average values because series that demonstrated more or less completely different phases in development were often rather young or rather old. This phenomenon is related to the age ranges of the cohorts in the Nymegen Growth Study from which all illustrations of dental casts are taken.[162] *An asterisk indicates that the pertinent dental cast does not belong to the series but serves as a substitute. The age indicated is adapted to the other ages in the series. Substitutes were used mainly because the length of the series was often too short to present the complete picture.*

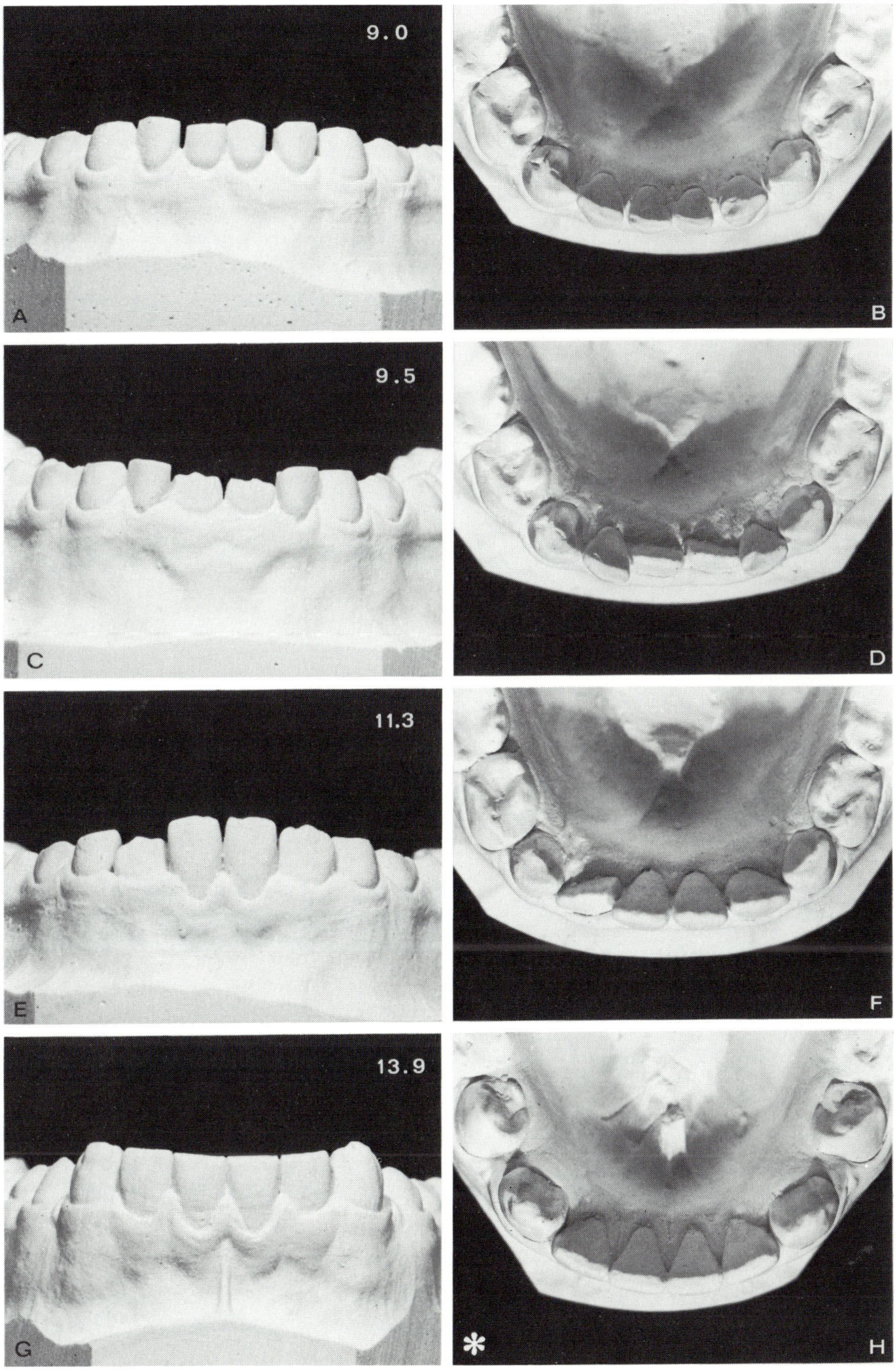

Figure 2-7

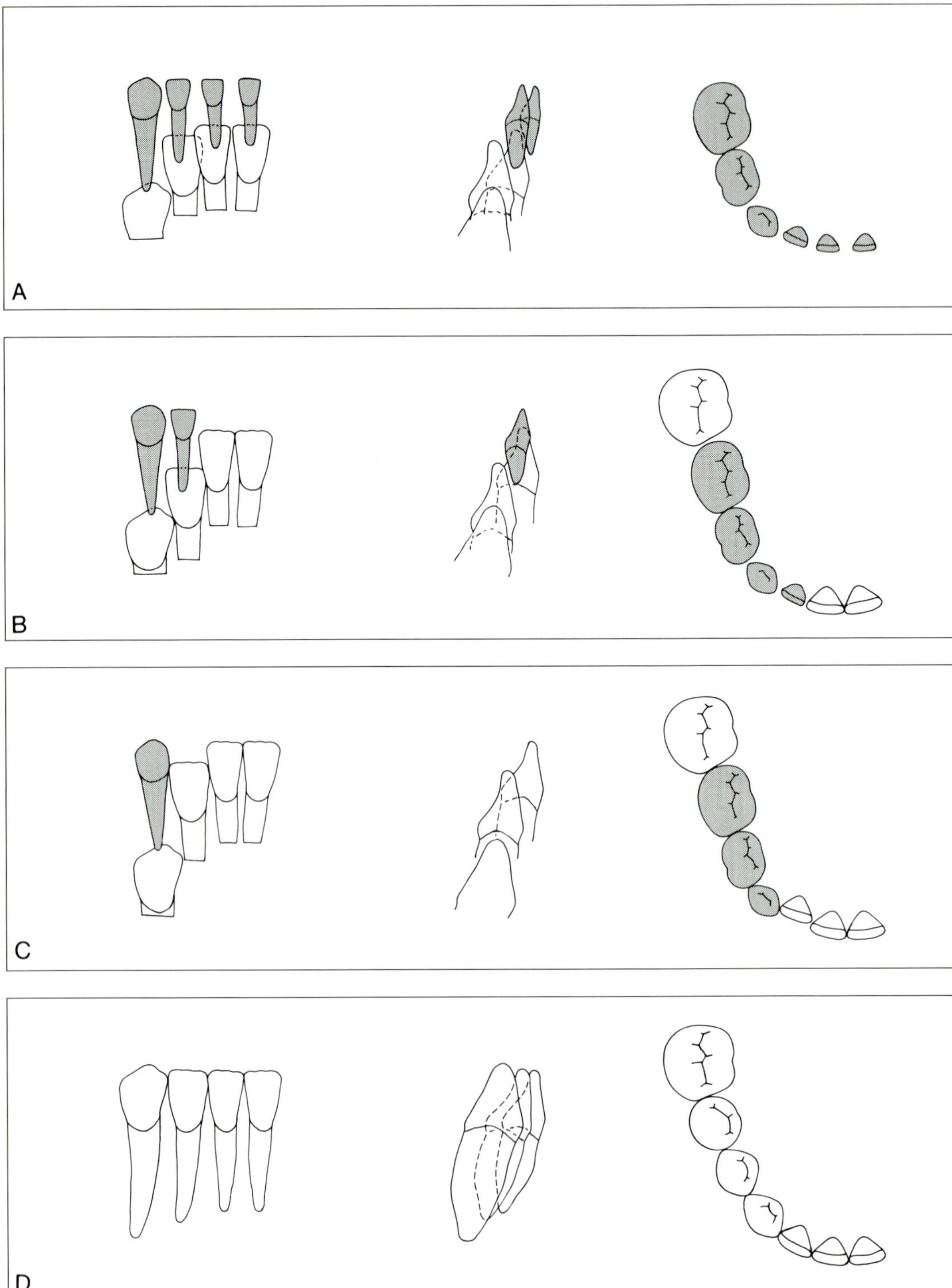

Figure 2-8

Fig. 2-8 Schematic drawings of frontal, lateral, and occlusal views of the Mandibular Incisor Transition Pattern A characterized by emergence of the central and lateral permanent incisors in nonrotated or only slightly rotated positions in a medium anterior section of the apical area.

A Diastemata between the anterior deciduous teeth. No contact between the crown of the central permanent incisor and the root of the adjacent lateral deciduous incisor. The central permanent incisor is less lingually inclined.
B After emergence, the incisal edge of the central permanent incisor moves labially. The crown of the lateral incisor is no longer overlapped.
C The erupting lateral incisor has displaced the deciduous canine distally and laterally and contact exists between the latter and the first deciduous molar. Sufficient space becomes available for the lateral incisor to move labially to the proper position within the dental arch.
D After completion of the transition of the posterior teeth, the apex of the lateral incisor is able to move distally as more space becomes locally available within the jaw.

more lingually than where their predecessors were located. In their subsequent eruption they move labially and their incisal edges attain a more labial position than that of their predecessors.

When sufficient space is available, the arch form will be harmonious after the mandibular incisors are fully erupted and the labial movements performed. In crowded situations the labial displacement of lateral incisors cannot be completed.

In extremely crowded conditions a lateral deciduous incisor may become prematurely resorbed and be exfoliated before the adjacent central permanent incisor emerges. A deciduous canine may experience a comparable process and become exfoliated when the lateral permanent incisor emerges. Subsequently, the latter can move labially and consequently the space in the dental arch, available later on for the permanent canine, will be reduced further. In addition, the intercanine distance will not increase as normally occurs when the distoincisal corner of the erupting lateral permanent incisor makes contact with the mesial surface of the root of the deciduous canine. Premature loss of the mandibular deciduous canine frequently occurs unilaterally and without preceding premature loss of a mandibular lateral deciduous incisor. In that situation often a midline shift occurs.

2.5.2 Mandibular Incisor Transition Pattern B

Emergence of the mandibular central permanent incisor in distolingually rotated position (Figs. 2-9 and 2-10). Depending on the space available locally and the increase in intercanine distance, the initially rotated central incisor will attain a normal position within the dental arch. The same holds true for the lateral permanent incisor. Further, the rotation of the central incisor may be corrected prior to the emergence of the lateral incisor.

In a large or medium anterior section of the apical area, correction of the initially rotated permanent incisors usually takes place before loss of the deciduous canines. In a small anterior section of the apical area the space needed to correct the rotations is lacking and does not become available or only in a limited extent during further development. Premature loss of lateral deciduous incisors and canines associated

Fig. 2-9 Longitudinal series of dental casts of a medium anterior section of the apical area, showing on the right side the Mandibular Incisor Transition Pattern B, characterized by distolingually rotated emergence of the central incisor and mesiolingually rotated emergence of the lateral incisor.

A, B *No diastemata are present in the anterior region between the deciduous teeth.*
C, D *The mandibular right central permanent incisor has emerged in a distolingually rotated orientation. During the preceding eruption no favourable contact existed between that tooth and the root of the adjacent lateral deciduous incisor, unlike the situation on the left side.*
E, F *The right lateral permanent incisor has emerged in a mesiolingually rotated orientation. In the preceding eruption contact existed with the root of the adjacent deciduous canine, leading to a distal and lateral displacement of the latter. The rotation of the right central permanent incisor improved with continuing eruption.*
G, H *The initial rotation of the two permanent incisors on the right side is eliminated. In this case alignment of the four incisors has utilised part of the leeway of the posterior teeth. The premature loss of both mandibular second deciduous molars may have had a favourable effect on the alignment of the incisors.*

with the emergence of the adjacent permanent incisor may not occur because the initially rotated teeth occupy less space than they would otherwise have done. The lack of contact between the distoincisal corner of the lateral permanent incisor and the mesial surface of the root of the deciduous canine excludes the possibility of distal and lateral displacement of the canines based on this contact. Absence of a corresponding contact between the central permanent incisor and the lateral deciduous incisor will, in an earlier phase, exclude comparable increase in space for the emerging central permanent incisor.

2.5.3 Mandibular Incisor Transition Pattern C

Emergence of the mandibular central permanent incisor in mesiolingually rotated position and of the lateral incisor in nonrotated or only slightly distolingually rotated position (Figs. 2-11 and 2-12). When sufficient space is available, the rotation of the mandibular central permanent incisor usually corrects during the postemergence eruption phase. A nonrotated or only slightly distolingually rotated lateral incisor usually has adequate contact with the root of the adjacent deciduous canine before emergence, resulting in a distal and lateral displacement of the latter. This change may not happen when the lateral permanent incisor is rotated distolingually to a considerable extent.

In a medium anterior section of the apical area, the space available for alignment of the permanent incisors is usually too limited for complete correction before the transition of the posterior teeth. The improvement that takes place during the second transitional period is usually limited and depends on a number of factors that will be explored in Chapters 3 and 4.

In a small anterior section of the apical area, little or no improvement will take place before transition of the posterior teeth.

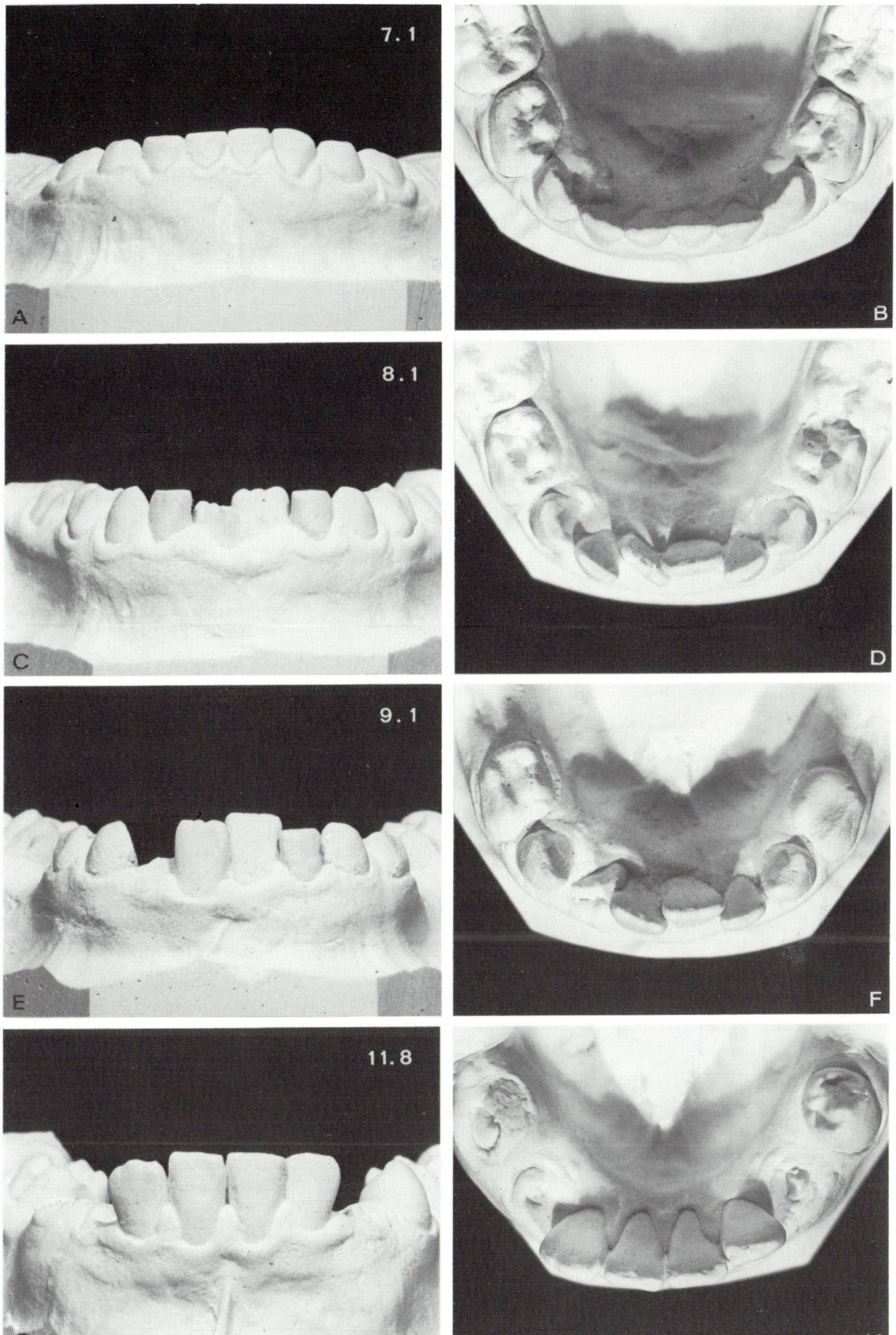

Figure 2-9

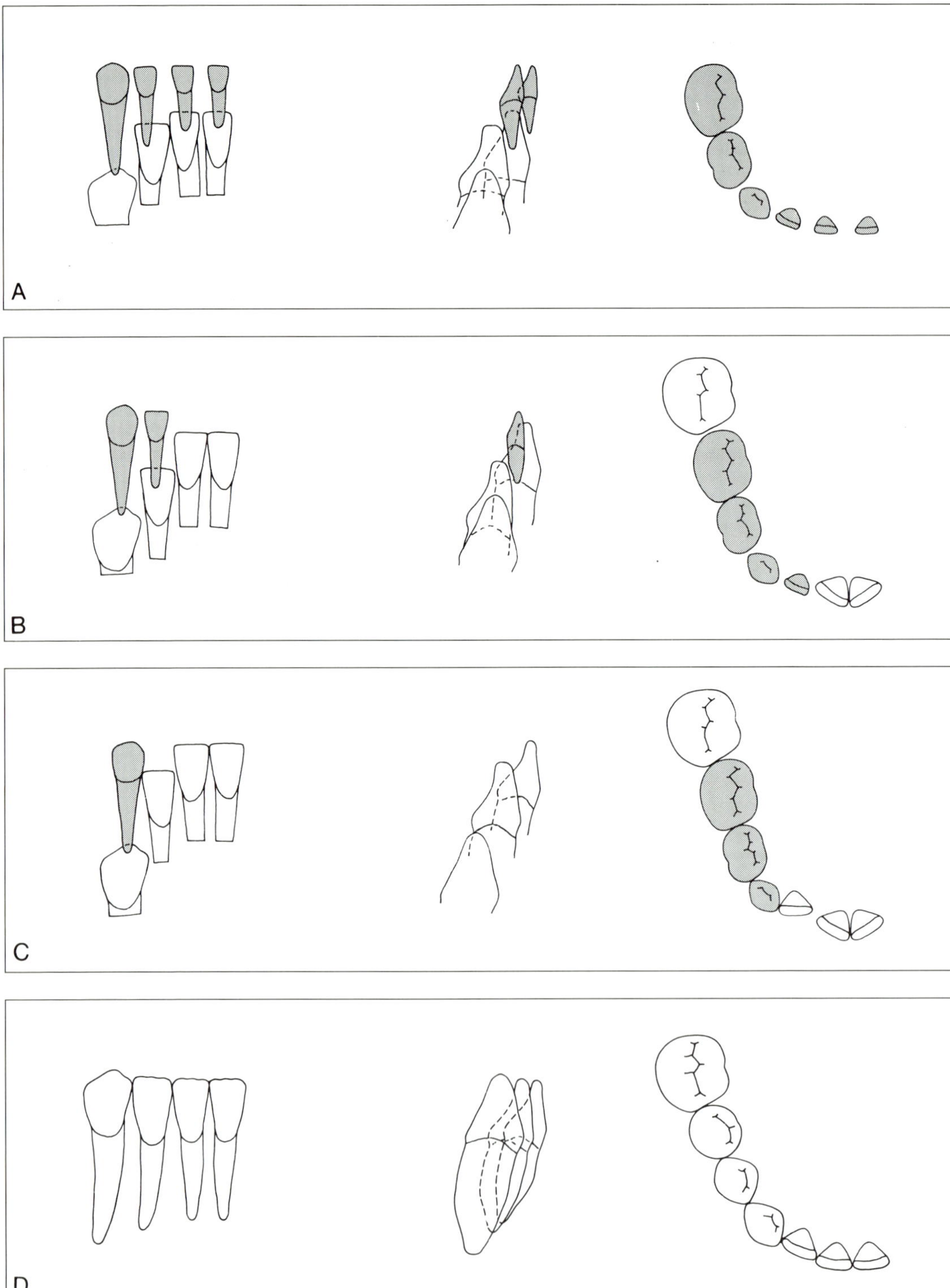

Figure 2-10

Fig. 2-10 Schematic drawings of the Mandibular Incisor Transition Pattern B characterized by distolingually rotated emergence of the central incisor and mesiolingually rotated emergence of the lateral incisor, in a large anterior section of the apical area.

A Large diastemata between the anterior deciduous teeth. The rotated position of the central and lateral permanent incisors is associated with an absence of overlapping at the incisal edges of these teeth.
B The continuing eruption of the central permanent incisor is accompanied by labial movement of its incisal edge, particularly its distal part, and partly by correction of its rotation.
C Before emergence of the lateral permanent incisor, contact existed between its distoincisal corner and the mesial surface of the root of the adjacent deciduous canine, leading to a distal and lateral displacement of the latter. The diastema mesial to the mandibular first deciduous molar has disappeared. After emergence the rotated lateral permanent incisor also moves labially with its mesial incisal corner and the rotation is gradually corrected.
D The end of the transition of the posterior teeth. All incisors may be well aligned by the time eruption is concluded. It may also occur that the correction of the rotation is completed during the second transitional period.

Fig. 2-11 (see page 48) Longitudinal series of dental casts of a medium anterior section of the apical area demonstrating bilaterally the Mandibular Incisor Transition Pattern C, characterized by mesiolingually rotated emergence of the central incisor and nonrotated or only slightly distolingually rotated emergence of the lateral incisor.

A, B Some small diastemata in the anterior region between the deciduous teeth.
C, D Both central permanent incisors have emerged in a mesiolingually rotated orientation; some space is present between the two crowns.
E, F During the postemergence eruption the mesial sides of the central incisors moved labially and the rotations became corrected. The lateral permanent incisors emerged nonrotated.
G, H The erupting right permanent canine has affected the position of the adjacent lateral incisor. The distal corner of the latter has moved lingually. In this respect the conditions have been more favourable on the left than on the right side.

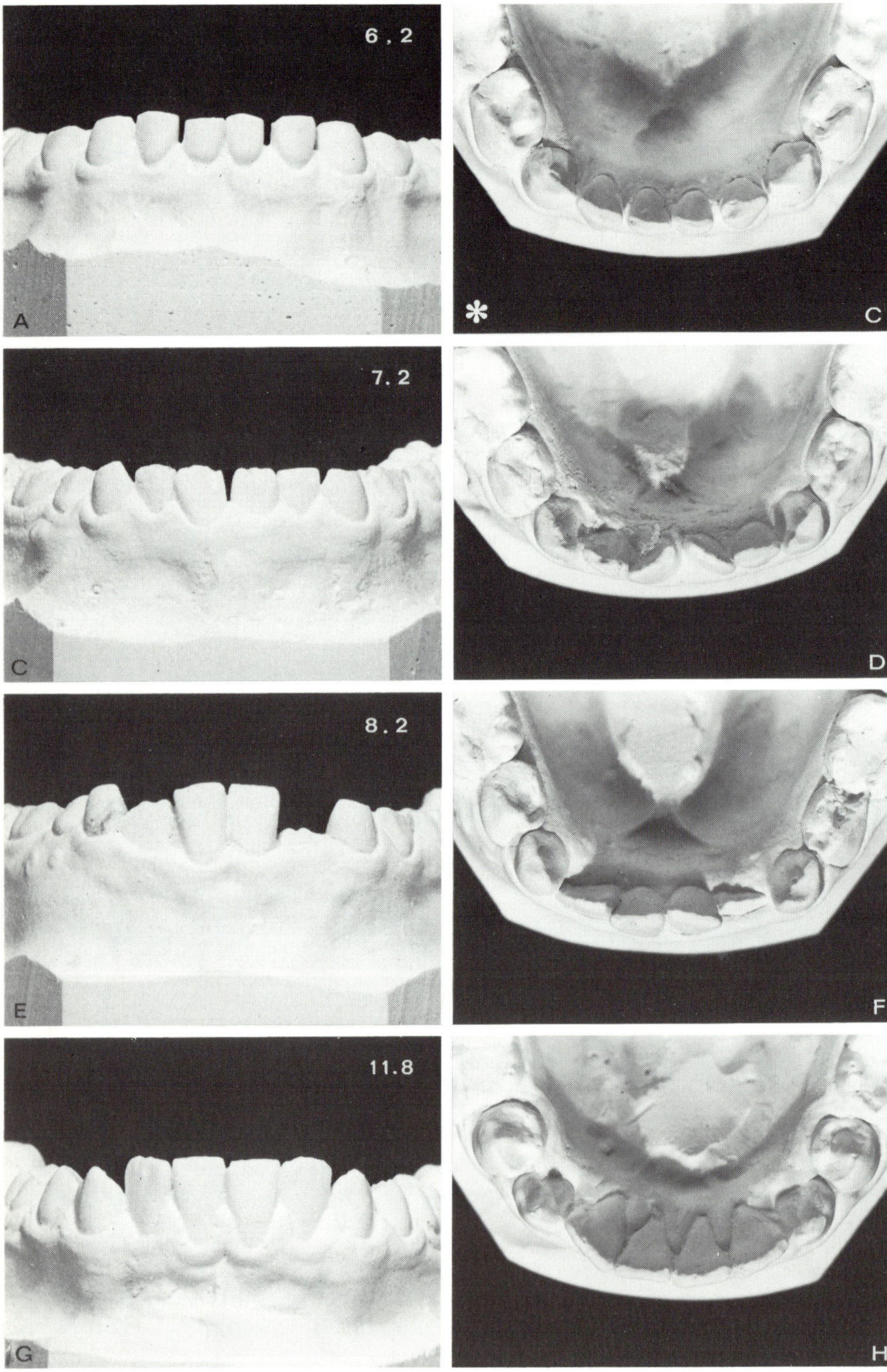

Figure 2-11

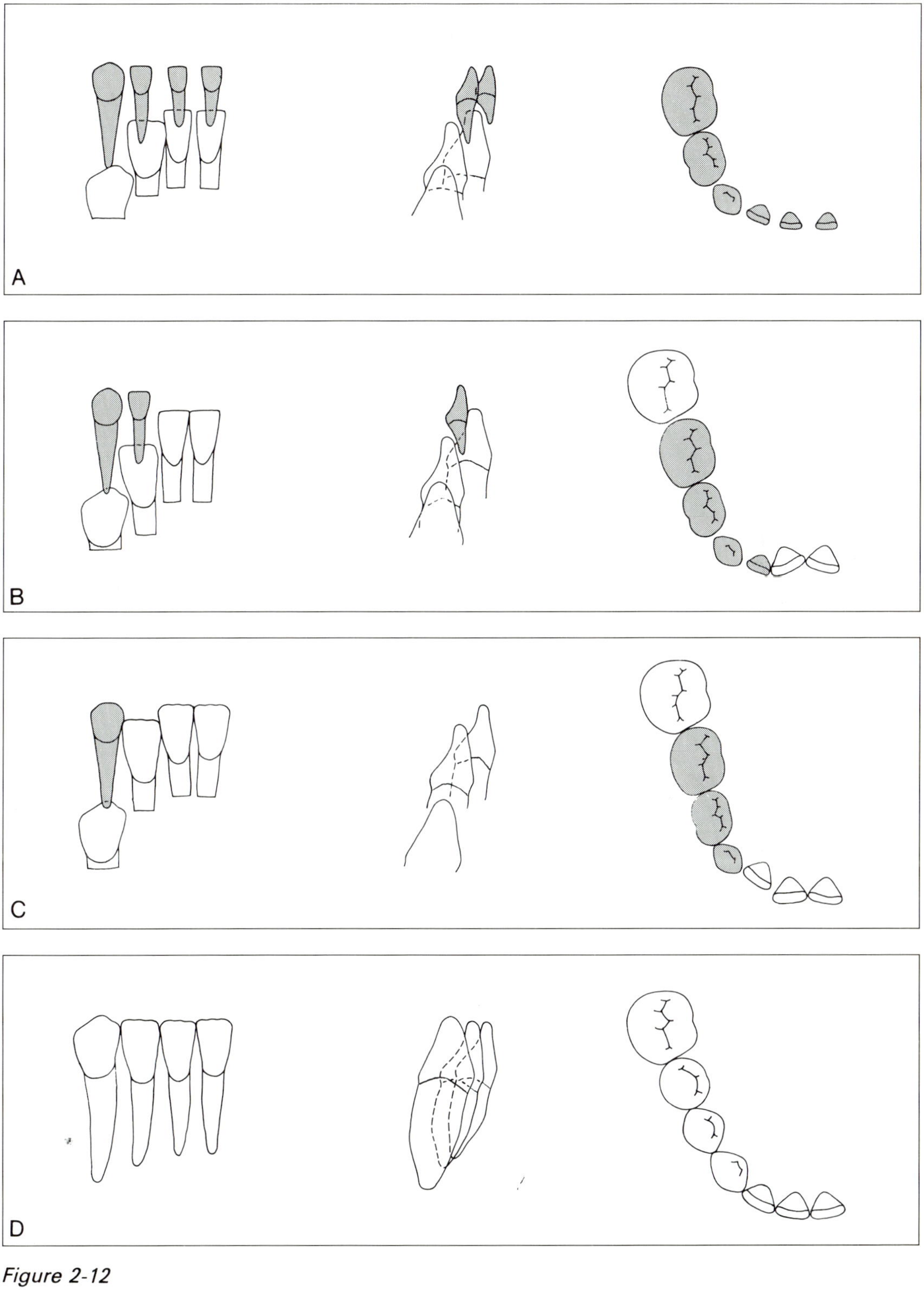

Figure 2-12

Fig. 2-12 (see page 49) Schematic drawings of the Mandibular Incisor Transition Pattern C characterized by mesiolingually rotated emergence of the central incisor and nonrotated or only slightly distolingually rotated emergence of the lateral incisor, in a large anterior section of the apical area.

A Large diastemata between the anterior deciduous teeth. Sufficient space for the rotated central permanent incisors. Limited overlapping of the lateral incisor by the central incisor.
B During and after the postemergence eruption the rotations of the central permanent incisors are corrected. When the lateral incisor erupts, further contact will develop with the root of the adjacent deciduous canine, resulting in a distal and lateral displacement of the latter.
C The lateral permanent incisor has emerged lingually and continues to erupt in that direction until tongue pressure moves it in line with the other teeth of the dental arch. Sufficient space becomes available for this displacement that frequently takes place after the tooth has reached the level of the occlusal plane.
D Completion of the transition of the posterior teeth.

2.6 Supplementary remarks

Transition of the mandibular incisors and their final location depend mainly on the size of the anterior section of the apical area. Distinct variations exist in the position of the four permanent incisors before eruption begins. Normally, the lateral incisors are situated lingual to the central incisors and are aligned approximately in comparable arch shapes. However, morphogenesis may also start in rotated positions, leading to an initially deviating orientation of one or more mandibular incisors.

No data are available to indicate that initial rotations of mandibular permanent incisors are a sign of crowded conditions. It may very well be that these two variables are independent of each other, at least before emergence. Initial rotations correct spontaneously after emergence, if spatial conditions permit this to occur.

A differentiation must be made between initial rotations and those that develop secondarily. Eruption of an adjacent permanent canine may change the position of a lateral incisor. Similarly, changes may occur in a later period of the development of the dentition, leading to improved or worsened positioning of one or more teeth. The changes in the position of the mandibular incisors that may take place in association with the transition of the posterior teeth will be discussed in Chapter 10.

Contacts between the crowns of erupting permanent teeth and roots of the adjacent deciduous teeth lead to changes in dental arch dimensions and particularly to an increase in the intercanine distance. If this increase occurs and to what extent depend mainly on the size of the anterior section of the apical area. A lack in increase in intercanine distance during the transition of the incisors caused either by unfavourable or missing contacts or by premature loss of deciduous teeth will probably not be caught up or will only be slightly caught up later on.

Chapter 3

Variations in Transition of Mandibular Posterior Teeth*

3.1 Introduction

The space available in the dental arch for transition of the posterior teeth is bounded by the distal surface of the lateral permanent incisor crown and the mesial surface of the first permanent molar crown. The sum of the mesiodistal crown dimensions of the mandibular deciduous molars and canine exceeds that of their successors. The first premolar usually has a mesiodistal crown width similar to that of its predecessor or slightly smaller. The second premolar has a considerably smaller mesiodistal crown dimension than its predecessor. The reverse situation is common for the canines. These differences in mesiodistal crown dimensions of the corresponding deciduous and permanent posterior teeth are responsible for some typical features of the transition.

Distinct differences exist between the two jaws regarding the transition of the posterior teeth. These differences are associated with the relatively large middle section of the apical area in the mandible and the small one in the maxilla. Mandibular permanent canines and premolars erupt from spacious conditions in the middle section of the apical area to more limited ones in the dental arch. In the maxilla the space for the crowns of the corresponding teeth increases when they move from the middle section of the apical area to the dental arch.

The transition of the mandibular posterior teeth is discussed in relation to the space available for the permanent canine and premolars in the middle section of the apical area and in the dental arch. The variation in location of the permanent canine and the premolars and their relation to their predecessors and the adjacent lateral permanent incisor and first molar are indicated. The differences in emergence sequence and associated preemergence and postemergence behaviour are discussed. Nine transition patterns are distinguished, five of which are presented in detail.

* Reproduced from: "Transition of the lower posterior teeth" by Hein J.W. Wassenberg, Paul J.M.R. Bakker and Frans P.G.M. van der Linden. In: *Transition of the human dentition.* Monograph No. 13. Craniofacial Growth Series., Pg 39-62. Ed. Frans P.G.M. van der Linden. Center for Human Growth and Development. The University of Michigan, Ann Arbor, U.S.A., 1982.

3.2 The middle section of the apical area and the arrangement of the permanent canine and premolars before emergence

The anterior section of the apical area is bounded laterally by the mesial surfaces of the permanent canines (see page 28). The dimensions in the deciduous dental arch are of limited relevance for the size of the anterior section of the apical area, because the correlation between the mesiodistal crown dimensions of the corresponding deciduous and permanent anterior teeth is rather low. The space that is initially available in the dental arch is usually less than that required for the arrangement of the four mandibular permanent incisors in good alignment. During the transitional process the space available will increase as the canines move distally and laterally.
The situation is different for the canine-premolar region, where normally the interdental arch dimension from the distal surface of the crown of the lateral permanent incisor to the mesial surface of the first permanent molar does not increase but decreases with the transition of the posterior teeth. This dimension is slightly larger than the combined mesiodistal crown widths of the permanent teeth that emerge there. A lack in overall space does not normally exist and the middle section of the apical area is accordingly adequate in size. However, problems may arise when some of the excess space is utilised for an improved alignment of the incisors and when the emergence sequence is unfavourable. Premature loss of deciduous tooth material due to decay or extraction may considerably influence the course of events and the result of the transition of the posterior teeth.
The size and shape of the middle section of the apical area vary on the basis of *(1)* the overall morphology of the mandible, *(2)* the location of the permanent canine within the jaw and its relation to the adjacent lateral permanent incisor, and *(3)* the position of the first permanent molar. The latter depends on the mesiodistal crown dimensions of the deciduous molars and the molar's location during formation. Its subsequent mesiodistal position in the dental arch is mainly determined by its relation to the distal surface of the adjacent second deciduous molar.
Invariably the permanent canines are initially formed closer to the lower border of the mandible than the second premolars and particularly the first premolars. In the preeruption phase the forming parts of the premolars are closer to the level of the occlusal plane than of the canine, which becomes the longest tooth in the mandible. The tip of the canine crown is located lingual to the apex of its predecessor. However, the buccal aspect of its crown bulges out and is easily palpable. The premolars are formed between the roots of their predecessors. Prior to eruption the distal surface of the permanent canine crown is in contact with or in close proximity to the mesial side of the cementoenamel junction of the first premolar.
Considerable variation can exist in the relation between the permanent canine crown and the root of its predecessor, as has been discussed and demonstrated in Chapter 2. Also, the relation between the premolars and their predecessors can vary markedly, more so in the mesiodistal than buccolingual direction.
The size of the middle section of the apical area in relation to that of the anterior section depends partly on the positions of the permanent canine and adjacent lateral incisor and partly on the labiolingual inclination of the anterior alveolar process. As for the anterior region, large, medium, and small sections of the middle apical areas are distinguished (Figs. 3-1 to 3-3).

The differences in the sum of the mesiodistal crown dimensions of the two deciduous molars and canine and that of their successors are crucial. A marked difference can therefore exist between the mesiodistal crown dimensions of deciduous molars and canines and that of their successors, particularly for the canines. The differences in crown width of the corresponding individual teeth together with the sequence of emergence play an important role in the transition process of the posterior teeth.

3.3 Eruption before emergence

The sequence of emergence in the transition of the posterior teeth is not uniform as in the incisal region. The arrangement of the premolars and permanent canine within the jaw and their relation to the roots of the deciduous teeth and adjacent permanent teeth allow a variation in emergence sequence. The spatial conditions may also allow the two premolars and permanent canine to emerge simultaneously. Particularly in a large middle section of the apical area, one tooth does not need to emerge prior to its neighbour to create the space for the latter to erupt, as is typical for the incisor region. In most instances the mandibular permanent canine emerges first. In its preemergence eruption phase it passes the first premolar, which is initially closer to the occlusal plane. The canine has the longest distance to travel in its eruption; the first premolar the shortest. The second premolar, generally the last one to emerge, is initially located at a vertical level somewhere between those of the two other teeth. It therefore assumes an intermediate position regarding the length of the eruption path. The variation in initial direction of eruption and the subsequent eruption behaviour are greater in a large and also in a small middle section of the apical area than in a medium-sized area. It would appear that in a large middle section of the apical area the crowns have the freedom to be arranged in varying ways. In this situation the premolars can erupt in diverse directions. In a medium middle section of the apical area the canine and premolar crowns are situated in restricted spatial conditions, allowing less variation in their orientation. In a small middle section of the apical area the canine and premolar crowns are arranged in crowded conditions with the accompanying deviations in orientation.
In Fig. 3-4 the process of transition of the mandibular and maxillary posterior teeth is illustrated and explained for the most frequently observed sequences of emergence. In Fig. 3-5 some variations in the sequence of emergence of the posterior teeth, including the second permanent molar, are indicated. The moment of emergence of the latter in relation to the transition of the posterior teeth and particularly to the loss of the second deciduous molar is important with regard to the amount of mesial migration of the first permanent molar associated with the transition of the posterior teeth. The first permanent molar will become more mesially displaced when the second permanent molar emerges prior to the loss of the second deciduous molar than if it emerges after that event.[222]
Deciduous molars are rarely resorbed prematurely in association with erupting adjacent permanent teeth. The crowns of the premolars are located more or less between the roots of their predecessors and seldom extend mesially or distally beyond the approximal crown surfaces of their predecessors. Shortage of available space for the eruption of the permanent canine is usually associated with an exaggerated mesial

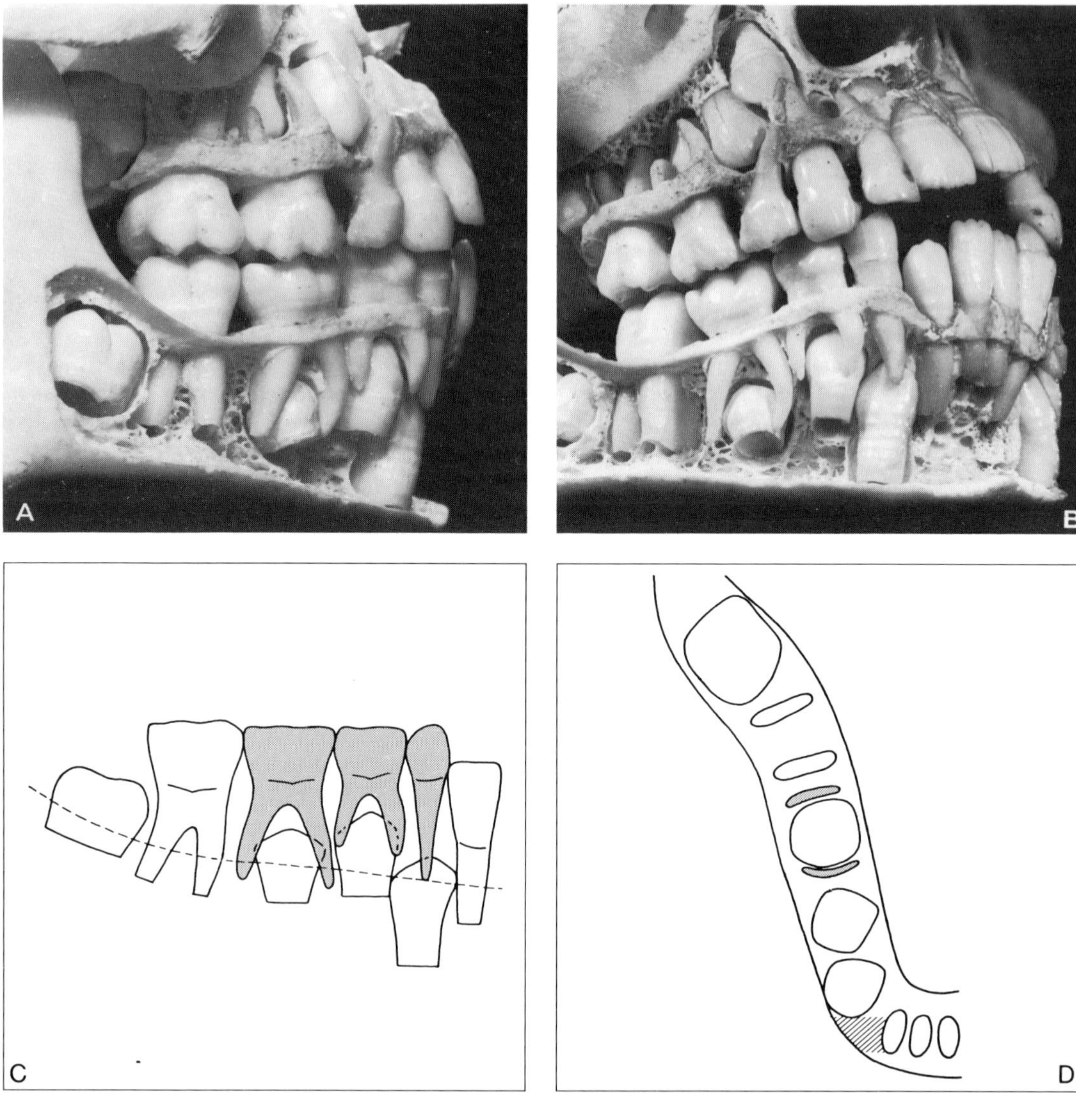

Fig. 3-1 *Large middle section of the apical area in the mandible. The position of the permanent canine, the differences in mesiodistal crown dimensions of corresponding teeth, and the size and shape of the middle section of the apical area in the mesiodistal direction are favourable.*

- *A* *The mesiodistal crown width of the mandibular second deciduous molar is considerably larger than that of its successor. The latter is at some distance from the mesial root of the first permanent molar. The mandibular permanent canine is only slightly mesially angulated.*
- *B* *Between the crowns of the premolars is a space of about 3 mm. However, the mesial surface of the first premolar is in contact with the distal corner of the permanent canine crown. The latter is slightly distal to the apex of its predecessor and distal to the root of the lateral incisor.*

C Schematic drawing with a dotted line indicating the section presented in D. Note the relation between the permanent canine crown and the root of the lateral incisor.

D Excess space is available between the mesial root of the first permanent molar and the distal surface of the root of the lateral incisor for the crowns of the premolars and permanent canine. Note the size of the indicated area between the permanent canine and the lateral incisor and particularly its sagittal dimension.

(Legend 3-2 continued)

C The crown of the permanent canine is mesial to the apex of its predecessor. Note the relationship between the permanent canine crown and the lateral incisor root.

D The space available between the mesial root of the first permanent molar and the distal surface of the root of the lateral incisor is sufficient but critical. The crown of the permanent canine must move distally to establish a good contact with the crown of the lateral incisor. Extra space is required, and it is questionable if that extra space can be provided from the distal side. The size of the indicated area between the permanent canine crown and the root of the lateral incisor is critical, particularly in a sagittal direction.

(Legend 3-3 continued)

B The differences in mesiodistal crown width of the canines and the first deciduous molar/premolar are unfavourable and overrule the favourable difference in that respect for the second deciduous molar/premolar. The crowns of the premolars are close together; the distal surface of the permanent canine crown lies approximately in the same plane as the distal surface of the root of its predecessor.

C The crowns of the permanent teeth that must still erupt are close together and crowded. The mesial surface of the permanent canine overlaps more than half of the root of the lateral incisor.

D To establish a harmonious contact between the crown of the lateral incisor and that of the permanent canine, the latter must move distally over a considerable distance, which is in fact impossible. The space available in the dental arch between the mesial root of the first permanent molar and the distal surface of the lateral incisor is too small to accommodate the permanent canine and premolars without crowding. The indicated area between the permanent lateral and permanent canine and particularly its sagittal dimension is a clear sign of the unfavourable conditions in that region.

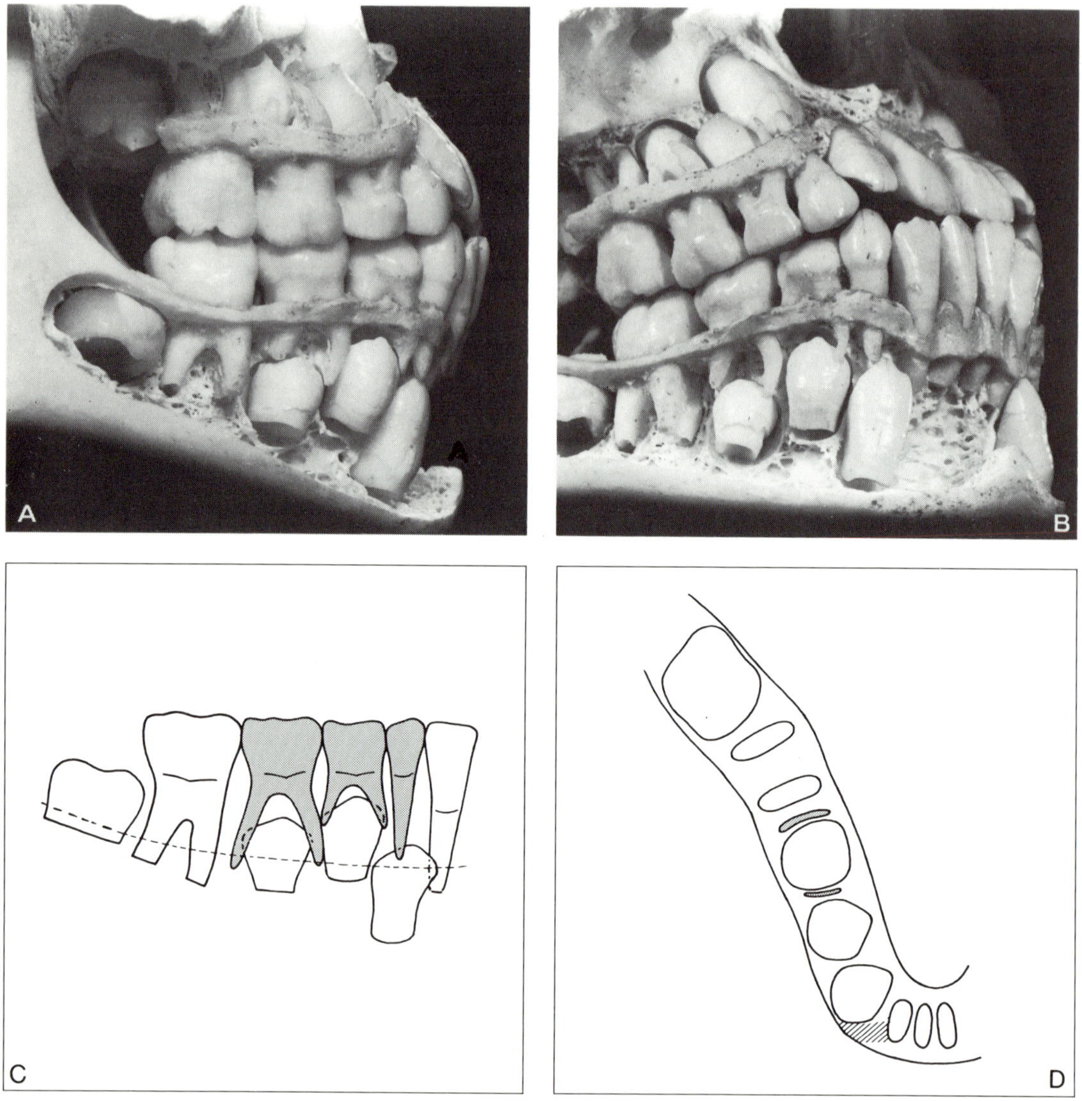

Fig. 3-2 Medium middle section of the apical area in the mandible. The position of the permanent canine, the differences in mesiodistal crown dimensions of the corresponding teeth, and the size and shape of the middle section of the apical area are critical.

A The mesiodistal crown width of the second deciduous molar is only slightly larger than that of its successor. The latter is rather close to the mesial root of the first permanent molar. The permanent canine is mesially angulated.

B Between the crowns of the premolars is a space of approximately 1 mm. The mesial surface of the first premolar is in close proximity to the distal surface of the permanent canine. The mesial side of the crown of the latter overlaps the root of the lateral incisor.

(Legend continues on page 55)

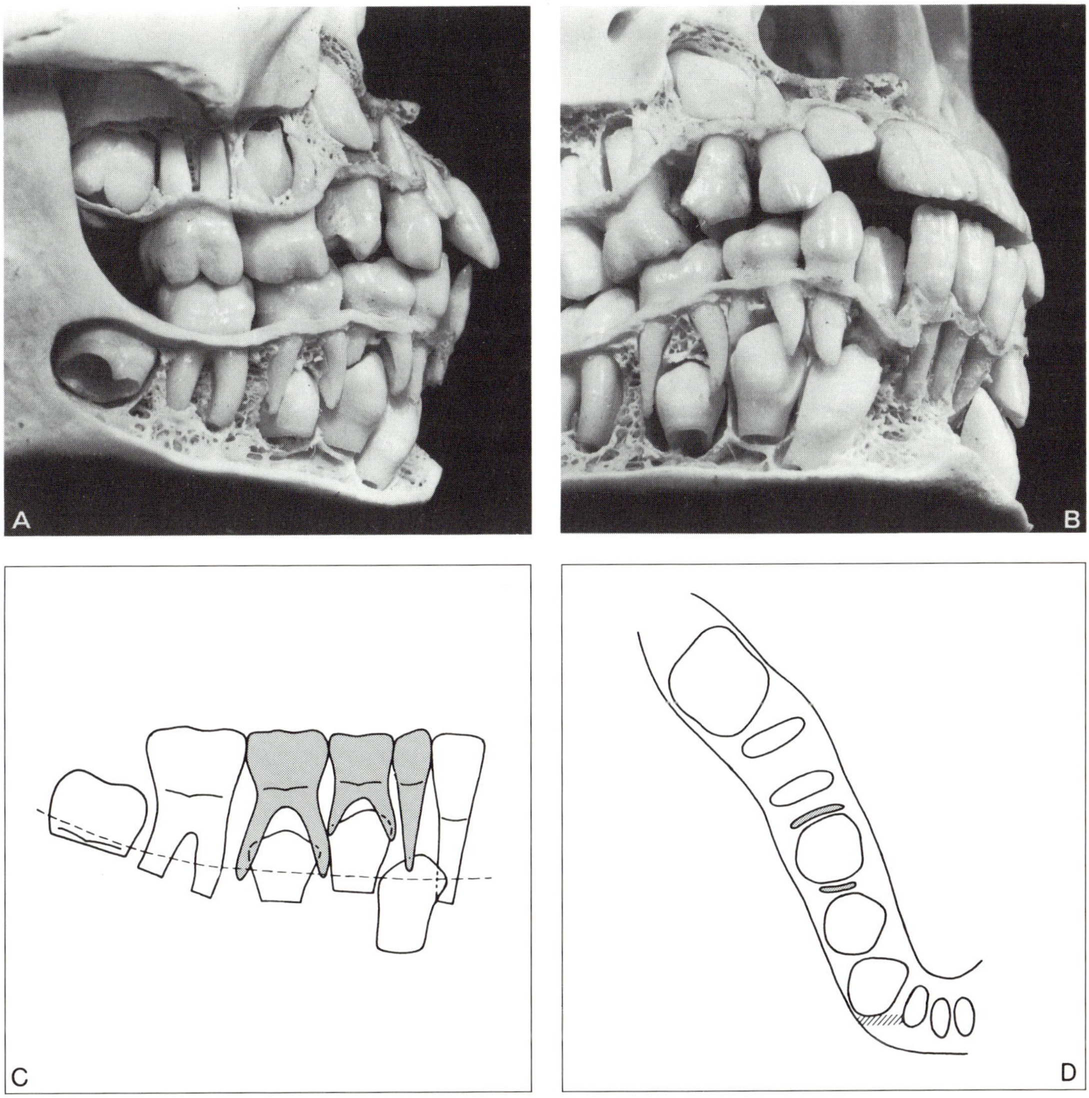

Fig. 3-3 Small middle section of the apical area in the mandible. The position of the permanent canine, its relation to the lateral incisor, the differences in mesiodistal crown dimensions of the corresponding teeth, and the size and shape of the middle section of the apical area are unfavourable.

A Some space exists between the distal surface of the crown of the second premolar and the mesial roots of the first permanent molar. However, the canine is distinctly mesially located and angulated.

(Legend continues on page 55)

Fig. 3-4 Schematic presentation of the transition of the mandibular and maxillary posterior teeth and the emergence of the second permanent molars.

A The premolar crowns are located between the roots of their predecessors, which resorb concomitantly with the eruption of the premolars. In both jaws the occlusal surface of the permanent canine is initially at a greater distance from the occlusal plane than that of the first premolar. In this illustration the mandibular canine has already started to erupt and is at the same level as the first premolar. Both mandibular premolars are approximately perpendicularly oriented in relation to the occlusal plane. The permanent mandibular canine is slightly mesially angulated. In a large middle section of the apical area in the mandible some space may exist between the canine and first premolar crown. The mandibular permanent second molar is mesiolingually oriented in accordance with its initial position.
In the maxilla the first premolar is initially the closest to the occlusal plane and normally maintains that condition and emerges as the first one of the three teeth involved. The distal corner of the permanent canine crown is situated close to the mesial-cervical region of the first premolar. As in the mandible, the second premolar takes an intermediate position regarding the distance between the crown and the occlusal plane. Both maxillary premolars are slightly mesially angulated, the canine somewhat more. The maxillary permanent second molar is distobuccally oriented in accordance with its initial position and the local spatial conditions in the tuberosity region.

B The mandibular canine emerges shortly after the loss of its predecessor and has left the adjacent premolar behind. The diastema originally present between the deciduous canine and first deciduous molar provides the extra space required to accommodate the wider permanent canine crown within the dental arch. In the maxilla the first premolar has erupted more than the two adjacent teeth.

C The mandibular first premolar emerges shortly after the canine. Sufficient space is available. In the maxilla the first premolar also emerges with adequate space.

D The mandibular second premolar emerges into an excess of space in accordance with the differences in mesiodistal crown dimensions involved. In the maxilla a comparable situation is found, though with less excess space.

E The mandibular premolars are fully erupted and the excess space is reduced mainly by mesial migration of the mandibular first permanent molar. In the maxilla the canine emerges as the last of the three.

F The second permanent molars have emerged and attained occlusion. In the maxilla the permanent canine has taken up its position within the dental arch. The extra space required for the wide permanent crown was obtained from the remaining diastemata in the incisal region and the excess remaining after the emergence of the premolars. The maxillary second permanent molar has emerged and occludes with the mandibular molar.

On the average the process of transition of the posterior teeth only lasts about 1 to 1.5 years, but it may take considerably longer. The sequence of emergence can differ markedly and all theoretically possible sequences occur. The maxillary permanent canine usually does not emerge prior to the first premolar unless excess space is available in that region, or when it is positioned buccally. Emergence of the second permanent molars can occur during transition (most frequent) or after transition of the posterior teeth. (From Van der Linden.[223])

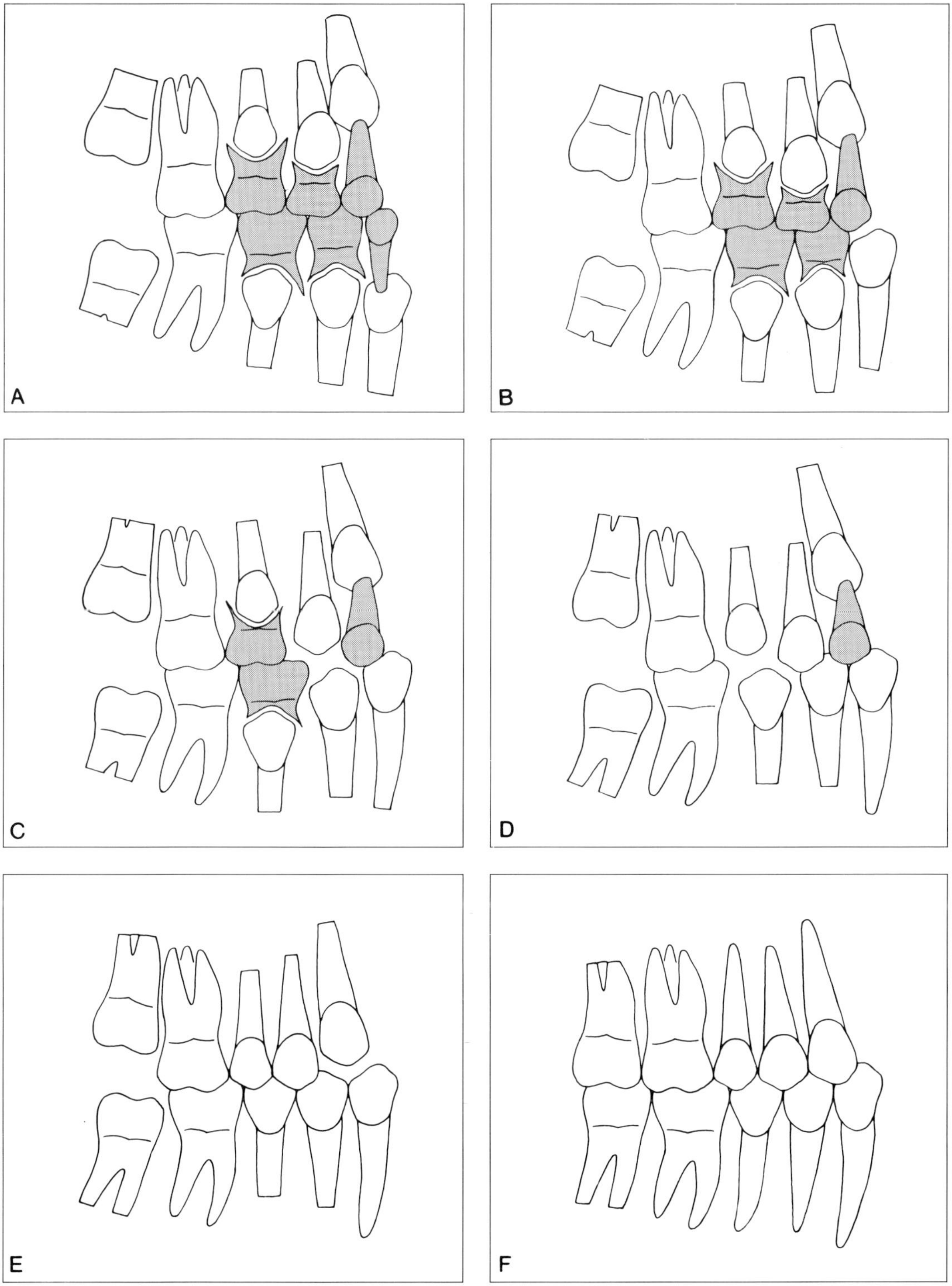

Figure 3-4

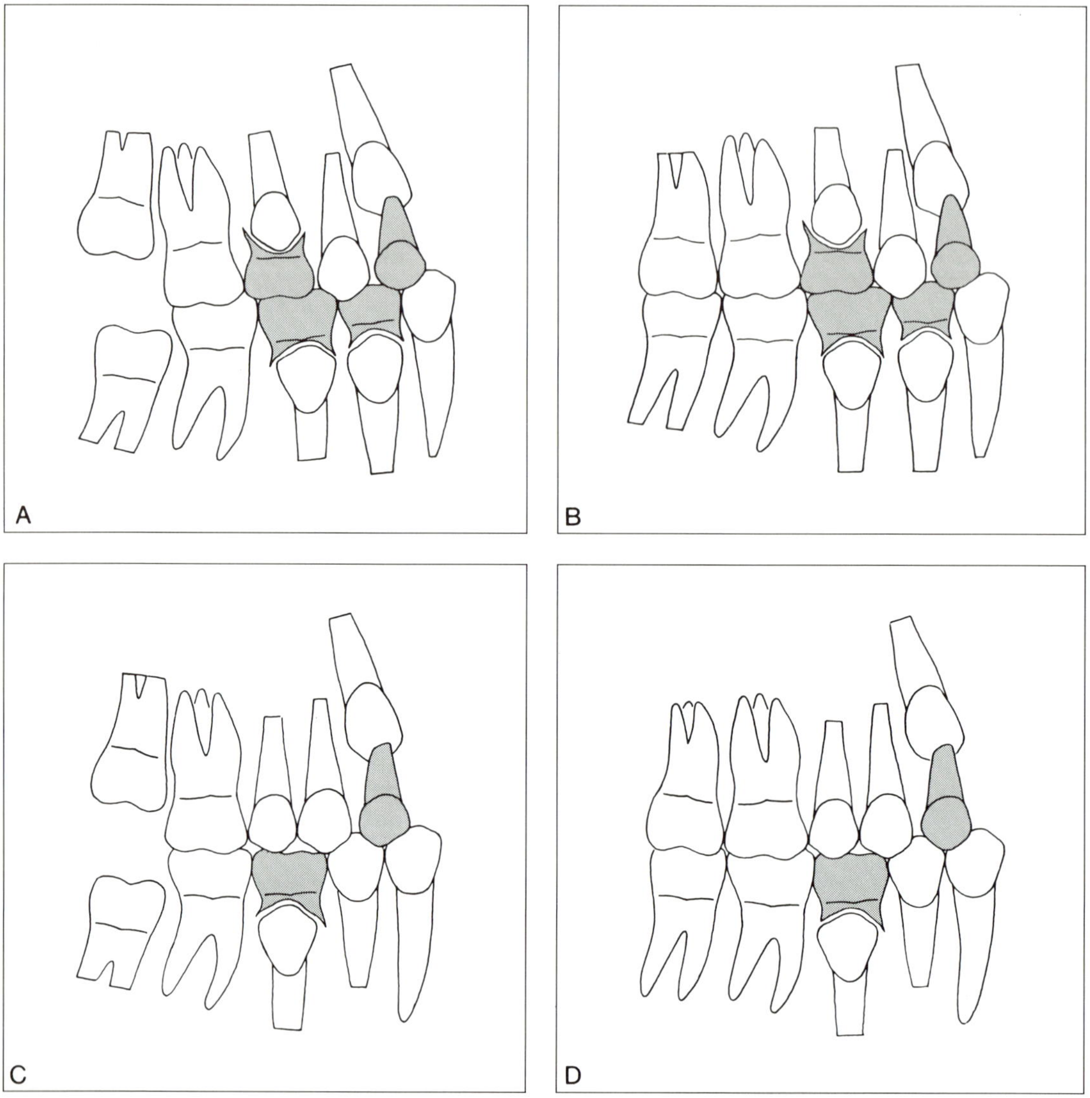

Fig. 3-5 Schematic presentation of some variations in the sequence of emergence of the posterior teeth, including the second permanent molars. (From Van der Linden.[223])

A The mandibular permanent canine and the maxillary first premolar have emerged at approximately the same time. The second permanent molars in both jaws have not yet emerged.

B Emergence of the second permanent molars has taken place during or shortly after the transition of the mandibular canine and the emergence of the maxillary first premolar.

C The mandibular first premolar and permanent canine have emerged simultaneously. The same holds true for the two maxillary premolars. The second permanent molars have not yet emerged.

D The mandibular and maxillary second permanent molars have emerged before complete transition of the posterior teeth. The maxillary deciduous canine and mandibular second deciduous molar have still to be replaced.

positioning and angulation of that tooth and an overlapping of the adjacent lateral incisor. Upon emergence, the canine will take up a corresponding position in the dental arch. There will be insufficient space for the canine and it will overlap the lateral incisor labially. This will be the case particularly when the permanent canine emerges prior to the exfoliation of the first deciduous molar. The extra space provided by the difference in mesiodistal crown dimensions of the premolars and their predecessors, is not available at the time required by the canine. The eruption and emergence of the second premolar normally are not influenced by the size and shape of the middle section of the apical area because it is placed between and below the roots, and at a later stage, below the crown of its predecessor.

A marked difference exists between the incisors/canines and the deciduous molars/premolars regarding the time that elapses between the loss of the deciduous tooth and the moment of emergence of its successor. As a rule, a premolar emerges prior to the loss of the crown of its predecessor, in contrast to the situation for the canines and incisors. Premolars emerge under the crowns of their predecessors. The loss of deciduous molars does not take place before but after their successors emerge. Thus the gingival tissue does not need to be pierced. An erupting premolar displaces the crown of its predecessor usually lingually and brings it into supraposition. It is pushed back to the appropriate occlusal level when contact with the opposing teeth is established. The buccal cusp of a premolar usually emerges slightly lateral to the buccal surface of its predecessor, especially in the maxilla. After the deciduous molar crown is exfoliated, the occlusal surface of the premolar becomes exposed.

3.4 Eruption after emergence and subsequent change in orientation

The direction of the postemergence eruption and subsequent location of the premolars are determined mainly by the contact that develops between the opposing teeth. This holds particularly true for the buccolingual orientations and to a lesser extent for the mesiodistal ones. Regarding the latter, the emergence sequence, the spatial conditions in the dental arch, and the contacts with adjacent teeth are most important. However, the direction of the postemergence eruption of the canine and its subsequent location in the buccolingual direction are mainly influenced by conditions in the same dental arch, such as the contact relations with the adjacent teeth. The forces exerted by the tongue and the buccal musculature seem to play a secondary role in that respect.

The vertical and buccolingual variation in positioning for the premolars and permanent canine is limited and is different from that of the incisors. The ultimate vertical position of the premolars is determined by the occlusal contacts with the antagonists. That is also the case for the canines, although less rigidly so, because the vertical contact relation of these teeth is not as definite as that of the premolars.

Particularly the mandibular permanent canine, which generally erupts first, can emerge under unfavourable conditions. Its mesial surface will then usually overlap the lateral incisor crown labially. However, this contact may improve later, depending on the differences in mesiodistal crown dimensions of the deciduous molars/premolars and the sequence of emergence.

When the canine does move distally from its crowded position and occupies some of the space orginally utilised by the first deciduous molar crown, the first premolar

subsequently can run into problems. This movement of the canine, probably partly caused by the buccal musculature, can take place before the first premolar has had the chance to erupt fully. However, when both deciduous molars are lost almost simultaneously, and the same conditions exist for the permanent canine, the situation is more favourable because the first premolar is able to erupt freely and can move distally and does act less as restriction for the distal movement of the canine. It can be an obstacle if the first premolar has reached full occlusion prior to the loss of the second deciduous molar. Then the canine cannot readily benefit from the excess in crown width of the second deciduous molar. How far a mandibular permanent canine that emerged under crowded conditions will be able to improve in position depends also on its original orientation before emergence and on its subsequent contact with the lateral incisor crown.
The mandibular first premolar, like the permanent canine, has a slight tendency to erupt in a mesial direction. The mandibular second premolar often erupts in a slightly distal direction.[99]
Problems usually arise in cases of crowded conditions for the premolars, which may result from the premature loss of crown material of their predecessors, particularly in combination with unfavourable emergence sequence and relatively early emergence of the second permanent molars.[122,172] The first premolars then have a tendency to erupt in a more buccal direction and the second premolars in a more lingual direction.

3.5 Patterns in transition of the mandibular posterior teeth

To distinguish patterns in the transition of the incisors, their rotational position serves as a parameter. For the transition of the posterior teeth the leeway space is of major

TABLE 3-1
Survey of nine combinations in the transition of the mandibular posterior teeth based on three emergence sequences and the size of the leeway space. Combination based on emergence sequences (5, 3, 4; 5 (3, 4); and 5, 4, 3) are not incorporated so as to reduce the complexity of the presentation. The five patterns demonstrated by means of photographs of longitudinal series of dental casts and by schematic drawings are labeled A, B, C, D, and E. The ones marked with an X-sign are discussed in combination with the patterns demonstrated.

leeway space / sequence of emergence	large $> +1.1$ mm	medium $+1.1$ to -1.1 mm	small < -1.1 mm
3, 4, 5	A	B	C
(3, 4) 5	X	D	X
3 (4, 5)	X	X	E

NB. The use of ( ) indicates simultaneous emergence.

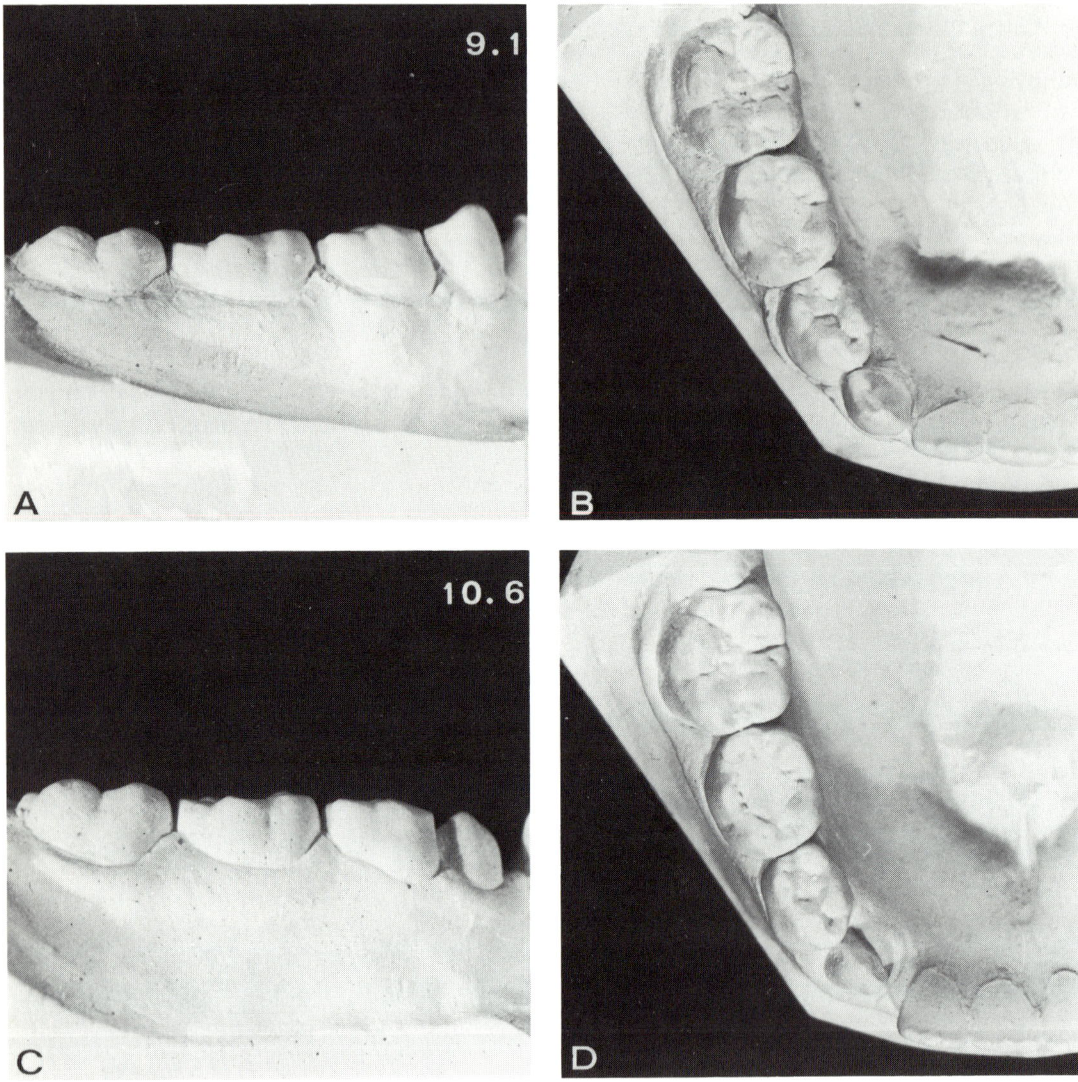

Fig. 3-6 Lateral and occlusal views of a longitudinal series of dental casts of the Mandibular Posterior Teeth Transition Pattern A, characterized by the emergence sequence 3, 4, 5 and a large leeway space.

A, B A harmoniously shaped dental arch with a diastema between the lateral permanent incisor and the deciduous canine.

C, D The permanent canine has emerged and sufficient space is available. Note that the second deciduous molar has only a slightly larger mesiodistal crown width than the first molar.

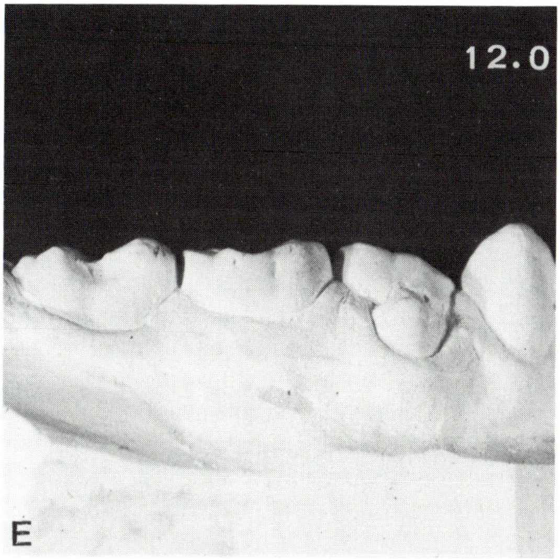

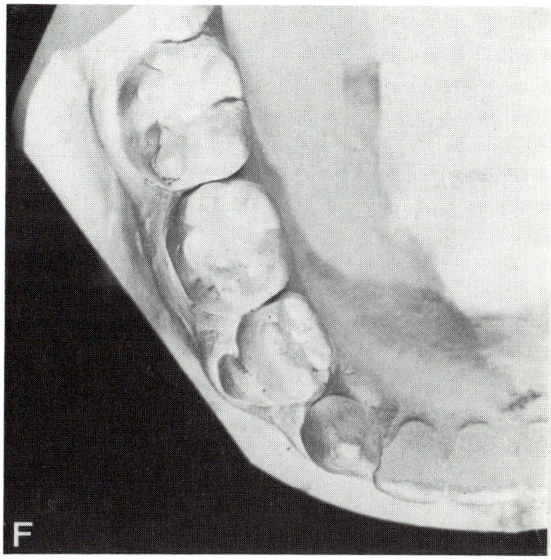

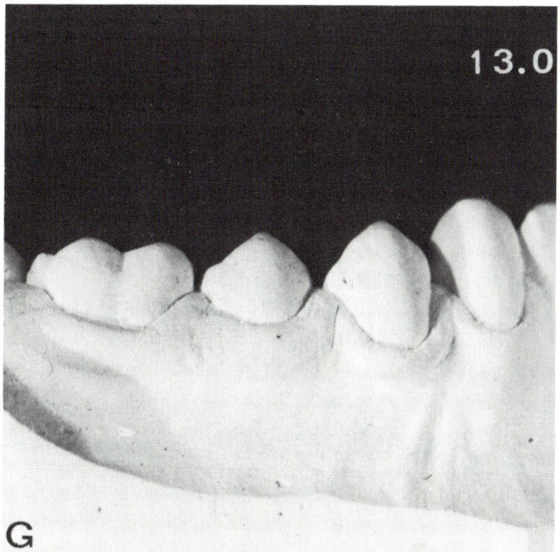

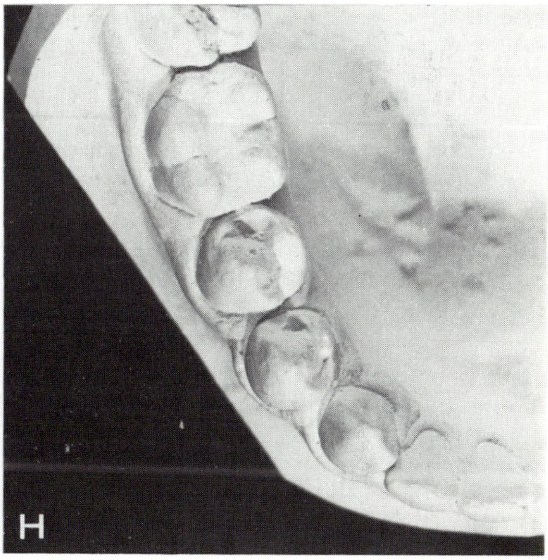

E, F *The first premolar has emerged in a buccal direction and has pushed its still present predecessor lingually. The permanent canine has completed its eruption and has established an acceptable contact with the lateral incisor.*

G, H *The second premolar has emerged. Some space is still present between the premolars. The permanent canine has moved lingually, particularly its mesial side, and the contact point with the lateral incisor has become less acceptable. It is unlikely that this change in canine position is related primarily to changes within the mandible. It is probably caused by the development of an unfavourable occlusal contact with the maxillary teeth. The first premolar has moved into a good transverse position. The permanent second molar emerged after the transition of the posterior teeth was completed.*

importance and is used for this purpose. Further, the leeway space is easier to estimate than the size of the middle section of the apical area and is more useful for clinical purposes.

Dividing the transition of the mandibular posterior teeth into patterns is not only based on size of the leeway space but also on differences in the emergence sequence. Table 3-1 presents a survey of the nine patterns; five of them will be demonstrated by means of photographs and schematic drawings. The remaining four will be discussed briefly in connection with the others.

The difference in mesiodistal crown dimension between the second deciduous molar and its successor plays a dominant role in the transition process in critical situations. It seems to determine more than the size of the leeway space what is going to happen in the canine and first premolar region. It makes quite a difference in comparable critical cases with a similar leeway space whether a relatively large mesiodistal crown dimension of the second deciduous molar is associated with small values in this respect for the deciduous canine and first deciduous molar or vice versa. In the latter instance the leeway space can be utilised more effectively than in the former case, in which the emergence sequence is more crucial. In cases with a large leeway space the size differences between the corresponding deciduous and permanent teeth are of limited importance. A relatively large mesiodistal second deciduous molar crown will then not endanger the course of events of the transition of the posterior teeth.

The changes associated with the transition of the mandibular posterior teeth frequently do not take place symmetrically. That holds true not only for the timing but also for the manner of the transition itself.

In the presentation of the transitional patterns the eruption of the second permanent molar is not usually taken into account. Some aspects related to the time of emergence of the second permanent molars in relation to the transition of the posterior teeth will be discussed in Chapter 4.

Fig. 3-7 Schematic lateral and occlusal views of Mandibular Posterior Teeth Transition Pattern A, characterized by the emergence sequence 3, 4, 5 and a large leeway space.

A Diastemata on both sides of the deciduous canine. Harmoniously shaped dental arch often accompanied by a slight eversion of the four incisors. Sufficient space was available within the jaw for the permanent canine to pass the first premolar during eruption.

B The canine has emerged with sufficient space in the dental arch, followed shortly thereafter by the first premolar. The crown of the first deciduous molar may be lost at a moment when the canine can benefit from the resulting space. This aspect can be important if a large difference exists in mesiodistal crown dimension between the deciduous canine and its successor.

C The first premolar has emerged and a comparable situation exists in relation to the crown of the second deciduous molar, as explained under B, for the canine in relation to the crown of the first deciduous molar. The extra space provided in the arch by the replacement of the second deciduous molar by the second premolar can lead to a distal migration of the first premolar and the teeth mesial to it.

D The space remaining in the arch can be closed mainly from the mesial aspect, particularly when the second permanent molars have not yet emerged. The incisors can become more upright and the anterior section of the dental arch flattened.

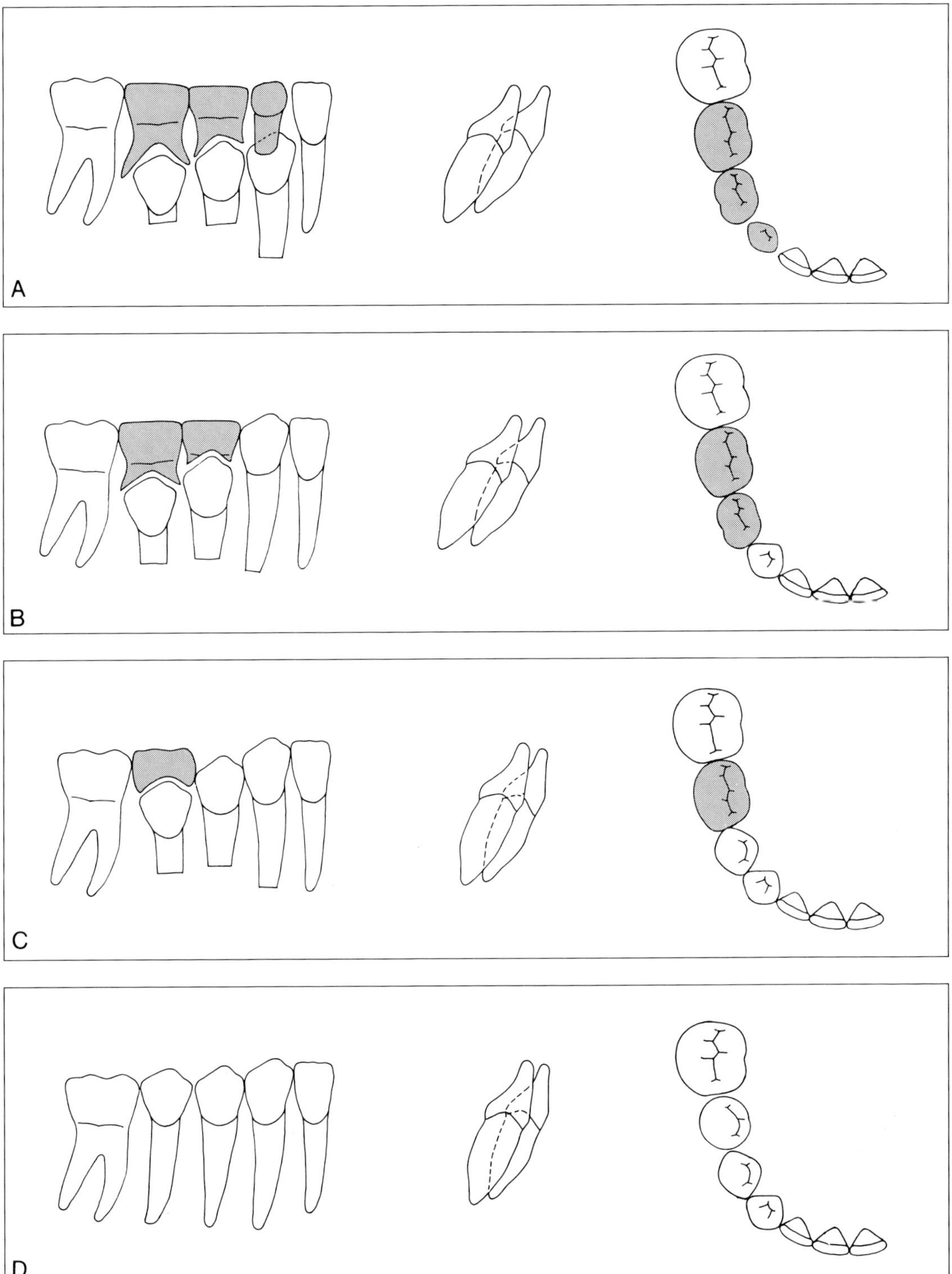

Figure 3-7

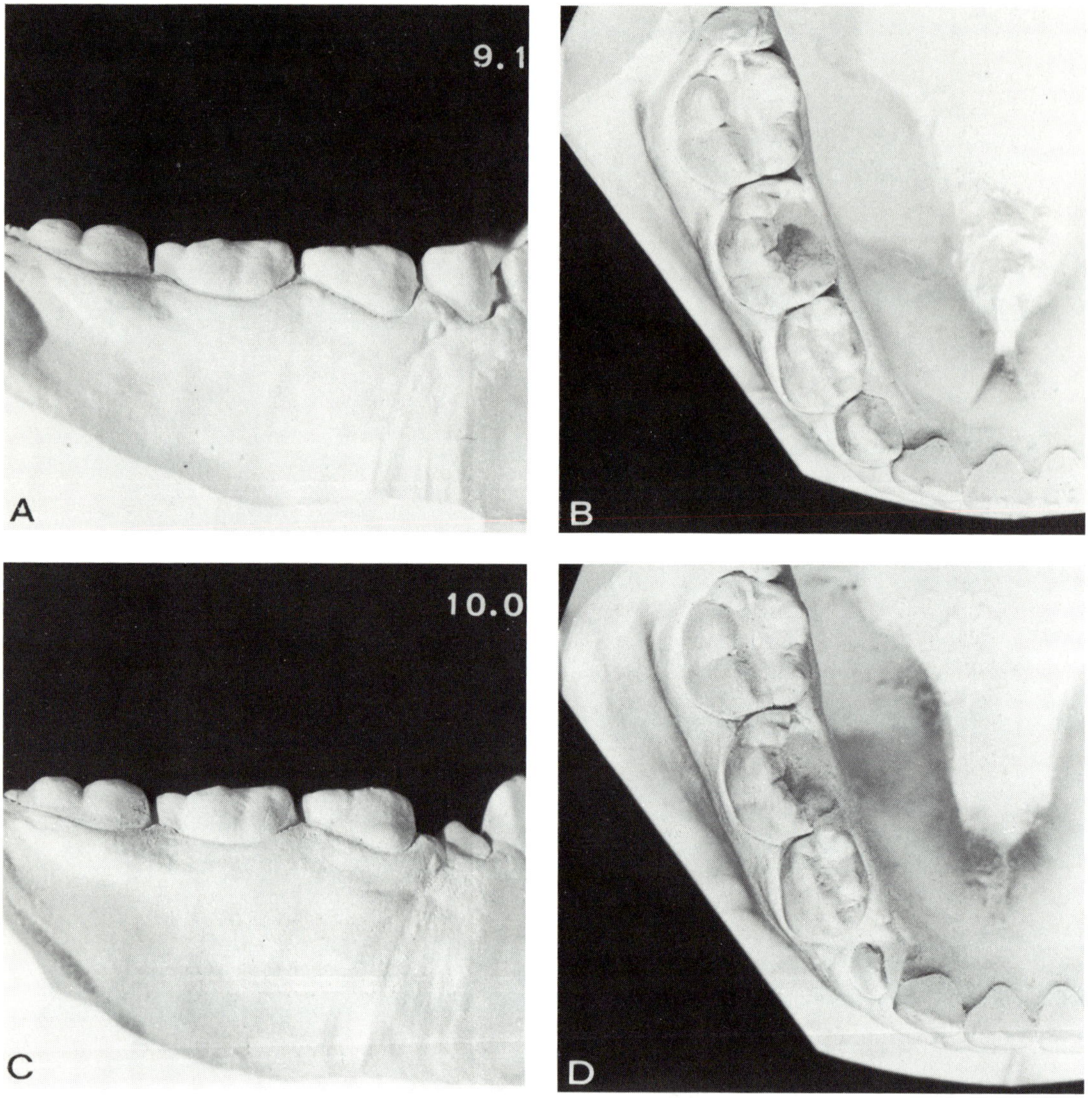

Fig. 3-8 Longitudinal series of dental casts showing the Mandibular Posterior Teeth Transition Pattern B, characterized by the emergence sequence 3, 4, 5 and a medium leeway space.

A, B A harmoniously shaped dental arch with good contact points and without diastemata. Note that the mesiodistal crown dimensions of the second and first deciduous molars are only slightly different. The dimension of the latter is about 2 mm larger than that of its successor.

C, D The permanent canine emerges in a proper relation with the lateral incisor. However, the space available is limited and the tooth erupts with a distolingual rotation.

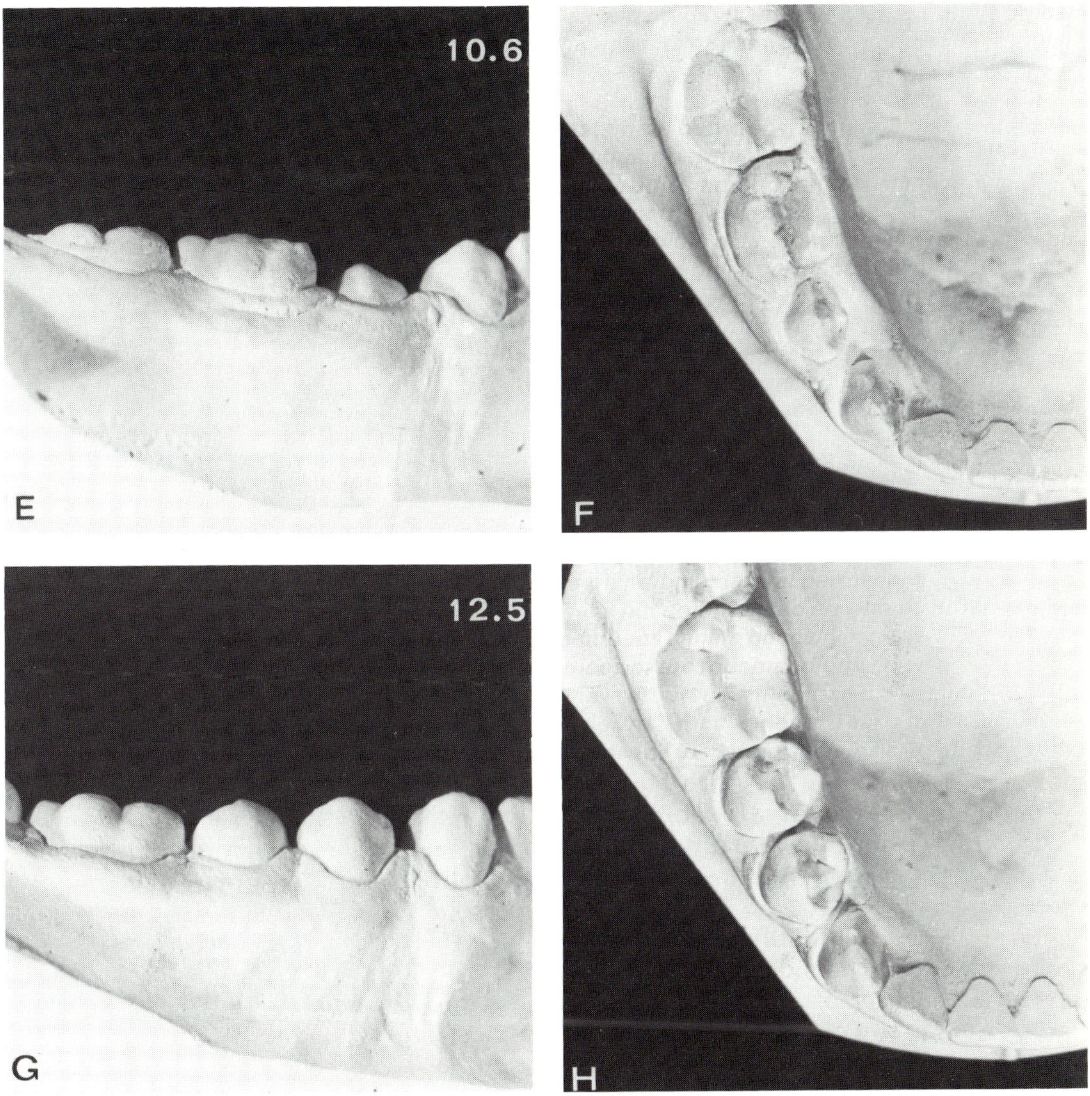

E, F Loss of the first deciduous molar prior to the completion of the eruption of the permanent canine allows the latter to move distally and utilise some of the available excess space.

G, H After the loss of the second deciduous molar the first premolar can move distally, particularly when the second premolar erupts in a distal direction. Enough space is now available in the posterior region. However, the distolingual rotation of the canine, related to its original orientation in the jaw, a rotational movement that may be associated with the limited space available upon eruption, or the combination of both, is not corrected. It is questionable how far this will happen later on. Pattern B may result in good contacts between all teeth involved or with some limitation in that respect, as shown here.

3.5.1 Mandibular Posterior Teeth Transition Pattern A

Pattern A is characterized by the emergence sequence 3, 4, 5 and a large leeway space (Figs. 3-6 and 3-7). The transition sequence allows the development of good contact relations between the lateral incisor and the permanent canine and also between the other teeth involved. Maximum use can be made of the leeway space for a good alignment of the posterior segment. The mandibular first permanent molar migrates only slightly mesially. The mandibular incisors tend to move lingually.

3.5.2 Mandibular Posterior Teeth Transition Pattern B

Pattern B is characterized by the emergence sequence 3, 4, 5 and a medium leeway space (Figs. 3-8 and 3-9). The transition sequence is the same as in Pattern A, with the added advantage that it allows an optimal use of the space that becomes available, particularly when the second permanent molar does not emerge before the transition is completed. The mandibular first permanent molar migrates then only slightly mesially. When favourable conditions are present in the initial location of the teeth prior to emergence, the permanent canine crown can, upon emergence, establish a good contact with the lateral incisor. The same holds true for both premolars and their contacts with each other and the adjacent teeth.

3.5.3 Mandibular Posterior Teeth Transition Pattern C

Pattern C is characterized by the emergence sequence 3, 4, 5 and a small leeway space (Figs. 3-10 and 3-11). The space available in the jaw for the crowns of the permanent canine and both premolars is limited. This shows up particularly in the position and angulation of the permanent canine and its relation to the lateral incisor root. The permanent canine usually emerges buccally and overlaps the often rotated lateral incisor crown labially. Subsequently, the canine can utilise some of the space that has

Fig. 3-9 Schematic drawing of the Mandibular Posterior Teeth Transition Pattern B, characterized by the emergence sequence 3, 4, 5 and a medium leeway space.

A Harmoniously shaped dental arch without diastemata.
B The permanent canine has emerged with a shortage of space and overlaps the lateral incisor labially.
C Depending on the time elapsed between the loss of the first deciduous molar and the complete eruption of the first premolar, the permanent canine can migrate distally in its postemergence eruption phase. A good contact with the lateral incisor may be established. The first premolar undergoes a comparable process when, shortly after its emergence, the crown of the second deciduous molar is exfoliated and the eruption of the second premolar lags behind that of the first.
D The leeway space has been mainly utilised for the distal migration of the permanent canine and the premolars. Little mesial migration of the first permanent molar has occurred. This is more likely to happen when the second premolar erupts in a distal direction and the second permanent molar emerges after the transition of the posterior teeth is complete. Fortunately, both aspects seem to be evident in the majority of cases.

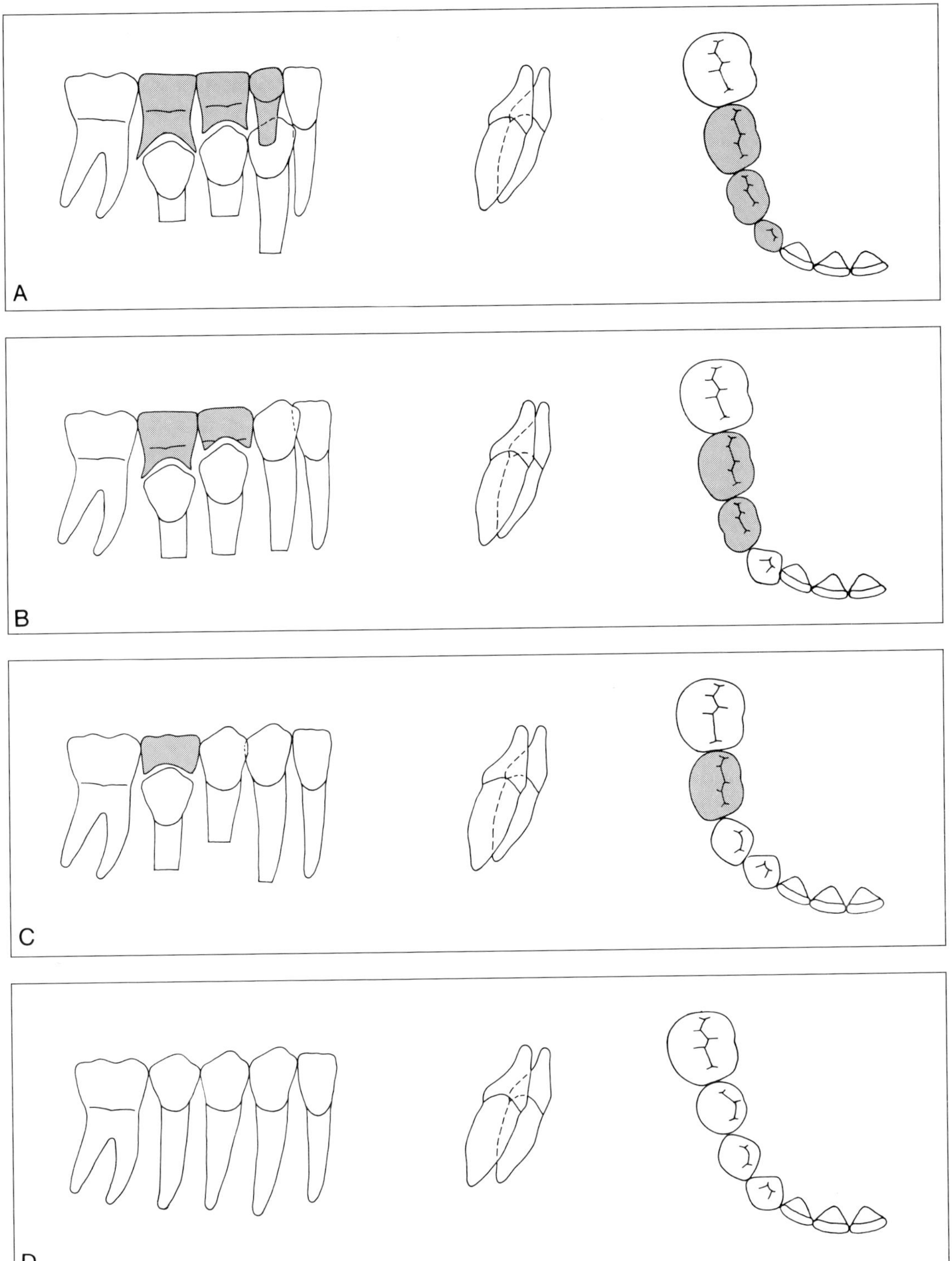

Figure 3-9

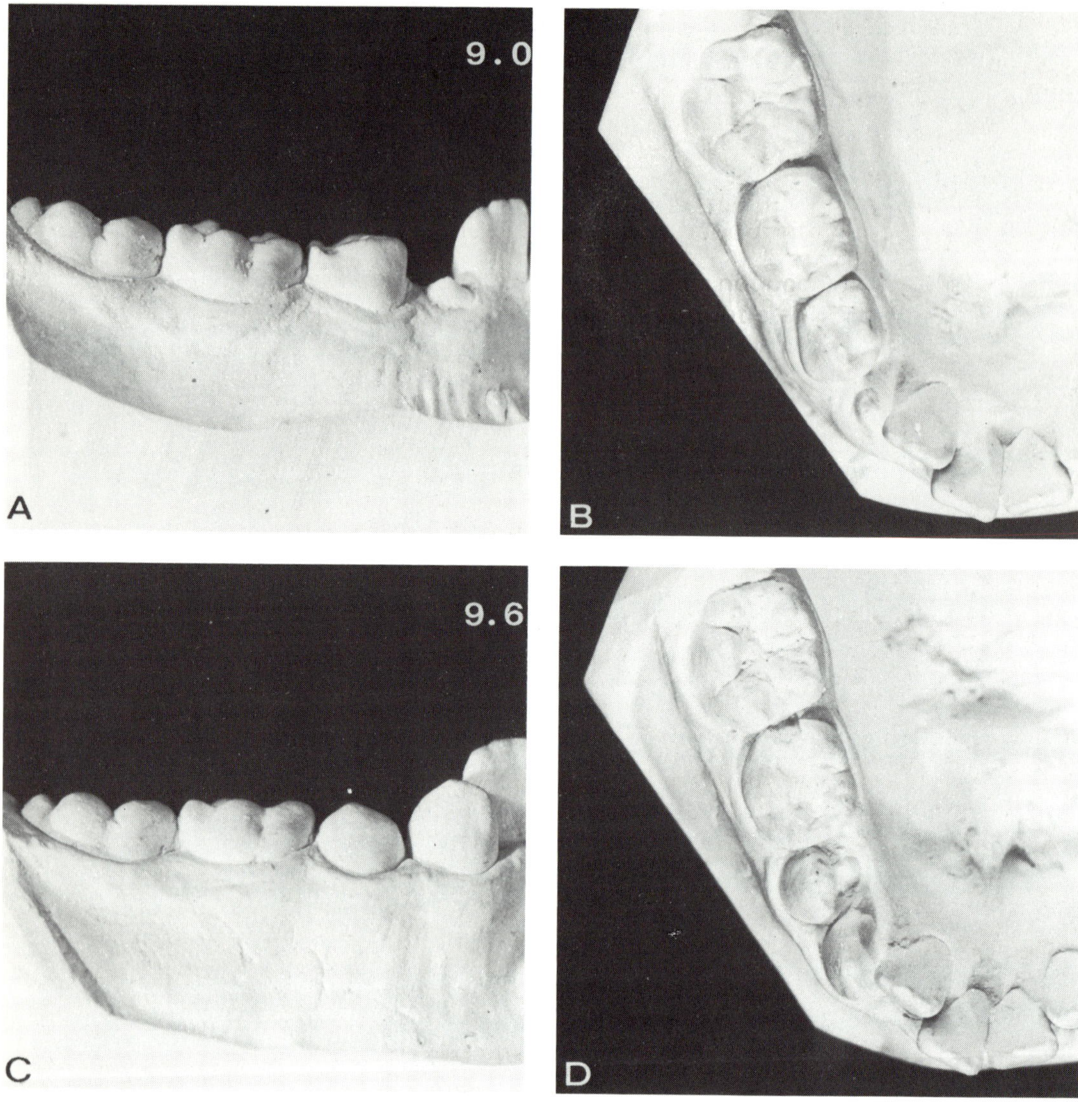

Fig. 3-10 Longitudinal series of dental casts showing the Mandibular Posterior Teeth Transition Pattern C, characterized by the emergence sequence 3, 4, 5 and a small leeway space.

A, B Crowding in the incisor region and a shortage of space for the emerging permanent canine.

C, D The first premolar has emerged after the canine, which has utilised some of the space previously occupied by the first deciduous molar. The canine erupts further and overlaps the lateral incisor. Insufficient space remained for the first premolar.

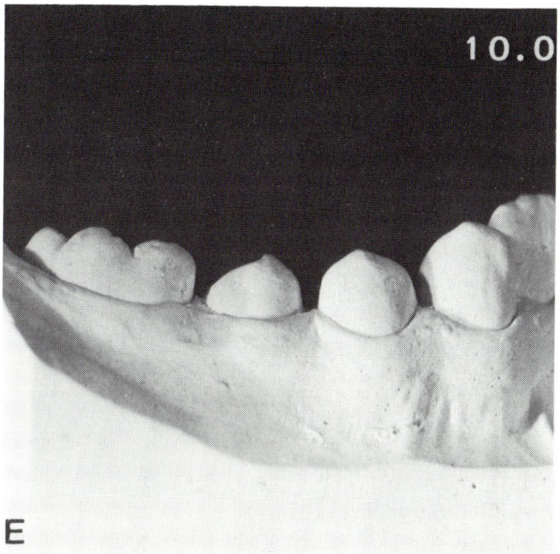

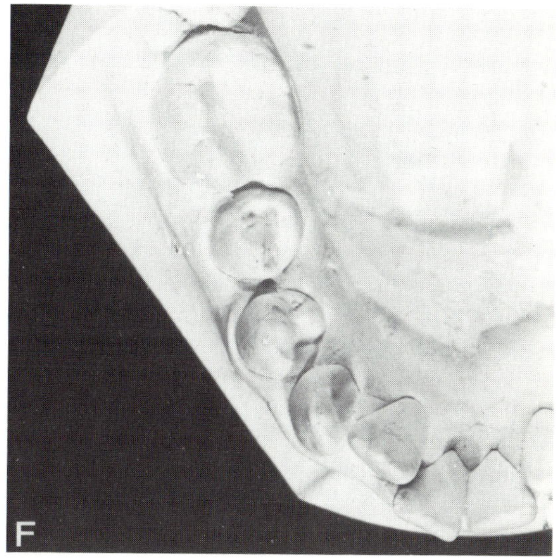

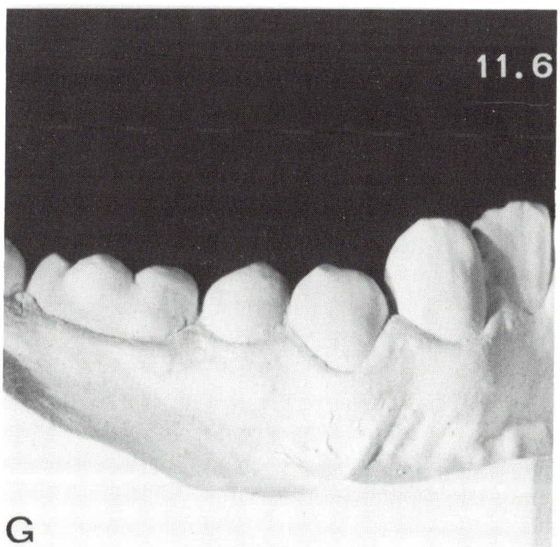

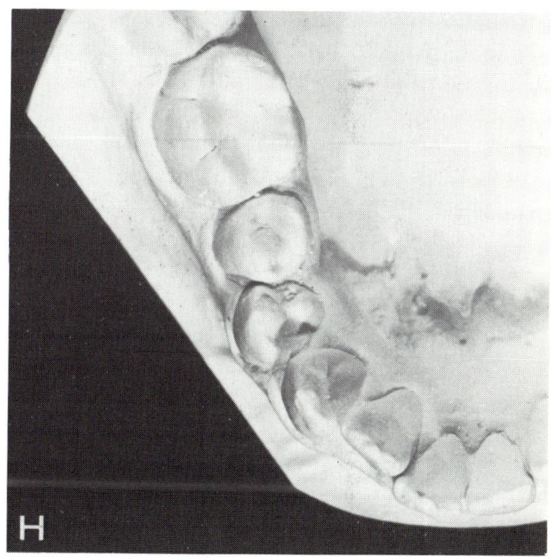

E, F *After loss of the second deciduous molar crown, the first premolar and also the canine will benefit from the extra space that becomes available. Note the difference in mesiodistal crown dimensions of the second deciduous molar and the second premolar.*

G, H *The position of the lateral incisor and its contact with the canine has improved. However, all contact points mesial of the permanent first molar leave something to be desired. The first permanent molar has probably moved somewhat mesially, and the extra space that became available for its successor after the transition of the second deciduous molar is not optimally used for relief of crowding.*

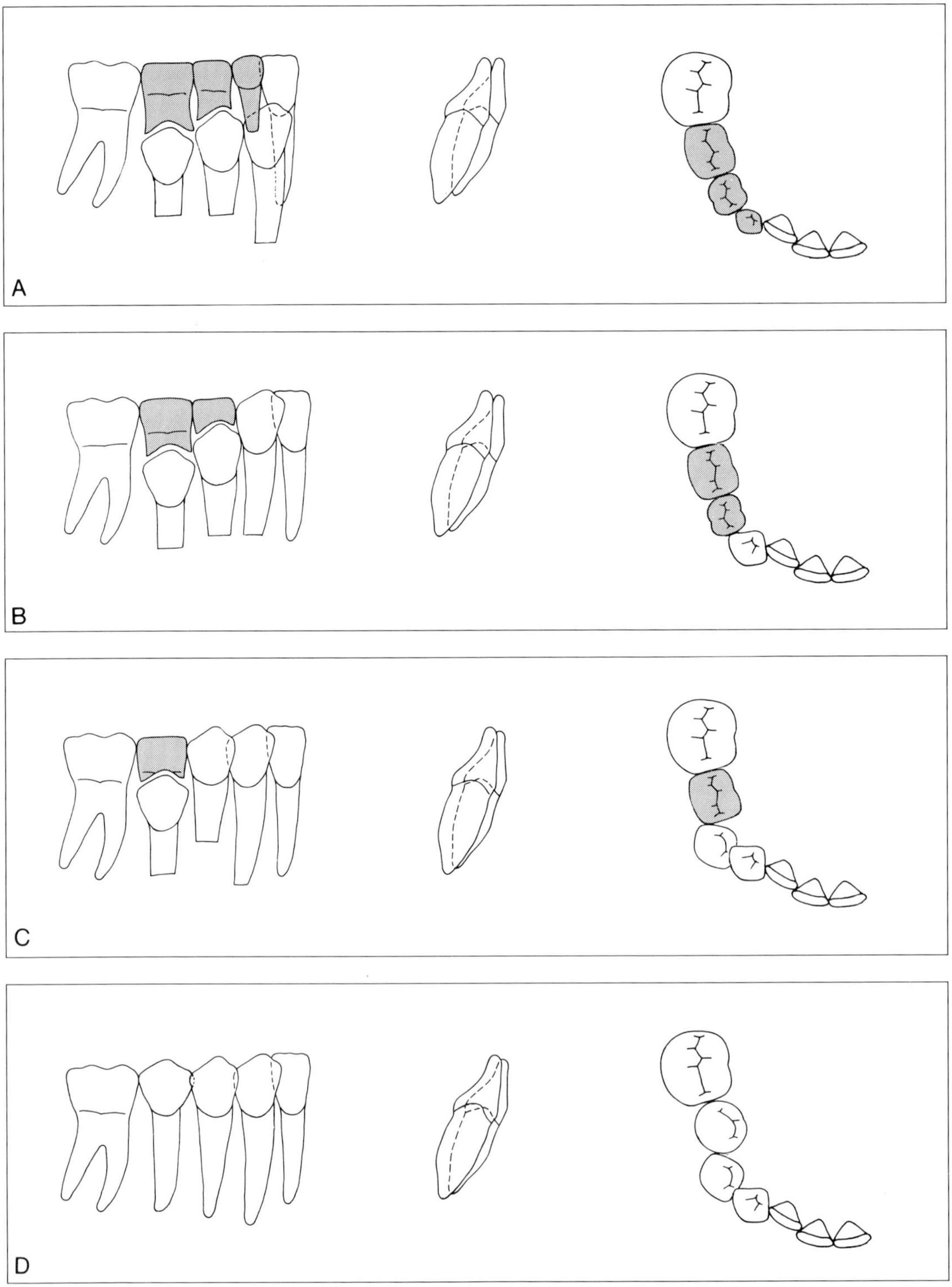

Figure 3-11

Fig. 3-11 Schematic drawing of the Mandibular Posterior Teeth Transition Pattern C, characterized by the emergence sequence 3, 4, 5 and a small leeway space.

A Crowding in the canine incisor region. The crowns of the permanent canine and both premolars are close together; the space available for them in the jaw is limited.
B There is insufficient space within the dental arch for the canine; it has erupted mesially and overlaps the lateral incisor crown. This situation will take place particularly when the mesiodistal crown width of the permanent canine is large compared to that of its predecessor.
C The canine may move somewhat distally when the first deciduous molar is exfoliated. This usually results in a lack of space for the already emerged first premolar, which may continue its eruption in a buccal direction.
D The first premolar in crowding may improve its position in the dental arch by utilising some of the space originally occupied by the second deciduous molar crown. The second premolar may become lingually positioned. Slipping contacts in the anterior section of the arch can become worse. As a rule the first permanent molar will not move mesially, or only slightly so, during transition of the posterior teeth.

been occupied by the first deciduous molar crown and move distally, thus improving the canine-incisor relation. Consequently, the first premolar will find its space reduced and may then also become located in a crowded situation. The replacement of the second deciduous molar by its successor may present some relief for the first premolar or canine. However, the crowding will not be eliminated completely. Usually, the distal migration of the first premolar and canine will be limited and only part of the extra space that becomes available after loss of the second deciduous molar will be utilised. A comparatively small mesiodistal crown width of the latter is favourable and will result in a better alignment of the canine and first premolar than otherwise.

3.5.4 Mandibular Posterior Teeth Transition Pattern D

Pattern D is characterized by the emergence sequence (3, 4)* 5 and a medium leeway space (Figs. 3-12 and 3-13). This transition sequence eliminates the favourable distal migration of the permanent canine that can occur when its emergence shortly precedes that of the first premolar. If a poor contact develops with the lateral incisor, the canine is more likely to move mesially than distally. The leeway space will then not primarily be utilised by distal migration of the premolars and canine but by mesial migration of the first permanent molar. However, when a favourable contact becomes established between the canine and the lateral incisor, the leeway space may be utilised primarily from the mesial aspect, and a normal arrangement of the teeth may be the end result.

* Use of ( ) indicates simultaneous emergence.

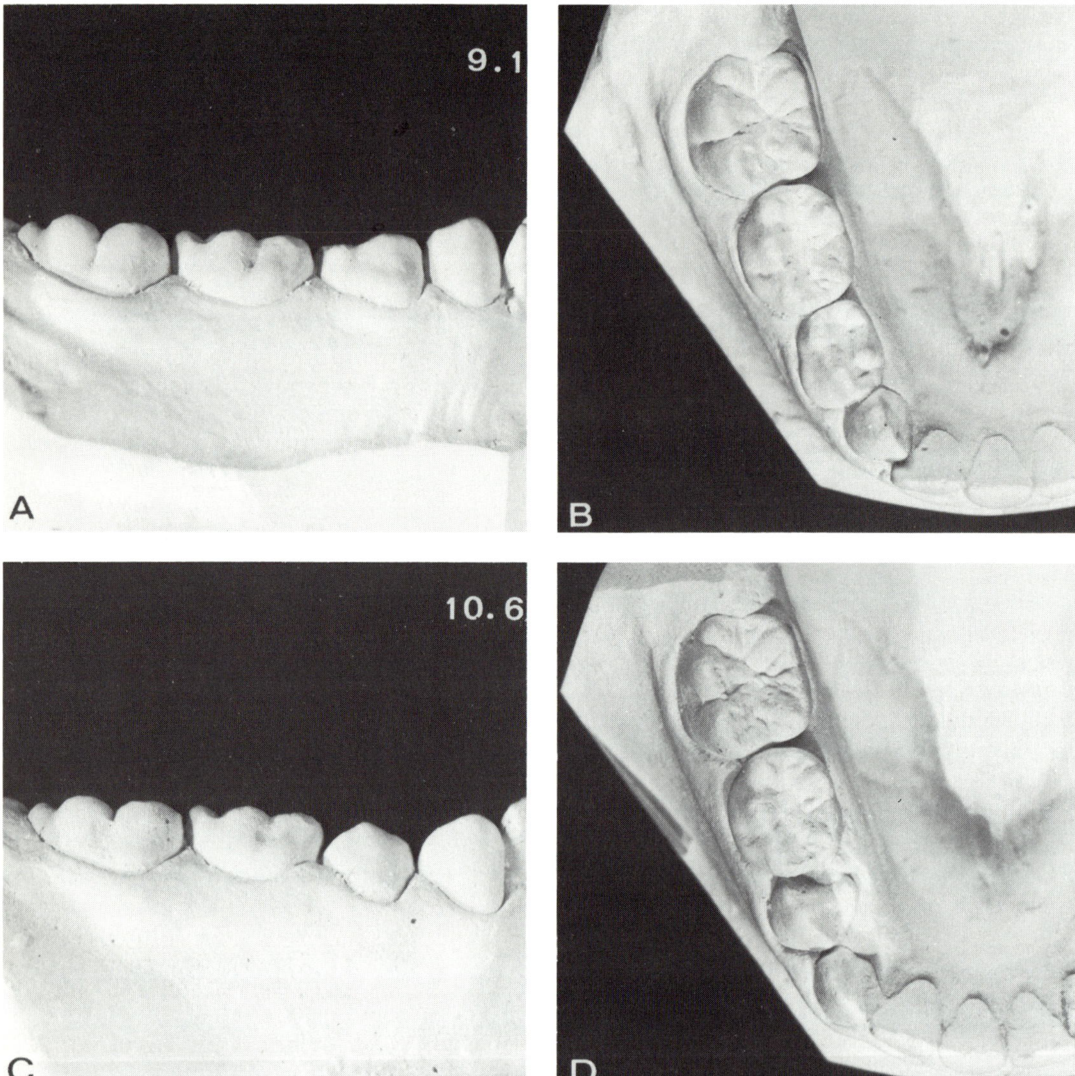

Fig. 3-12 Longitudinal series of dental casts showing the Mandibular Posterior Teeth Transition Pattern D, characterized by the emergence sequence (3, 4) 5 and a medium leeway space.

A, B The distal corner of the lateral incisor extends labially and distally over the deciduous canine crown. Some crowding exists in that region.

C, D After almost simultaneous emergence of the permanent canine and first premolar a good contact between the canine and lateral incisor seems to develop initially. The mesiodistal crown dimensions of the deciduous and permanent canine differ only slightly.

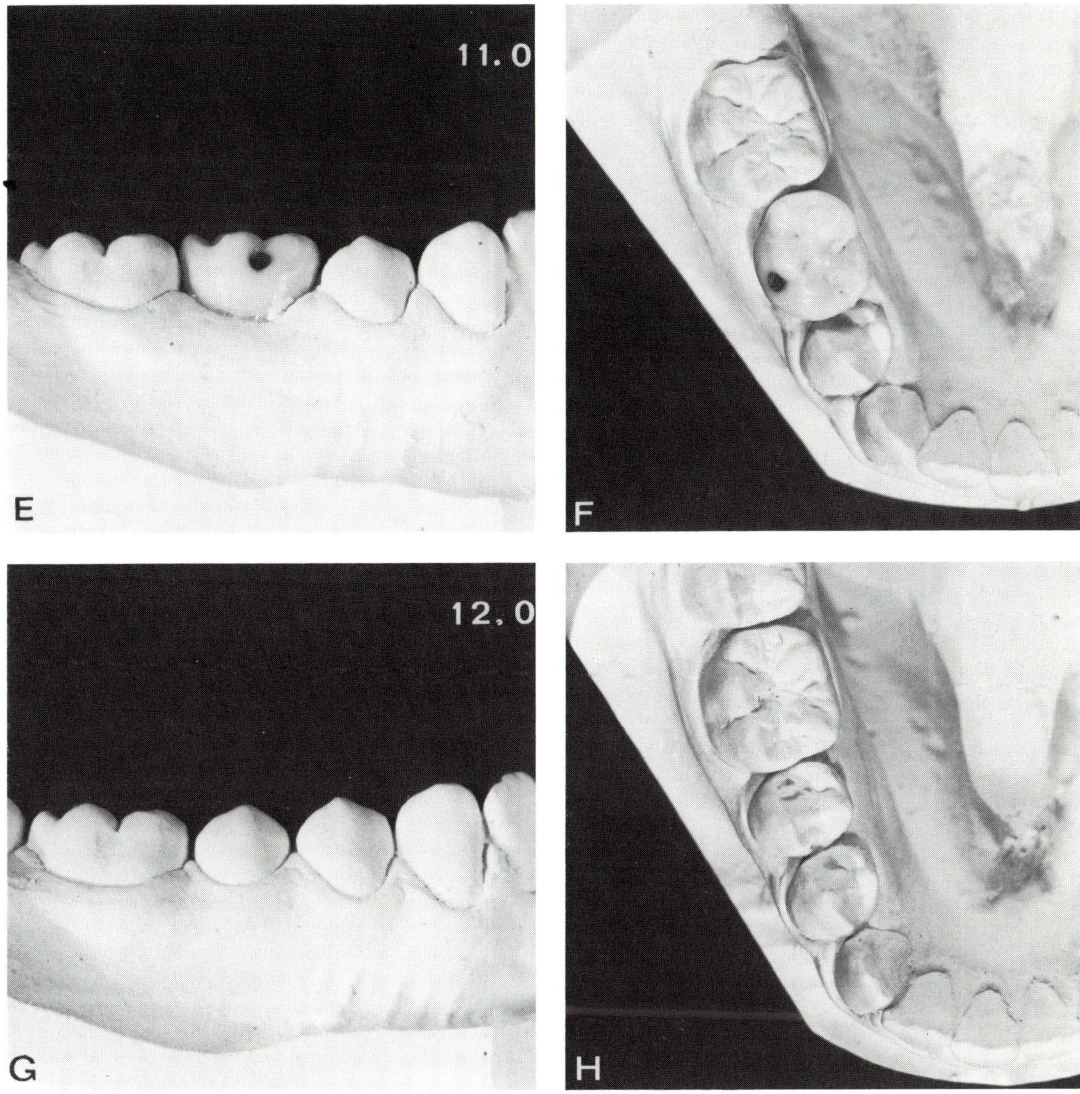

E, F *The first premolar maintained its infraposition. Its eruption probably slowed down prematurely because its distal marginal ridge established contact with the mesial surface of the second deciduous molar inferior to its most mesially located point.*

G, H *After loss of the second deciduous molar crown the first premolar erupted further and moved distally, occupying some of the extra space that became available. However, in the meantime, the mesial surface of the canine moved lingually in relation to the adjacent lateral incisor and the contact between the two deteriorated. It is not unlikely that occlusion with the maxillary teeth is responsible for this change.*

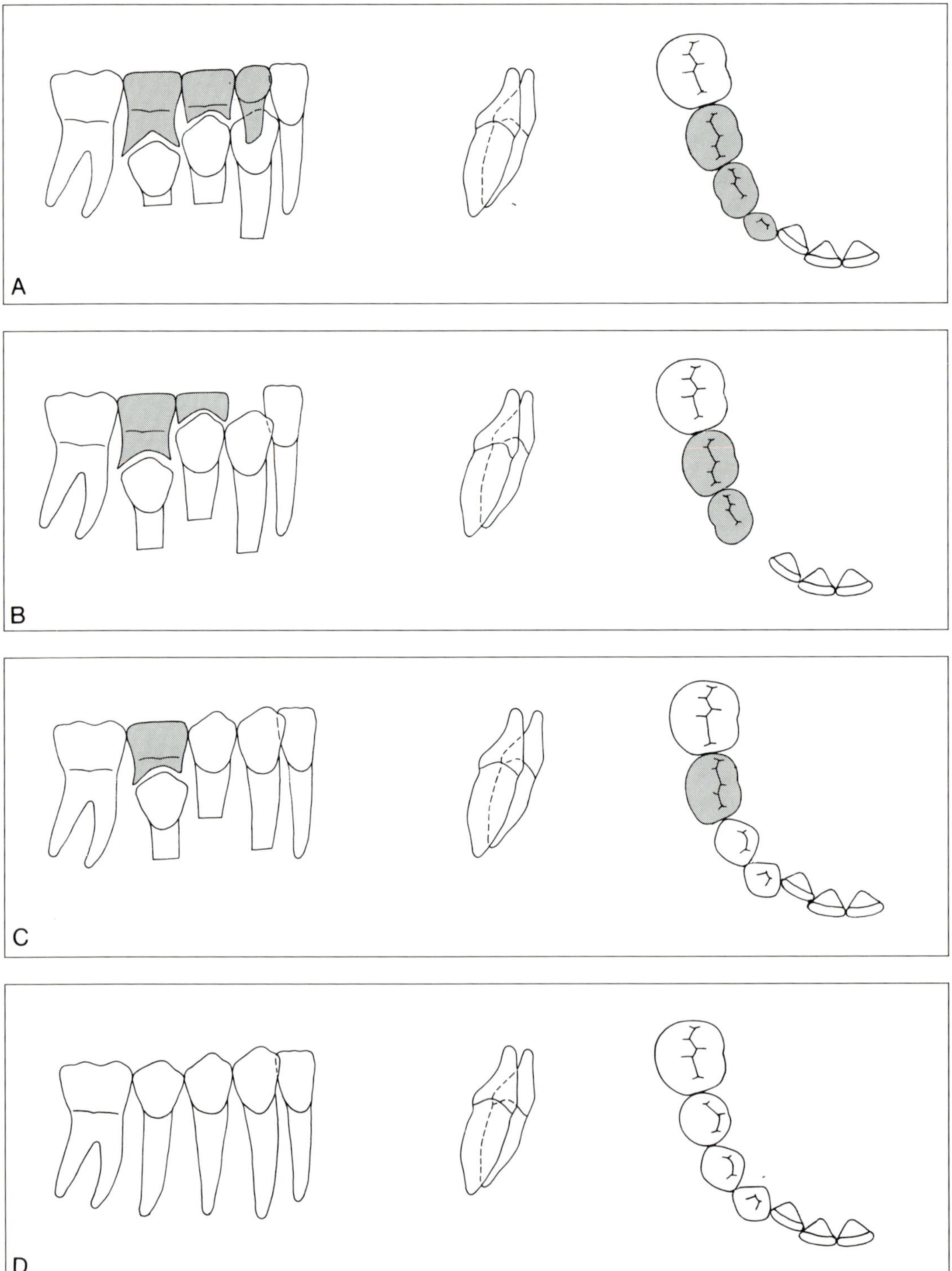

Figure 3-13

Fig. 3-13 Schematic drawing of the Mandibular Posterior Teeth Transition Pattern D, characterized by the emergence sequence (3, 4) 5 and a medium leeway space.

A A dental arch without diastemata and sometimes some crowding in the canine incisor region. The mesiodistal dimension of the crown of the deciduous canine is similar to that of its successor, a particularly favourable feature in this transition pattern.
B When the permanent canine and first premolar emerge simultaneously, the deciduous canine is usually exfoliated prior to the crown of the first deciduous molar.
C After the simultaneous emergence of the permanent canine and the first premolar, the former can move distally and occupy some of the space originally occupied by the first deciduous molar crown. The canine overlaps the lateral incisors, which have been moved lingually.
D The extra space that became available after the loss of the second deciduous molar crown may be used for a further alignment of the canine and first premolar. The extra space can also be utilised by a mesial movement of the first permanent molar. Some crowding in the incisor-canine region usually remains. The amount of mesial movement of the first permanent molar depends on the changes that took place in the dental arch during the transition and the emergence of the second permanent molar as well as the direction of the second premolar.

The position of the permanent teeth prior to emergence is presumably not the only factor that will determine whether an end result will be adequate or not. It is probably also related to the speed with which the changes take place and whether good or bad contacts between the lateral incisor, canine, and first premolar are to be realized. A distally erupting second premolar and emergence of the second permanent molar after the transition is completed favour a good development.

The emergence sequence (3, 4) 5 combined with a large leeway space will normally result in a harmonious dental arch. The favourable course of events described for Pattern A will, with a large leeway space, also take place with the emergence sequence (3, 4) 5.

The emergence sequence (3, 4) 5 combined with a small leeway space will give less good results than that described above for Pattern D when the circumstances are unfavourable. The simultaneously erupting permanent canine and first premolar are close together during the preemergence and postemergence eruption, leading to a more mesial positioning of the canine than would otherwise have been the case. Crowding initially present between the canine and incisors can become worse. However, it can also be reduced to some extent later on.

3.5.5 Mandibular Posterior Teeth Transition Pattern E

Pattern E is characterized by the emergence sequence 3 (4, 5) and a small leeway space (Figs. 3-14 and 3-15). This sequence of emergence seems favourable for improving the mesially erupting canine associated with a small leeway space. That holds particularly

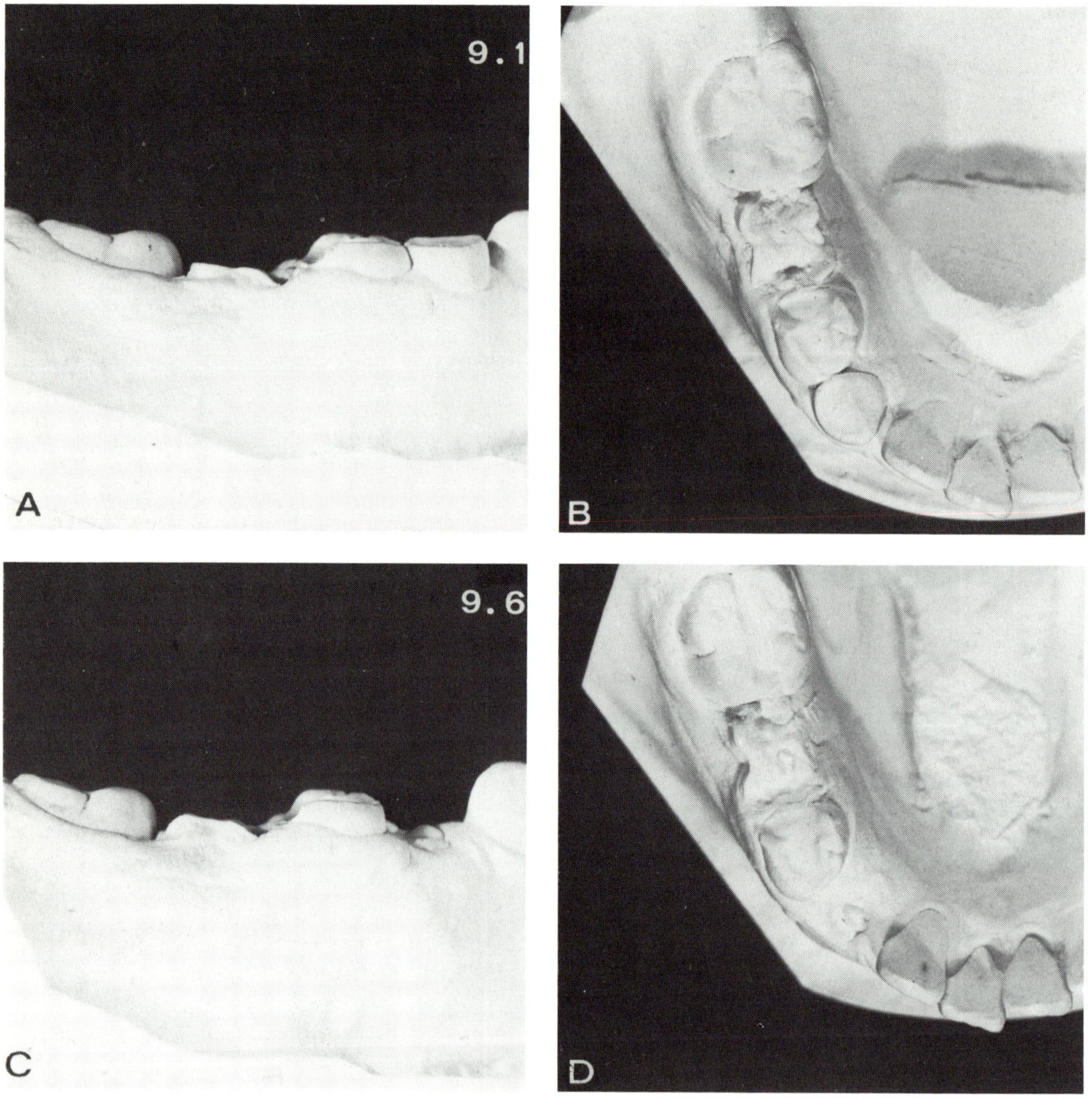

Fig. 3-14 Longitudinal series of dental casts of an exceptional case demonstrating the Mandibular Posterior Teeth Transition Pattern E, characterized by the eruption sequence 3 (4, 5) and a small leeway space. The case shown here is not a good example of the Pattern E because a diastema is present in the anterior region of the dental arch. However, it shows an extremely favourable course of events in the transition of the posterior teeth that occasionally may be found in Pattern E. The development illustrated here is more likely to be seen in cases with medium leeway space.

A, B *Harmonious dental arch form with a diastema mesial to the deciduous canine. Tooth material of the second deciduous molar is prematurely lost, though the amount of space available for the crown of its successor is probably maintained until the replacement.*

C, D *The permanent canine emerges and has adequate space in the dental arch.*

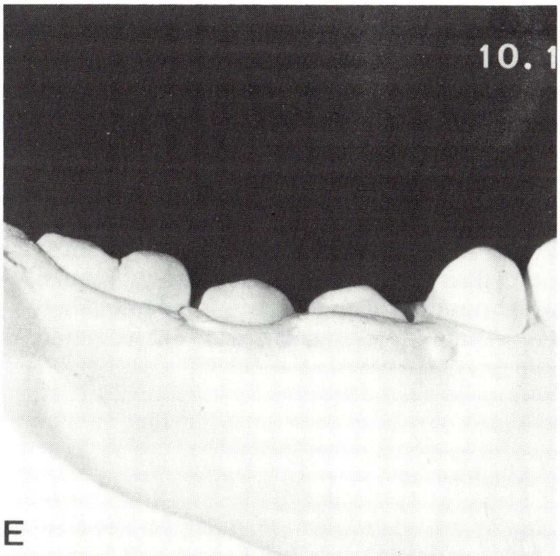

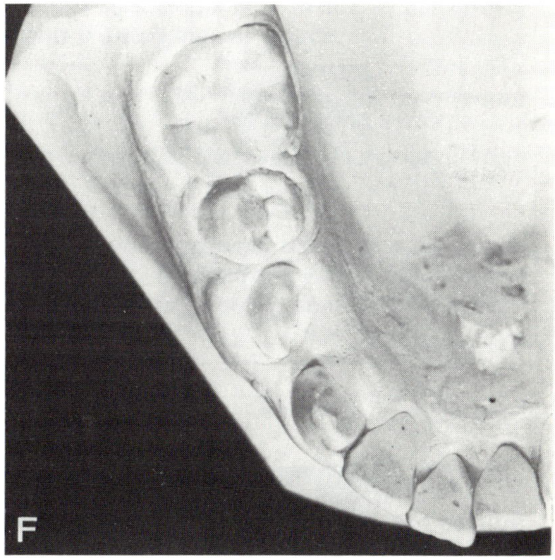

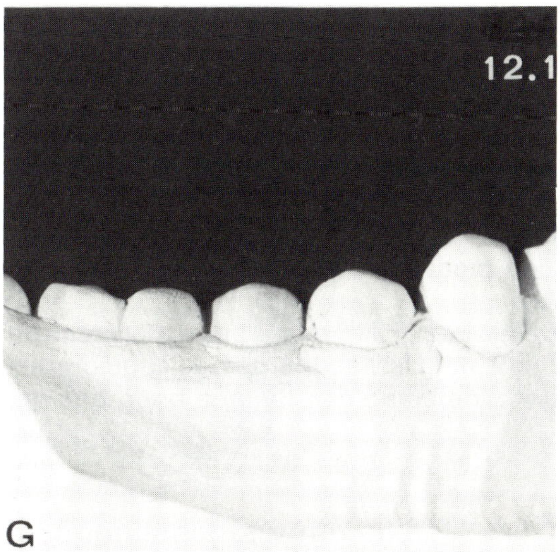

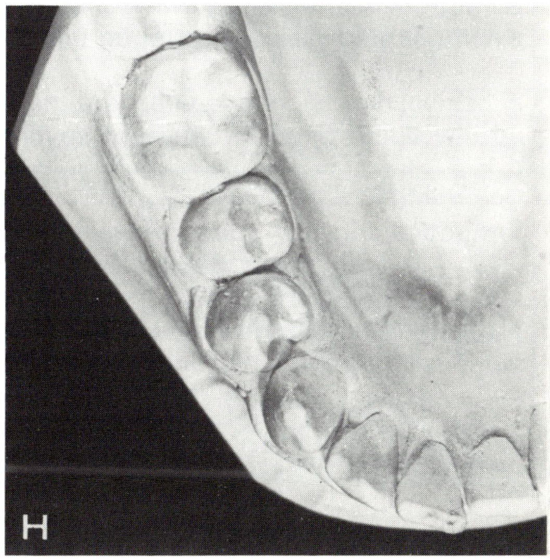

E, F *A good contact point is established between the permanent canine and the lateral incisor. Both premolars have emerged almost simultaneously and the second one has erupted in a distal direction and established contact with the first permanent molar prior to the emergence of the second permanent molar.*

G, H *Adequate end result. The first premolar, which emerged rotated, is still rotated and will probably maintain that orientation. A mechanism other than occlusal contact, which can improve a rotated premolar, is missing.*

In small leeway spaces crowding can easily develop. The ultimate location of the teeth and the amount of crowding depend largely on the sequence of emergence. In the sequence 3 (4, 5) crowding is more likely to be concentrated in the canine-first premolar region. In the sequence 3, 4, 5 the crowding will be more gradually distributed over the lateral incisor-canine-premolar region. The sequence (3, 4) 5 leads to a concentration of the crowding in the canine-lateral incisor region. The canine then becomes mesiobuccally rotated and overlaps the lateral incisor.
As has been previously explained, the difference in mesiodistal crown dimensions between the second deciduous molar and its successor is crucial in critical situations in the transition of the mandibular posterior teeth. When this difference is relatively small the sequence of emergence is less important than when this difference is large. A small leeway space with a comparatively small mesiodistal crown width of the second deciduous molar, associated with a relatively large mesiodistal crown dimension of the deciduous canine and first deciduous molar, will not usually lead to problems in the transition of the posterior teeth. The permanent canine and first premolar can emerge and attain a good position in the dental arch independent of the loss of the second deciduous molar. A small leeway space with a large crown width of the deciduous second molar compared to that of its successor (associated with relatively small mesiodistal crown dimensions of the deciduous canine and first deciduous molar) is most unfavourable.
This chapter does not deal with the effect of premature loss of deciduous molars on the transition and on the final position of the teeth. However, premature loss can have strong effects, particularly in cases with crowded situations and with small middle sections of the apical area. The reduction in leeway space that can be but does not always have to be the result of premature loss of deciduous molars, may be considerable. An originally large leeway space can become a small one by the abnormal mesial migration of the first permanent molar and/or the distal migration of the mesially positioned teeth. Then the premolar below the deciduous molar that was lost prematurely and also the adjacent teeth may not find enough space left over for their emergence into their proper positions in the dental arch. Well known in this respect are the lingually emerging mandibular second premolars. Under certain conditions reduction of the leeway space can be partly regained by an emerging second premolar that drives the first permanent molar distally, particularly when good contact points exist mesially. The effect of premature loss of deciduous molars will be treated in detail in Chapter 14.

Chapter 4

Changes in the Mandibular Incisor Region Associated With the Transition of Mandibular Posterior Teeth *

4.1 Introduction

Replacement of the deciduous canines and molars by their successors influences the position of the teeth distally and mesially of them. The first and second permanent molars will migrate more mesially. The extent of this migration depends on the alterations that take place during the transition. The changes in position of the incisors are more complex and thus justify separate discussion.
The relation between the size and shape of the anterior and the middle section of the apical areas is discussed. The orientation of and relations between the five most mesial permanent teeth before and after transition of the posterior teeth are described. Three patterns of changes in the mandibular incisor region associated with transition of the posterior teeth are presented. These patterns are distinguished on the basis of the spatial conditions in the anterior region before the transition of the posterior teeth. In addition, the changes involved are analysed with reference to the conditions that can be distinguished in the canine premolar region.

4.2 Relation between the size and shape of the anterior and middle sections of the apical area

The morphogenesis of the mandible and its subsequent growth, together with the position of the forming teeth, determine the shape and size of the apical area. The correlation of the apical area with the size of the deciduous and permanent teeth is limited. It seems that the ultimate size and shape of the apical area is determined by control mechanisms other than the size of the teeth.

* Reproduced from: "Changes in the lower incisor region associated with the transition of the lower posterior teeth" by Paul J.M.R. Bakker, Hein J.W. Wassenberg and Frans P.G.M. van der Linden. In: *Transition of the human dentition.* Monograph No. 13. Craniofacial Growth Series., Pg 63-73. Ed. Frans P.G.M. van der Linden. Center for Human Growth and Development. The University of Michigan, Ann Arbor, U.S.A., 1982.

The site where the permanent canines form determines the demarcation of the anterior and middle sections of the apical area. In further development this role is taken by the mesial side of the crown of the permanent canine before emergence and by that of its root and apex subsequently. In situations with anterior and middle sections of the apical area of standard size, a relative mesial position of the canine crown before emergence will consequently lead to a small anterior section of the apical area and a large middle section. A relatively distal position of the canine will result in the reversed situation. Generally, a large anterior section of the apical area is associated with a large middle section. However, a small anterior section of the apical area can occur in combination with a large middle section and the reverse.

4.3 Orientations of and relations between incisors, canine, and premolars before transition of the posterior teeth

The position of the mandibular incisors at the end of the first transitional period can vary considerably, as has been indicated in Chapter 2. The local conditions in the anterior segment and the manner of transition of the posterior teeth determine how the position of the incisors will alter in that respect. The position of the not-yet-emerged permanent canine and its relation to the adjacent lateral incisor are crucial. However, the relation between the canine and the first premolar is important too. This also applies to the position of the second premolar and the first and second permanent molars. Whether the extra space that becomes available with the transition of the posterior teeth is used for an improvement of the position of the incisors also depends on the sequence of emergence of the canine, both premolars, and the second permanent molar.

4.4 Conditions in the dental arch after transition of the posterior teeth

In the mandible the incisors are most susceptible to influences within and outside the dental arch. Rotations present at emergence usually correct subsequently, whenever space is available, as a result of pressures exerted by the tongue and lips. However, mandibular incisors seem to be the most vulnerable teeth regarding increases in malposition, crowding, and overlapping. This holds true for the development of the dentition and also applies to postadolescent changes in the position of teeth. With increasing age mandibular incisors that were originally perfectly aligned may begin to overlap. Existing crowded conditions can worsen. The combination of *(1)* the large susceptibility to influences originating within and outside the dental arch, *(2)* the relatively fragile contact points, and *(3)* the room within the jaws that allows the teeth to approximate to each other and to rotate leads to these undesirable changes in the position of the mandibular incisors.
Crowded conditions in the anterior region can improve by utilising the space that becomes available with the transition of the posterior teeth. The contacts between the incisors and the contact that will develop between the lateral incisor and permanent

canine are essential for changes associated with the transition of the posterior teeth. Favourable contacts can lead to considerable improvement; unfavourable ones lead to a worsening of the situation. A mesially angulated and erupting permanent canine can emerge mesially in the dental arch, labial to the lateral incisor. The lateral incisor cannot move labially, and its lingual position is maintained during the continuing eruption of the canine. Particularly in instances of small leeway space, the canine will be limited in its possible distal movement, leading to a continuation of the existing situation. The contact between the canine and the premolar is less important because the cross section of the the premolar is round, not flat. This applies even more to the contact between the two premolars, because the contact is formed by two rounded structures. The round section of the premolar crowns is, however, responsible for the fact that premolars emerged in a rotated position will not be corrected by pressures exerted by the tongue and buccal musculature. Occasionally, occlusal contacts can improve initially rotated premolars to some extent.

4.5 Patterns in changes in the mandibular incisor region associated with transition of the posterior teeth

Symmetry exists in the size and shape of both middle sections of the apical area. However, mandibular permanent canine crowns are not always formed in corresponding locations on the left and right sides. Their relation to the premolars and already emerged incisors will vary accordingly. In addition, positions of the incisors frequently are not symmetrical. Changes in the left and right side of the incisor region, usually evoked by the transition of the posterior teeth, are not independent of each other. Both sides interact in that respect.

The changes are divided into three patterns, based on differences in the space available in the incisor region. Special attention will be paid to the contact between the permanent canine and the lateral incisor. In addition, the influence of the early and late emergence of the second permanent molar will be dealt with.

Changes in the mandibular incisor region associated with the transition of the posterior teeth will be treated on the basis of the conditions present in the canine premolar region.

4.5.1 Mandibular Incisor Region Changes Pattern A

Pattern A is characterized by excess space available in the anterior segment of the dental arch (Figs. 4-1 and 4-2). More space is available for the four permanent incisors than is needed. Diastemata are present. The mandibular canine emerges without contacting the lateral incisor, the position of which is not affected. The middle section of the apical area and the leeway space are large. The premolars can emerge without spatial limitations. Diastemata between the permanent teeth anterior of the first permanent molar will be present initially; they gradually become reduced and in most instances interproximal contacts will develop between all teeth.

Emergence of the second permanent molar before or after completion of the transition will not affect the ultimate position of the teeth. In the first instance the first permanent

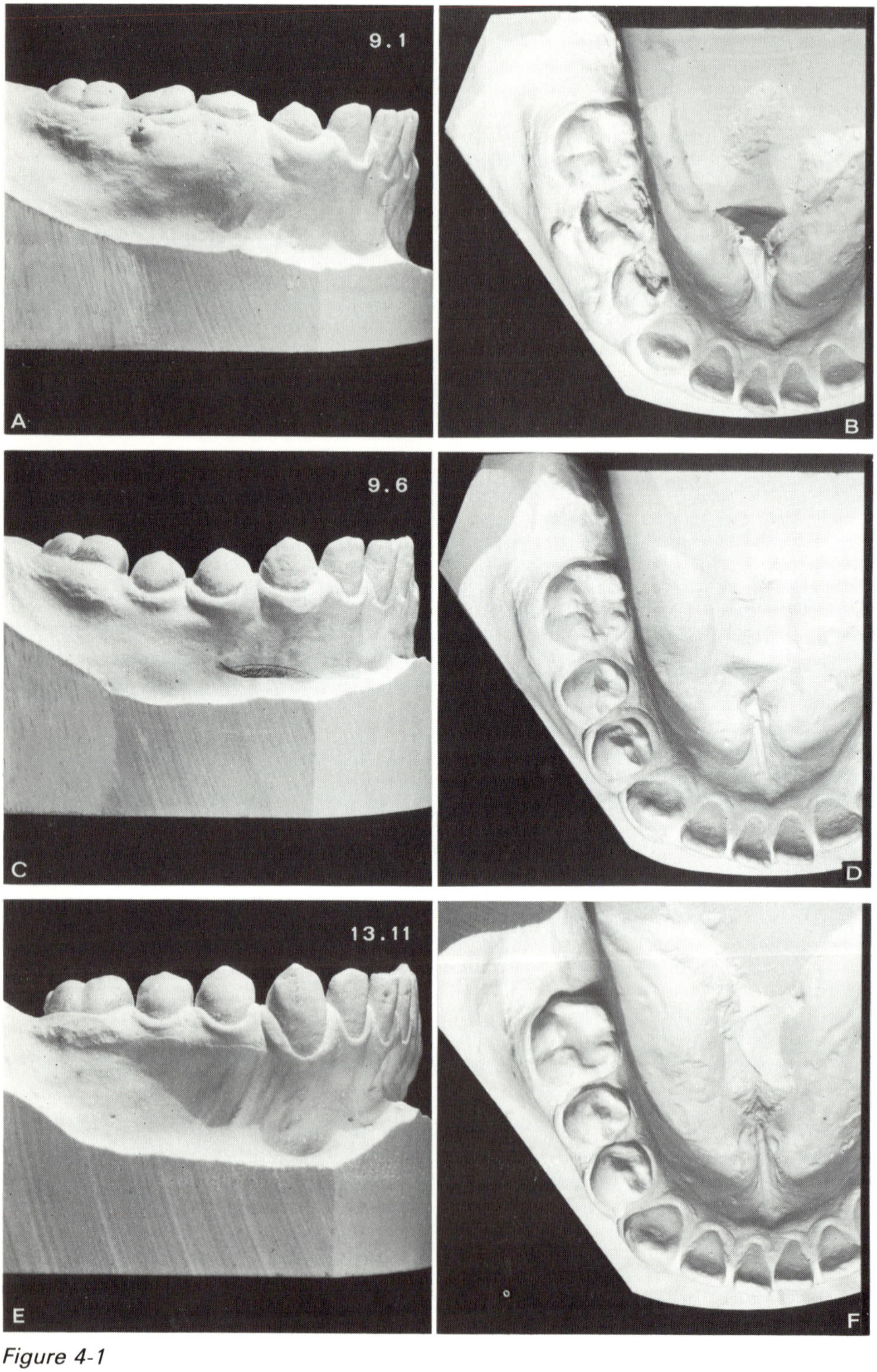

Figure 4-1

Fig. 4-1 Lateral and occlusal views of a longitudinal series of dental casts of the Mandibular Incisor Region Changes Pattern A, characterized by excess of space available in the anterior segment of the dental arch.

A, B *Diastemata are present between the four incisors, which are somewhat irregularly positioned. The permanent canine has emerged without contacting the lateral incisor. The distance between the distal surface of the incisor and the mesial surface of the first permanent molar is large, notwithstanding the reduction in crown width of the second deciduous molar and the associated mesial migration of the first permanent molar.*

C, D *Both premolars have emerged, the second one last. Large diastemata are present between all teeth.*

E, F *Contact is developing between the posterior teeth. Diastemata are still present between the mandibular incisors, which have improved in position. Note that the initial rotation of the canine has also been corrected. The second permanent molar will emerge after the transition is completed.*

Fig. 4-2 (see page 90) Schematic lateral and occlusal views of the Mandibular Incisor Region Changes Pattern A, characterized by excess of space available in the anterior segment of the dental arch.

A *Diastemata are present between the incisors, which are well aligned. The permanent canine has emerged without contacting the lateral incisor, the position of which is not affected. A large leeway space provides excess space for the premolars.*

B *The canine and first premolar have emerged without making mutual contact initially. Subsequently, the crowns of the two teeth establish contact. The second premolar emerges into excess space. The first permanent molar will migrate mesially and experience a spurt in this respect when the second molar emerges and attains occlusal contact. Prior to that change diastemata are generally present.*

C *All permanent teeth (except the third molar) are harmoniously positioned within the dental arch. The roots are approximately equally distributed in the alveolar process. The arch form often flattens in the anterior region. Diastemata are reduced or eliminated.*

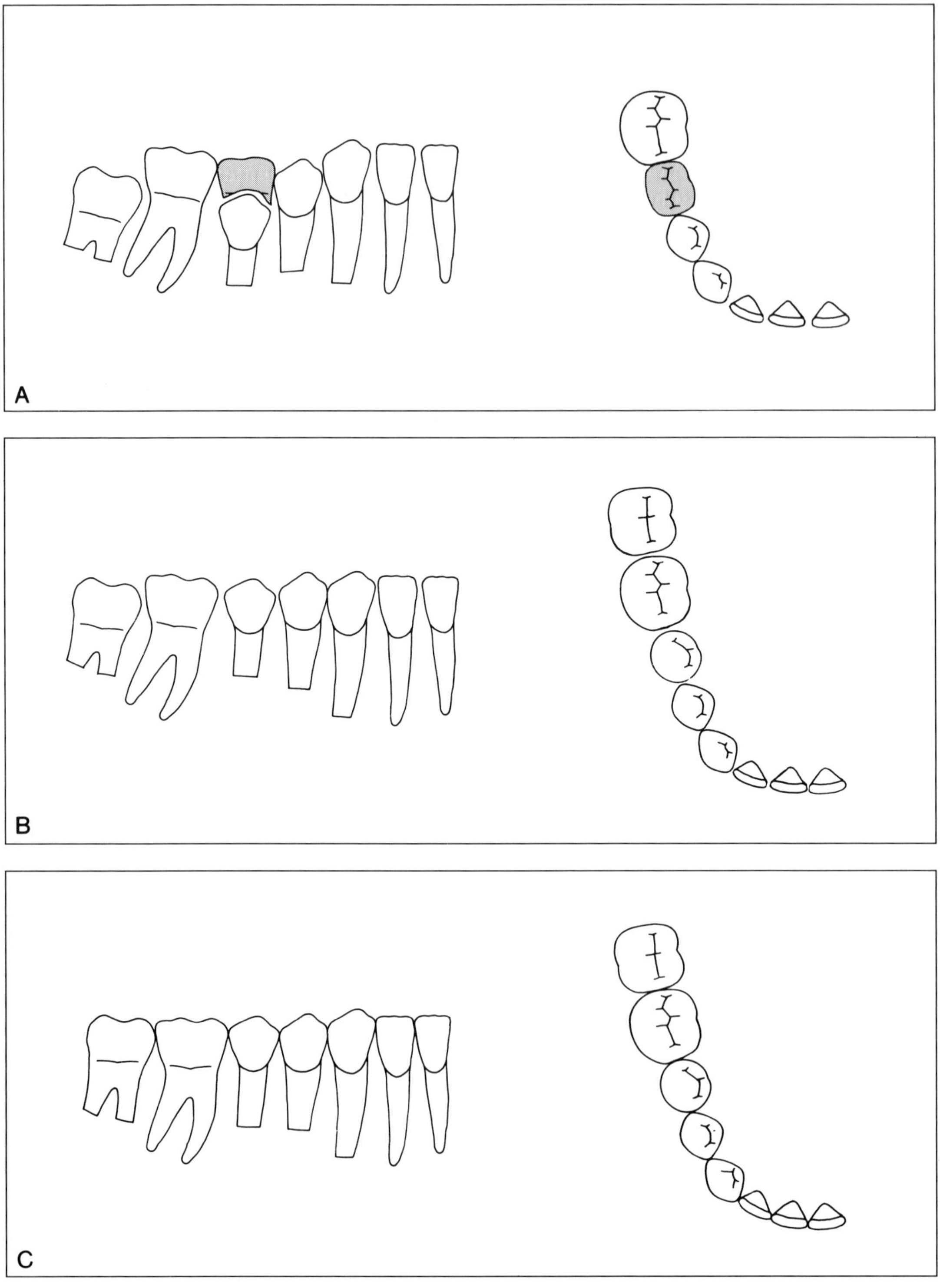

Figure 4-2

molar will migrate mesially earlier than in the second instance. The available space allows for this variation without resulting in complications.

4.5.2 Mandibular Incisor Region Changes Pattern B

Pattern B is characterized by a balance between the dental arch length required and available for the incisors (Figs. 4-3 and 4-4). The mandibular incisors are in contact and well aligned. The lateral incisor occupies a slightly lingual position. The permanent canine emerges in contact with the lateral incisor, without overlapping however. Depending on the situation in the posterior region, more or less extra space will become available after the deciduous molars are exfoliated. The canine can thus move distally and the incisor positions can subsequently change.
Early emergence of the second permanent molar may lead to an undesirable mesial migration of the first molar. Late emergence of the second permanent molar presents a more favourable condition for improved position of the incisors.

4.5.3 Mandibular Incisor Region Changes Pattern C

Pattern C is characterized by a shortage of available space in the anterior segment of the dental arch (Figs. 4-5 and 4-6). This pattern is the most critical and occurs in many instances when crowding is present in the mandibular anterior region after the transition of the posterior teeth. The shortage of available arch length can express itself in various ways. The incisors may overlap each other and the lateral incisor may be abnormally lingually positioned. The situation is particularly complicated when the deciduous canine has been resorbed prematurely. The incisors are then able to attain a better position at the sacrifice of the space destined for the permanent canine.
The canine usually emerges buccally, overlaps the lateral incisor, and is mesiobuccally rotated. The crowding of the incisors may increase. The sequence of emergence is critical. If the first permanent molar migrates mesially without the first premolar having had the opportunity to move distally, the crowded conditions and the position of the canine will not improve or only slightly improve. The size of the leeway space and the difference in mesiodistal crown width of the second deciduous molar and its successor are important factors. If a little extra space becomes available, only slight improvements can be expected. Substantial excess may result in considerable relief. However, the latter is seldom the case because a small anterior section of the apical area is usually associated with a small middle section and a small leeway space. Early emergence of the second permanent molar will reduce the chances for improvement.

4.6 Influence of conditions in the canine-premolar segment on the mandibular incisor region during transition of the posterior teeth

Three main factors associated with the transition of the posterior teeth play a role in the changes that take place in the incisor region: the size of the middle section of the apical area, the size of the leeway space, and the emergence sequence of the canine

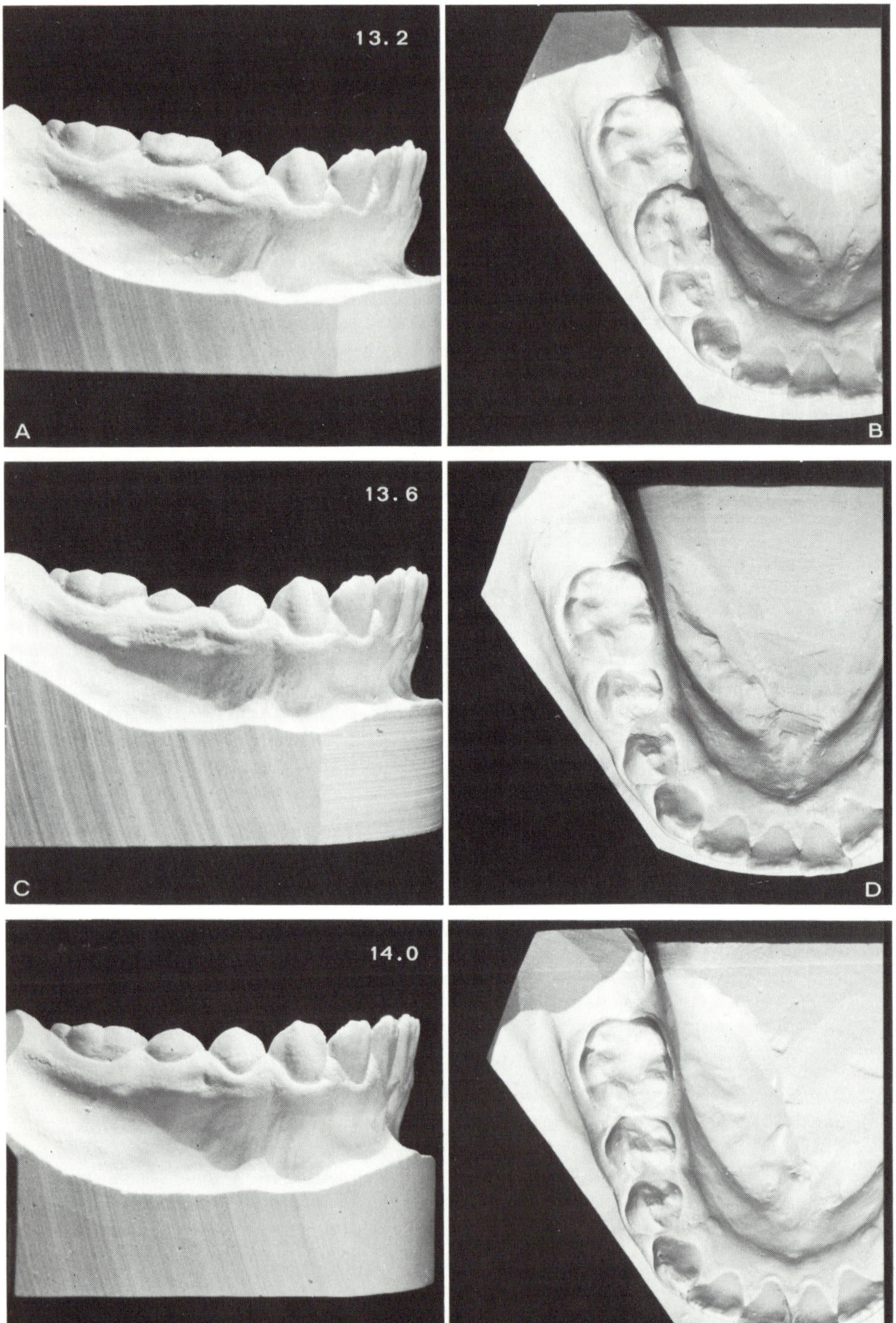

Figure 4-3

Fig. 4-3 Lateral and occlusal views of a longitudinal series of dental casts of the Mandibular Incisor Region Changes Pattern B, characterized by a balance between the required and available dental arch length for the incisors.

A, B The mandibular incisors are in contact with each other; the lateral incisor is slightly lingually positioned. The canine emerged in contact with the lateral incisor and slightly lingually. The first premolar has emerged after the canine and without an excess of space.

C, D The second premolar has emerged without contacting the adjacent teeth. The mesially located teeth can migrate distally and their individual positions can improve.

E, F The diastemata in the posterior region are closed. The incisors are slightly better aligned than at the beginning of the second transitional period. The contact between the canine and lateral incisor has improved. The late emergence of the second permanent molar is favourable.

Fig. 4-4 (see page 94) Schematic lateral and occlusal views of the Mandibular Incisor Region Changes Pattern B, characterized by a balance between the dental arch length required and available for the incisors.

A The incisors are in contact with each other and are well aligned. The lateral incisor may be slightly lingually positioned. The canine has emerged in contact with the lateral incisor without overlapping. The canine vertically overlaps the emerged first premolar. Its mesiodistal crown dimension is larger than that of its predecessor.

B After loss of the second deciduous molar the first premolar and canine can move distally and utilise some of the excess space available. The crowding in the canine region may be corrected. The position of the lateral incisor may improve.

C All permanent teeth (except the third molar) are in contact with each other and well aligned. The arch form usually does not flatten anteriorly. A late emergence of the second permanent molar works favourably in this pattern of changes.

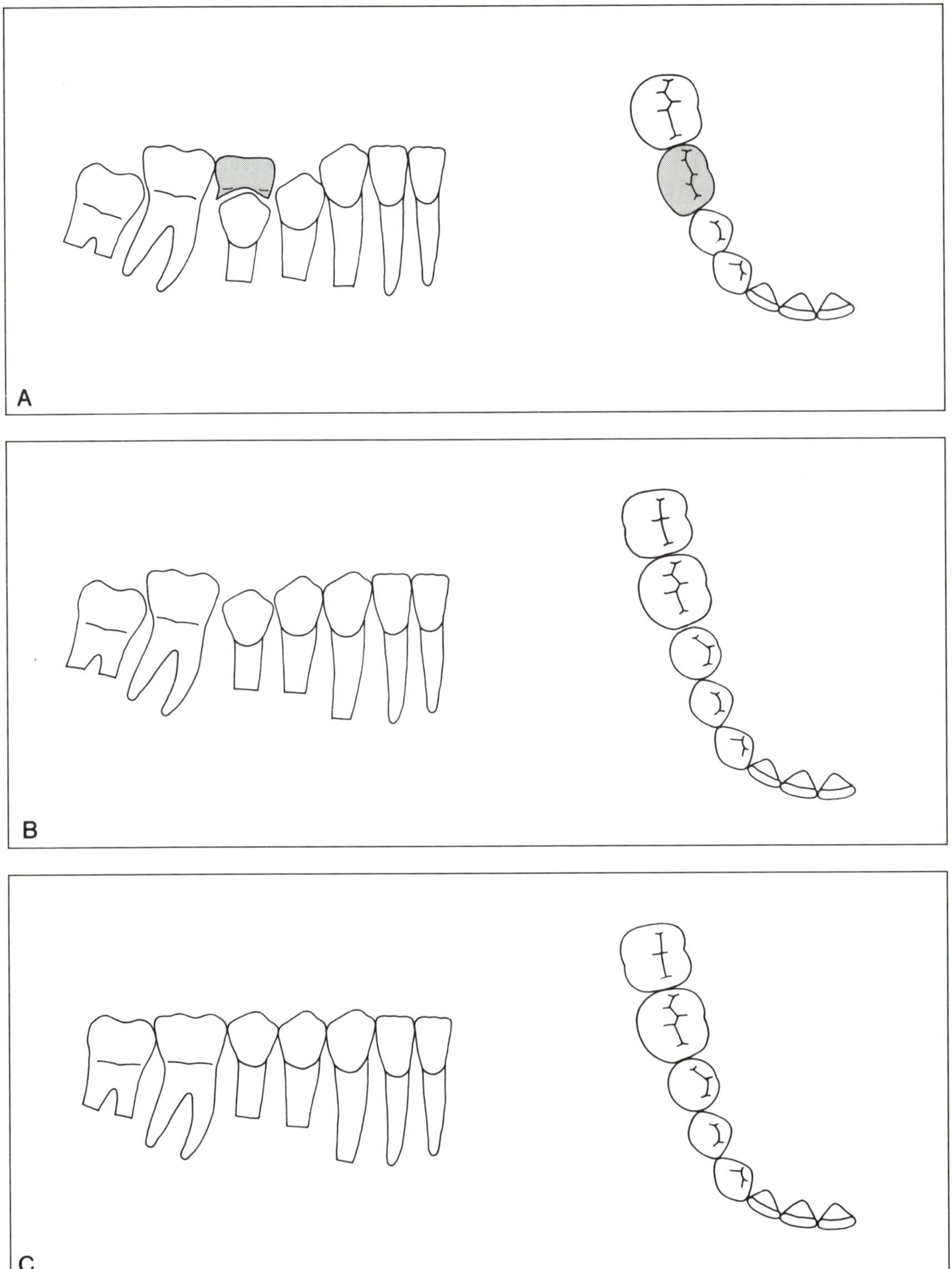

Figure 4-4

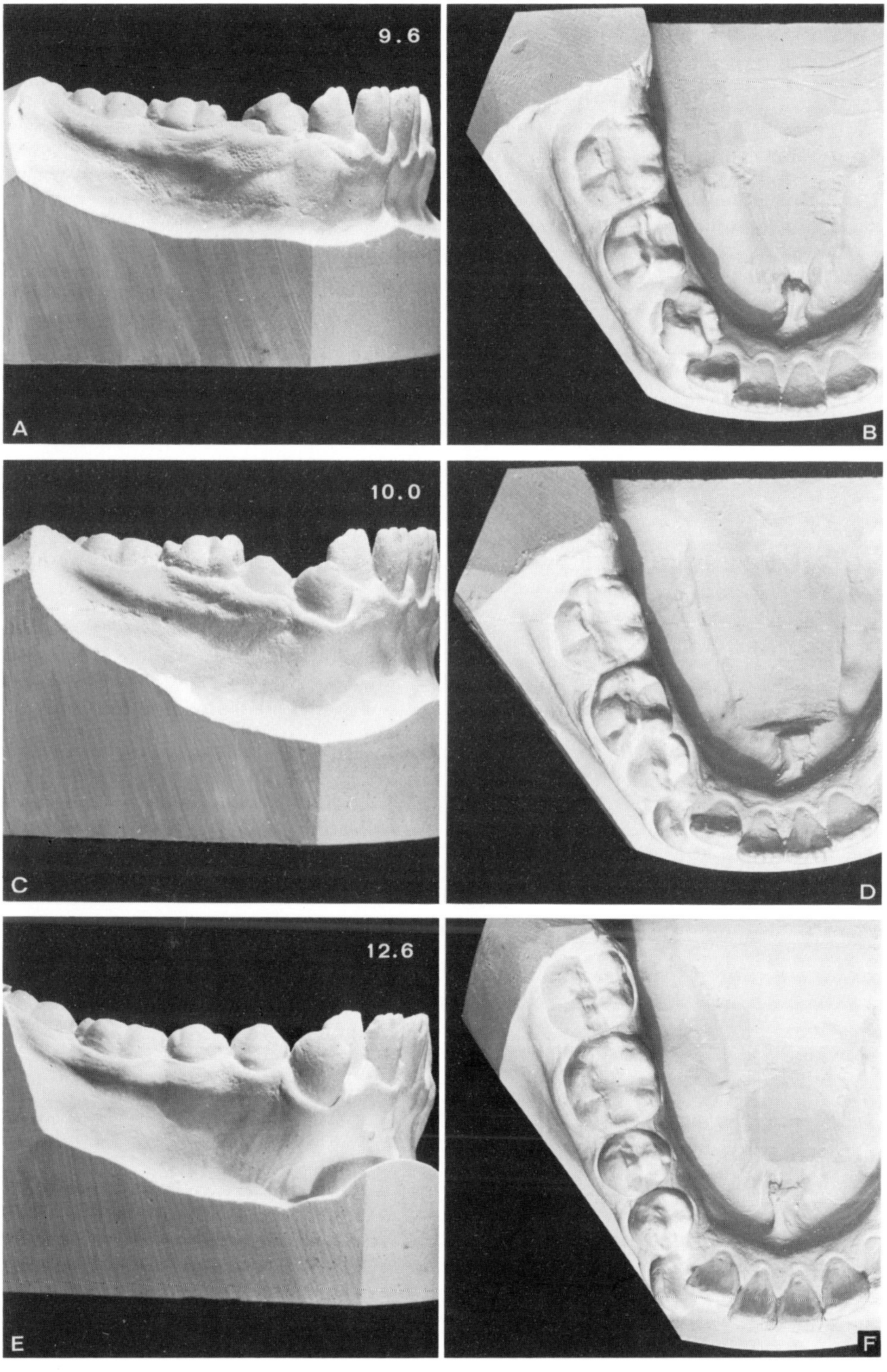

Figure 4-5

Fig. 4-5 *(see page 95)* *Lateral and occlusal views of a longitudinal series of dental casts of the Mandibular Incisor Region Changes Pattern C, characterized by a shortage of available space in the anterior segment of the dental arch.*

A, B *Crowding in the incisor region has led to premature resorption of the deciduous canine and temporarily improved incisor positions. However, the lateral incisor is still lingually positioned. The first premolar has already emerged. The position of the not-yet-emerged permanent canine can be detected on the plaster models.*

C, D *The canine emerged after the first premolar; this is indicative of a small middle section of the apical area and is unfavourable for the situation in the anterior region. In the meantime the first premolar moved distally. The canine overlaps the lateral incisor, is mesiobuccally rotated, and makes contact with the adjacent teeth.*

E, F *The excess in mesiodistal crown width between the second premolar and its predecessor did not improve the conditions mesial to it. Both premolars are properly positioned. The canine, however, has been displaced more buccally and the lateral incisor moved lingually. The second permanent molar has emerged and attained occlusion.*

Fig. 4-6 *Schematic lateral and occlusal views of the Mandibular Incisor Region Changes Pattern C, characterized by a shortage of available space in the anterior segment of the dental arch.*

A *Crowding in the incisor region. The canine has emerged buccally and overlaps the lateral incisor. The first premolar has emerged after the canine. The canine may also erupt later than the first premolar, or both teeth may emerge simultaneously.*

B *Crowding in the incisor region can increase. The canine will be displaced further buccally and becomes more mesiobuccally rotated.*

C *Even under the favourable circumstances illustrated here, the situation in the canine region will not improve. The canine may overlap the lateral incisor further and become even more buccally positioned. A more favourable development occurs when the first premolar can migrate distally. This development depends on the size of the leeway space, the sequence of emergence, and the time of emergence of the second permanent molar. The position of the canine can then improve.*

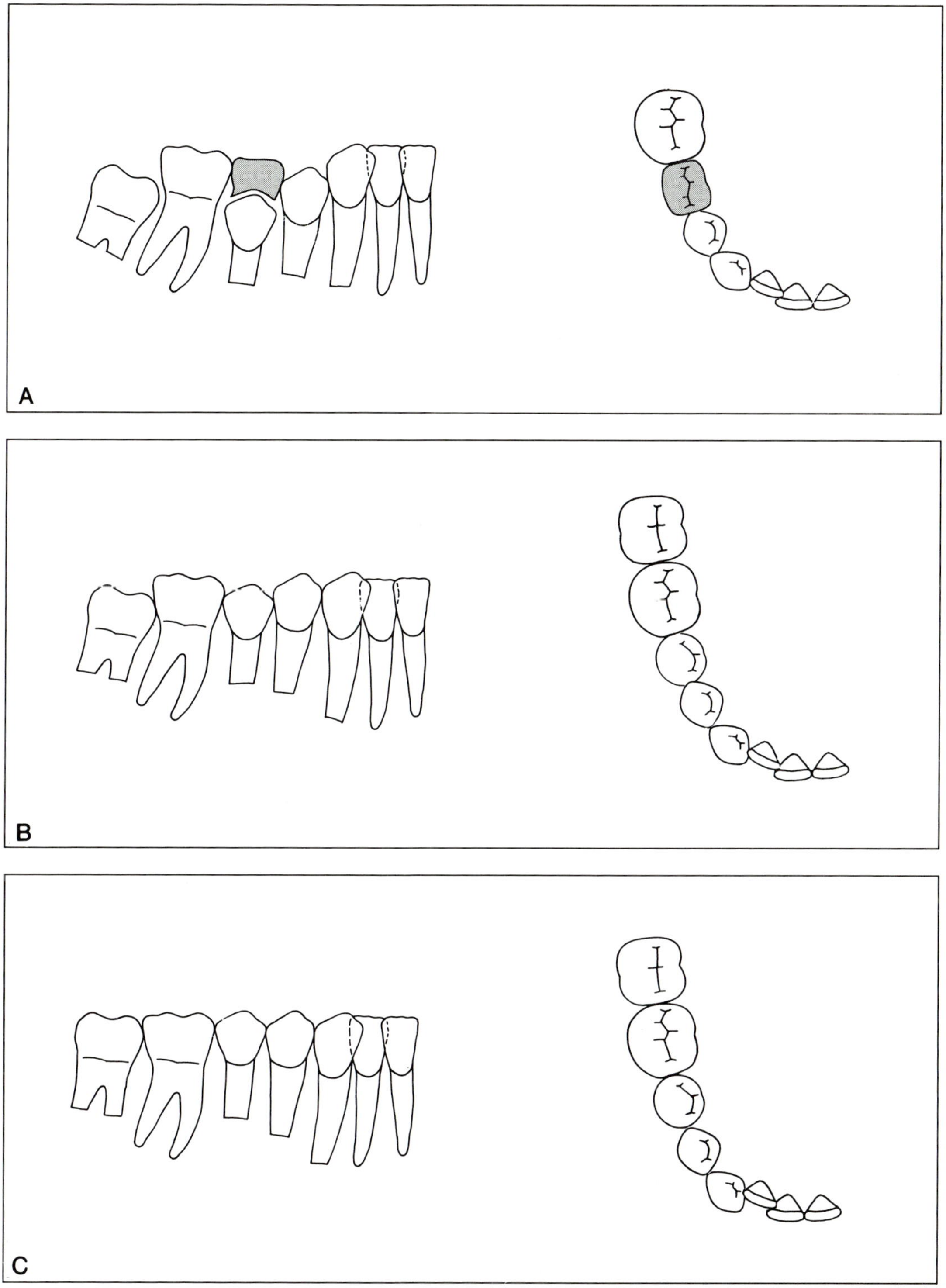

Figure 4-6

and premolars. An additional factor is the early or late emergence of the second permanent molar.

When excess space is available in the incisor region of the dental arch, these four factors are not essential and do not affect the end result. A small leeway space will not result in problems, particularly because the canine can move mesially and occupy some of the excess space in the incisor region. Either sequence of emergence will work out well. Early emergence of the second permanent molar will only serve to speed up the closure of diastemata.

Cases of a balance between the required and available dental arch length in the incisor region depend on a favourable combination of the four factors to result in a harmonious alignment of teeth. A small middle section of the apical area associated with a small leeway space can lead to a buccal and rotated emergence of the canine that will not correct later on. This situation may arise earlier when the permanent canine crown is abnormally large in relation to the crown of its predecessor. Emergence sequences in which the second premolar precedes the canine will limit the possibility for distal migration of the canine. Then the extra space is more likely to be utilised by mesial migration of the first permanent molar, particularly when the second molar emerges early. The most favourable sequence in eruption in this respect is canine, first and second premolar at the same time, and then the second permanent molar.

Cases of a shortage of available space in the incisor region of the dental arch depend even more on a favourable combination of the four factors under discussion. All remarks made above for cases of a balanced space condition for the incisors apply here in a stronger sense. A small middle section of the apical area and a small leeway space usually result in increased anterior crowding. The canine and incisors will overlap more, and lack of adequate contact support will aggravate the situation. The usual result is a canine that is not only tipped mesially to a marked degree but is also rotated mesiobuccally and located buccally to the dental arch. The premolars can still attain a proper position in the dental arch, because their crowns are equal in size or larger than those of their predecessors. In addition, the latter are not exfoliated before the premolars have emerged.

A large middle section of the apical area, large leeway space, favourable eruption sequence, and late emergence of the second permanent molar will usually not lead to total relief of marked incisor crowding. This crowding is primarily determined by the size of the anterior section of the apical area. When the distance between the left and right permanent canine crowns is small prior to emergence, then the distance between their apices will remain small after eruption is completed. Neither nature nor orthodontic therapy are able to permanently move mandibular canines laterally in the dental arch in cases of anterior crowding.[181,197] No rational explanation can be given for this phenomenon.

4.7 Supplementary remarks

What occurs in the mandible depends on the conditions within the dental arch and the pressures exerted by the tongue and buccal musculature. The occlusion with the maxillary teeth plays an essential role, particularly in changes in the posterior region.

Migration of posterior teeth and interlocking also determine the ultimate position of the mandibular canine and incisors. That also applies to the presence or absence of contact between the maxillary and mandibular incisors and canines.
The combination of a large middle section of the apical area, large leeway space, favourable angulation, direction of eruption of the permanent canine, and emergence of the second permanent molar after completion of the transition can lead to remarkable improvements in the position of the mandibular incisors. Lack of favourable conditions, however, will not lead to a relief of crowding and usually results in a poor contact between the permanent canine and lateral incisor.

Chapter 5

Variations in Transition of Maxillary Incisors*

5.1 Introduction

The morphology of the maxilla deviates markedly from that of the mandible. The maxilla is connected with other bones of the skull by sutures and does not act as a separate entity, as is the case for the mandible. Its shape and structure differ accordingly. Further, the maxilla can increase in size in the median plane because the intermaxillary suture maintains its growth potential until the development of the dentition is completed.
The space available within the maxilla for the permanent incisors before emergence is more limited than in the mandible. The amount by which maxillary permanent incisors exceed their predecessors in crown dimensions is greater than that for mandibular incisors. The crowns of maxillary permanent incisors are oriented within the jaw in a typical way; before emergence the spatial conditions in the maxilla allow a larger variation in the arrangement both vertically and sagittally of the permanent incisors than in the mandible. Consequently, the eruption process of maxillary incisors is characterized by a larger variation than that of mandibular incisors.
The transition of maxillary incisors is discussed in relation to the size and shape of the anterior section of the apical area. The variation in location of permanent incisors and canines before emergence and their relation to the adjacent deciduous predecessors are indicated. Eruption is treated in preemergence and postemergence phases. Five eruption patterns are presented by means of longitudinal records of dental casts and schematic drawings.

5.2 The anterior section of the apical area and the arrangement of anterior teeth before emergence

The location of the anterior section of the apical area in the maxilla is mainly determined by the size, shape, and anteroposterior orientation of the piriform

* Reproduced from: "Transition of the upper incisors" by Paul J.M.R. Bakker, Hein J.W. Wassenberg and Frans P.G.M. van der Linden. In: *Transition of the human dentition.* Monograph No. 13. Craniofacial Growth Series., Pg 75-99. Ed. Frans P.G.M. van der Linden. Center for Human Growth and Development. The University of Michigan, Ann Arbor, U.S.A., 1982.

aperture. A large variation exists in these respects. The forming canines are located in close proximity to the piriform aperture. As a result, the transverse distance between the two forming permanent canines can differ and their anteroposterior location can vary considerably. The central permanent incisors are formed in close proximity to the floor of the anterior part of the nose and with the intermaxillary suture in between. The morphology of the bony structure of the anterior part of the maxilla adjacent to the nose determines the space available in transverse and anteroposterior directions for the forming parts of the permanent incisors and canines and also the range available for location of the apices of these teeth upon complete eruption.

The anterior section of the apical area is bounded laterally by the location of the permanent canines and sagittally by the labial and palatal walls of the alveolar process. The space available for the roots of the deciduous teeth and crowns of the permanent teeth prior to their emergence is limited. Maxillary permanent central incisors have the widest crowns in relation to their roots. The anterior section of the apical area must accommodate these crowns together with the roots of their predecessors in a compartment that later will serve to contain the roots of the permanent incisors only. No other region of both jaws demonstrates such a comparatively large difference in space required in early and late stages of development of the dentition.

The maxillary permanent canine starts its formation lateral to the piriform aperture and at the largest distance from the occlusal plane.The permanent central incisor is formed near the midline and more anteriorly than the lateral incisor. The lateral incisor starts its formation at a more inferior level than the central edge incisor, consequently its incisal edge is located closer to the occlusal plane than the incisal edge of the central incisor, until the latter starts to erupt.

The cusp tip of the permanent canine and the cementoenamel junction of the adjacent lateral permanent incisor are more or less at the same level. However, some variation exists, depending on the differences in height of formation of the permanent incisors and canine and on the crown length of the lateral incisor.

The lateral permanent incisor is located palatal to the central incisor and canine. The permanent maxillary central incisor overlaps the lateral incisor (the amount of overlap depending on the space available for the lateral incisor, as determined by the intercanine distance, and on the crown size of the central and lateral incisors).

Before the maxillary permanent incisors emerge they show less frequent rotations than do mandibular incisors. This is probably related to differences in morphology between the anterior regions of the maxilla and mandible and differences in size and shape between the maxillary and mandibular permanent incisors. On the other hand, the maxillary permanent incisors with their relatively large mesiodistal crown dimensions show a larger variation when rotated than do mandibular incisors.

The relation between the space available and the space needed for arrangement of the tooth material within the anterior section of the apical area before the permanent incisors emerge shows a marked variation (Figs. 5-1 to 5-3). The anterior section of the apical area is of adequate size when the distance between the maxillary permanent canine crowns is large in relation to the mesiodistal crown dimensions of the maxillary permanent incisors. Frequently, a large anterior section of the apical area is associated with large diastemata in the deciduous dentition. There is no initial contact between the distal surface of the central permanent incisor crown and the root of the adjacent lateral deciduous incisor. Consequently, the distance between the maxillary deciduous

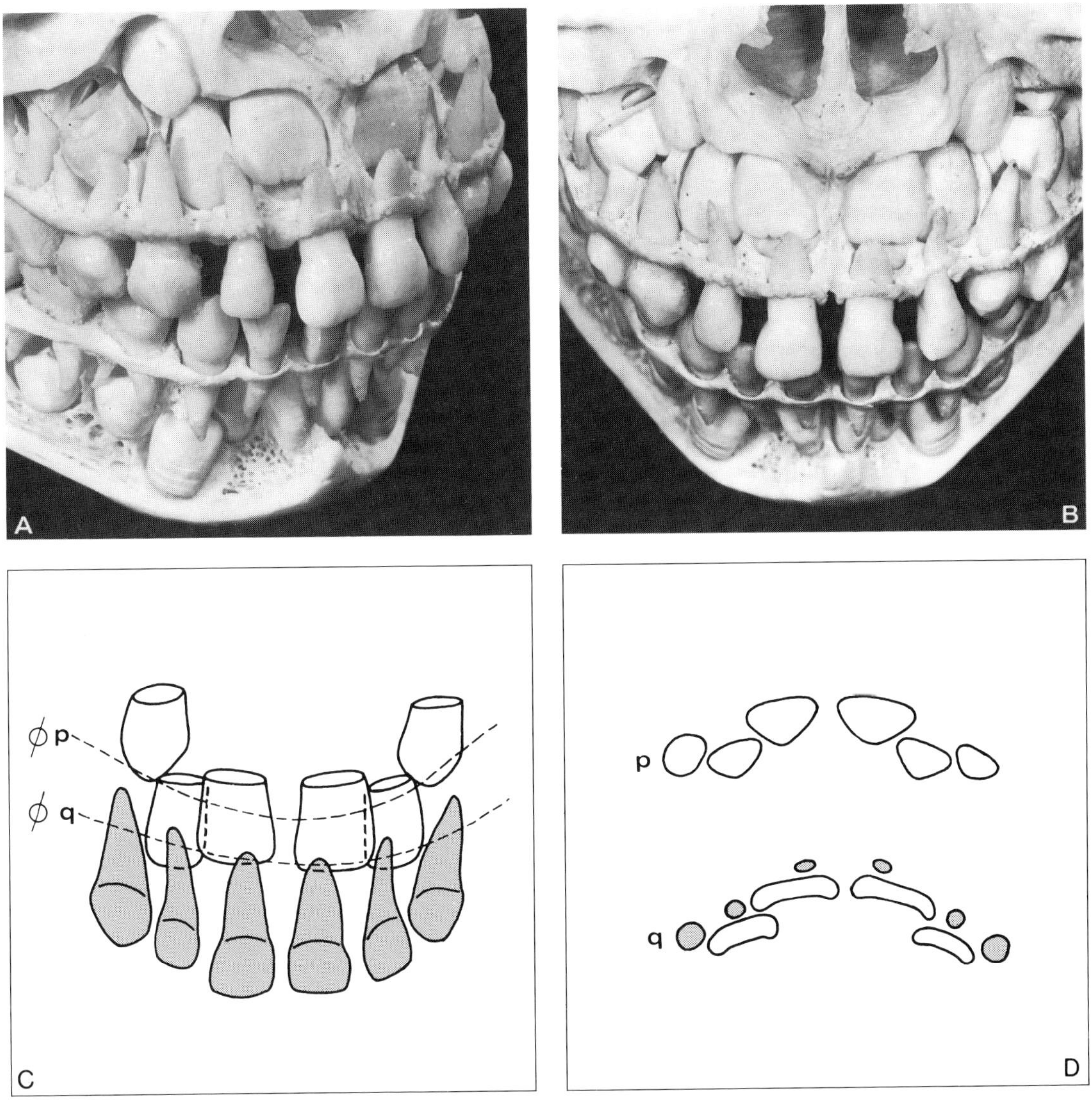

Fig. 5-1 Large anterior section of the apical area in the maxilla.

A, B Large diastemata between the crowns of the anterior deciduous teeth. The width of the piriform aperture and the associated distance between the crowns of both maxillary permanent canines are large. The permanent incisors show a more or less perpendicular mesiodistal angulation in relation to the occlusal plane. The crowns are not rotated. The central permanent incisor only slightly overlaps its neighbouring lateral incisor. Note the more caudal position of the incisal edge of the lateral permanent incisor than that of the central incisor.

(Legend continues on page 104)

(Legend 5-1 continued)

C *Schematic drawing of B with dotted lines indicating the sections presented in D. The distal surfaces of the crowns of the maxillary central permanent incisors do not contact the roots of the adjacent lateral deciduous incisors.*

D *In the region of the incisal borders of the permanent incisors (q) the lateral incisors are palatal to the central incisors. Note the relations between the roots of the deciduous teeth and the crowns of the permanent teeth. In the region of the cementoenamel junctions of the permanent incisors (p) the lateral incisors are also palatal to the central incisors. Note the triangular shape of the cross section of the roots of the permanent incisors.*

Fig. 5-2 *Medium anterior section of the apical area in the maxilla.*

A, B *The diastemata between the anterior deciduous teeth are medium-sized. The width of the piriform aperture and the associated distance between the crowns of both maxillary permanent canines are also medium-sized. The maxillary central permanent incisors are almost perpendicularly angulated in relation to the occlusal plane; they are not rotated. The permanent canine crown slightly overlaps the lateral incisor.*

C *The distal corners of the central permanent incisors contact the mesial surfaces of the roots of the adjacent lateral deciduous incisors.*

D *In the region of the incisal borders of the permanent incisors (q) a close proximity exists between the crowns of the permanent teeth and the roots of the deciduous teeth. Note the contacts described under C. In the region of the cementoenamel junctions of the permanent incisors (p) the teeth overlap. Note the close proximity between the permanent canines and the lateral permanent incisors.*

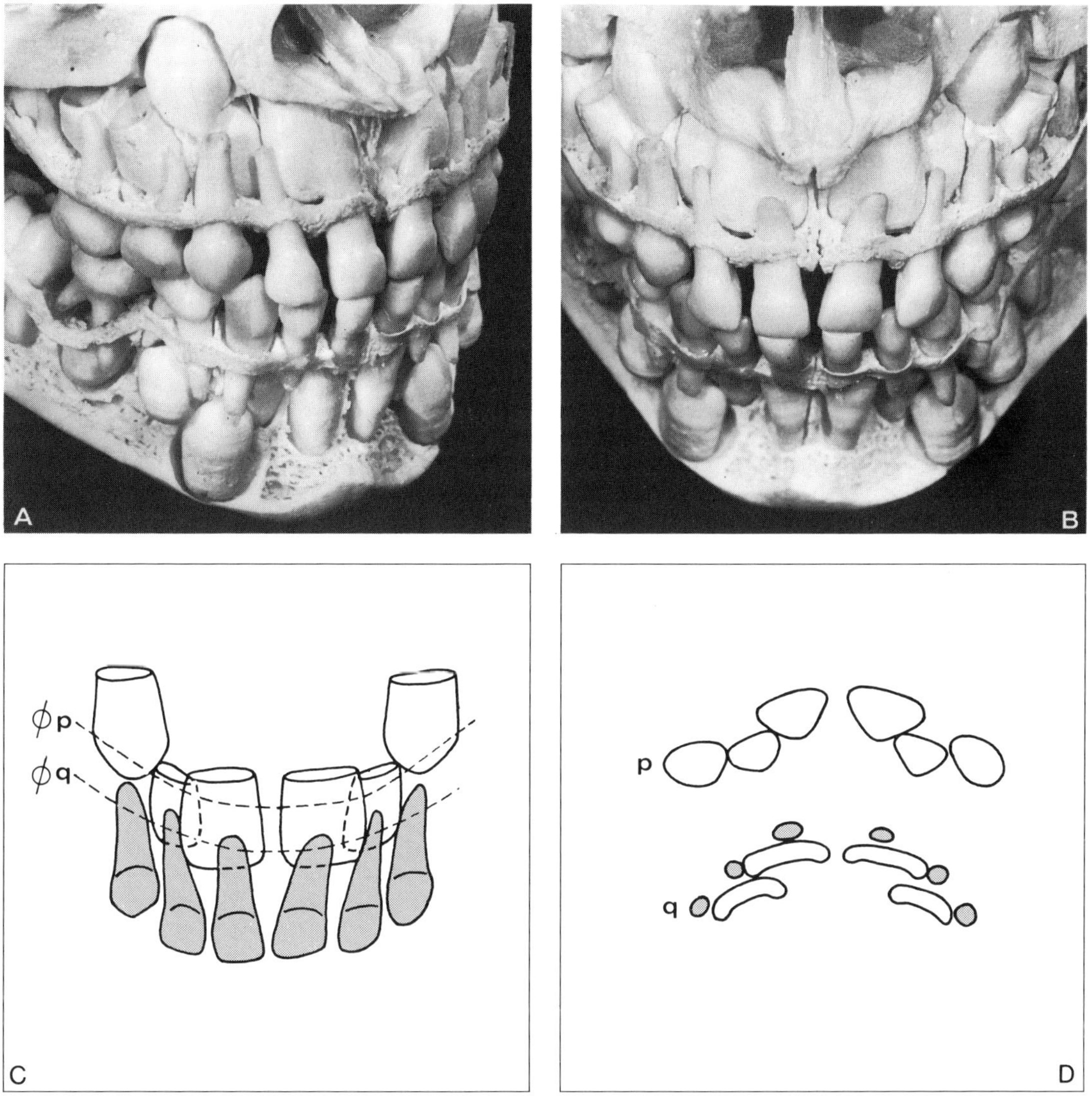

Figure 5-2

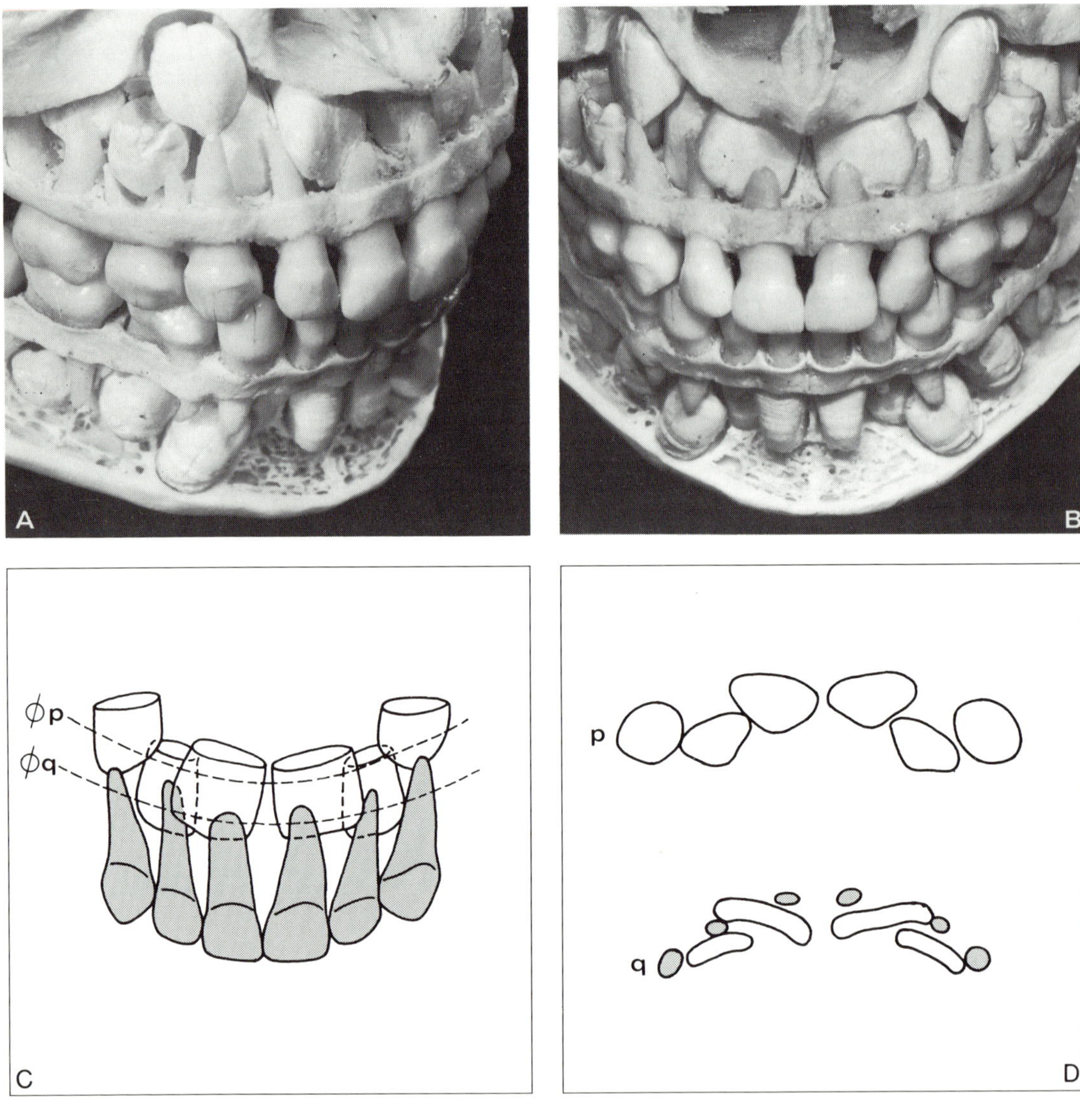

Fig. 5-3 Small anterior section of the apical area in the maxilla.

A, B *No diastemata between the deciduous incisors. The width of the piriform aperture and associated distance between both maxillary canine crowns is small. The distally angulated central permanent incisors are close together just below the floor of the nose. The close proximity between the formation area of a maxillary central permanent incisor and the median plane produced distally angulated crowns that are also mesiopalatally rotated. The central permanent incisors overlap the lateral incisors by approximately half their crown width. The permanent canine crown overlaps approximately one half the adjacent lateral permanent incisor.*

C *The distal corners of the crowns of the central permanent incisors contact the mesiobuccal surfaces of the roots of the adjacent lateral deciduous incisors.*

D *In the region of the incisal borders of the permanent incisors (q) the mesial incisal corners of the central incisors are abnormally palatally positioned. The contact between their distal incisal corners and the roots of the adjacent lateral deciduous incisors is not favourable. Close proximity exists between the central incisors in the region of the cementoenamel junctions of the permanent incisors (p). The space available for the arrangement of the permanent teeth is small.*

canines will not increase or will only slightly increase before and during emergence of the maxillary central permanent incisors. However, large diastemata in the maxillary anterior region are not always associated with a large anterior section of the apical area, and no or small diastemata are not always associated with a small anterior section. As for the mandible, only a limited correlation exists between the mesiodistal crown dimension of the maxillary incisors of the two dentitions.

5.3 Eruption before emergence

The transition of maxillary and mandibular incisors is illustrated and explained in Fig. 2-4 (page 34). Figure 5-4 shows six prepared skulls illustrating the transition of the maxillary incisors. This figure further shows the large variation in transition of maxillary incisors together with typical abnormalities.
In general, a central permanent incisor starts to erupt in the same direction as its orientation within the jaw. The descending central incisor passes the adjacent lateral incisor and the amount of overlap gradually reduces. As a rule, the overlapping has been fully eliminated before complete eruption of the central incisor, when its cementoenamel junction has reached the level of the incisal corner of the lateral incisor. Sufficient space is then available for the maxillary lateral permanent incisor to descend. In accordance with its original location within the jaw, the lateral incisor will then erupt in a more labial direction than the central incisor. When a permanent incisor erupts in a small anterior section of the apical area, not only the preceding deciduous tooth but also the adjacent deciduous tooth may become resorbed. A lateral deciduous incisor may be lost in association with the eruption of a permanent central incisor; a maxillary deciduous canine may prematurely exfoliate when the adjacent permanent lateral incisor erupts. The premature loss of one or two central deciduous incisors due to trauma (Fig. 5-5) will not result in disturbances in the development of the dentition, if the position and formation of their successors have not been affected.[101]

5.4 Eruption after emergence and subsequent change in orientation

The position of the maxillary permanent incisors becomes influenced after emergence by forces of the lips, tongue, and sometimes by factors of an abnormal nature, for

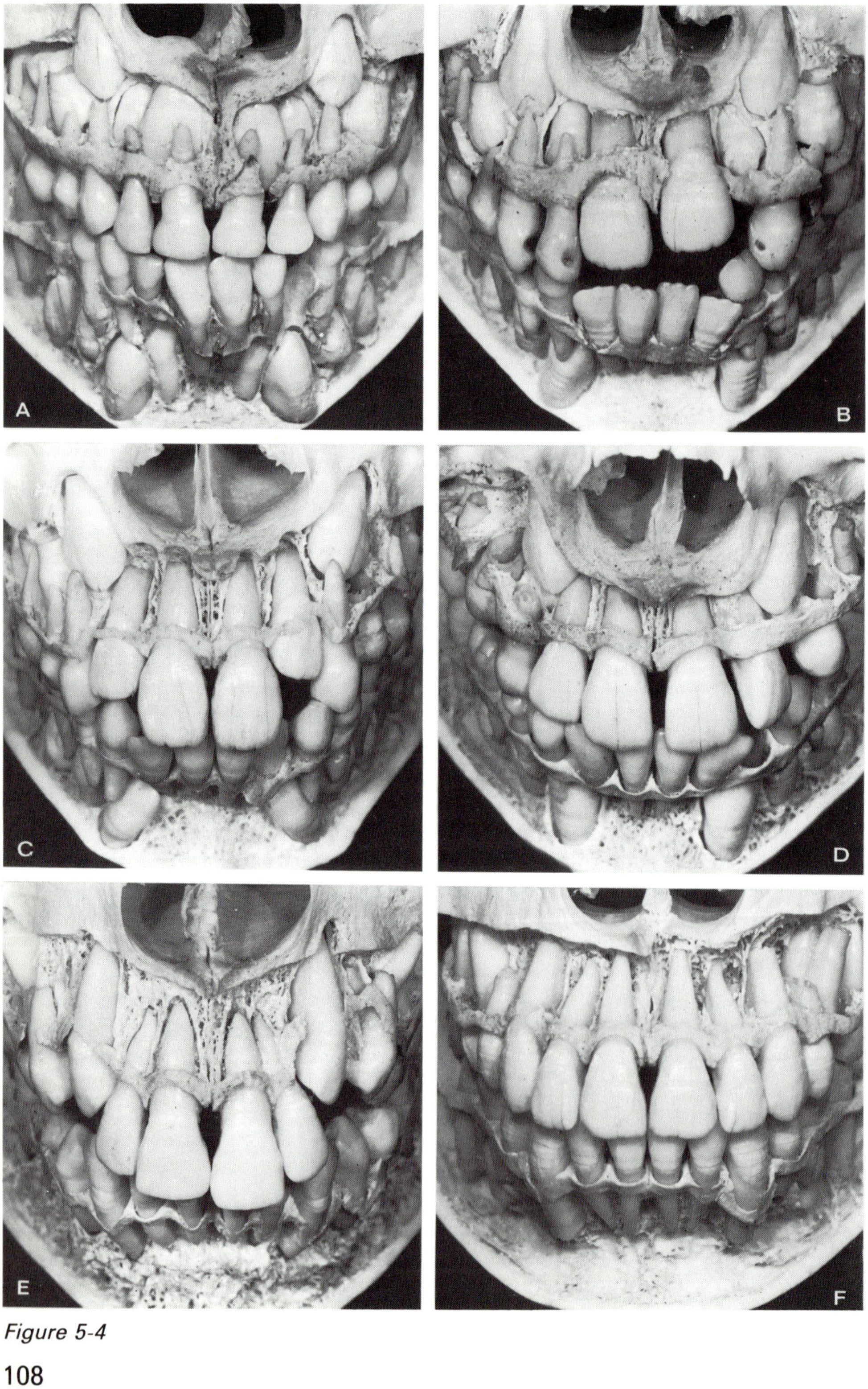

Figure 5-4

Fig. 5-4 Six preparations of human skulls with small and medium anterior sections of the apical area in the maxilla that demonstrate different aspects of and disturbances in the transition of the maxillary incisors and canines.

A Small anterior section of the apical area with all maxillary deciduous teeth still present. The mandibular central permanent incisors have already reached the level of the occlusal plane. The maxillary central permanent incisors have started their eruption and passed the adjacent lateral incisors. Note the contact between the distal corners of the crowns of the central permanent incisors and the lateral deciduous incisor roots. The asymmetry in the location of the maxillary central permanent incisors shows up in the morphology of the floor of the nose. No diastemata or only small diastemata are present between the anterior deciduous teeth. The width of the piriform aperture and the distance between the maxillary permanent canines are small. The central permanent incisors overlap approximately half the width of the crown of the adjacent lateral incisors.

B Small anterior section of the apical area, asymmetrically erupting central permanent incisors, and premature loss of the maxillary left lateral deciduous incisor. In the maxillary right quadrant contact exists between the central permanent incisor, the lateral deciduous incisor, and the deciduous canine. The distal and lateral movement of the deciduous canine, associated with the eruption of the central permanent incisor, can only take place on the right side and not the left. The maxillary lateral left permanent incisor has an abnormally shaped crown and is located in a rotated position.

C Medium anterior section of the apical area; maxillary central permanent incisors fully erupted and the lateral incisors partially erupted. The lateral incisors started to erupt and could move labially after the central incisors had descended. Note the difference in labial inclination between the central and the lateral incisors. The space between the root of the lateral incisor and the permanent canine crown is larger on the left than on the right side. The left lateral incisor will have more freedom to change in (mesiodistal) angulation during eruption than the right one.

D Small anterior section of the apical area with all four maxillary permanent incisors fully erupted. The maxillary left deciduous canine has been prematurely resorbed in association with the eruption of the adjacent lateral permanent incisor. The latter attains a more distal position in the dental arch than it otherwise would have done. Note the deviation in the midline of both dental arches.

E Medium anterior section of the apical area. The central and lateral incisors are fully erupted and their roots completely formed. The right permanent canine has emerged and erupted into contact with the crown of the lateral incisor. On the left side the canine has not erupted so far; the contact with the lateral incisor is not yet established. The roots of the central and lateral incisors are still close together. After the eruption of the canines the roots of the lateral incisors will be able to move distally.

F Medium anterior section of the apical area with fully erupted canines. The formation of their roots, however, is not yet completed. Some space exists between the roots of the lateral and the central incisors. Note the differences in labiolingual inclination between the central and lateral incisors. The apices of the lateral incisors are more palatally located than those of the central incisors. This difference is in accordance with the original sites of tooth formation and their subsequent position before eruption.

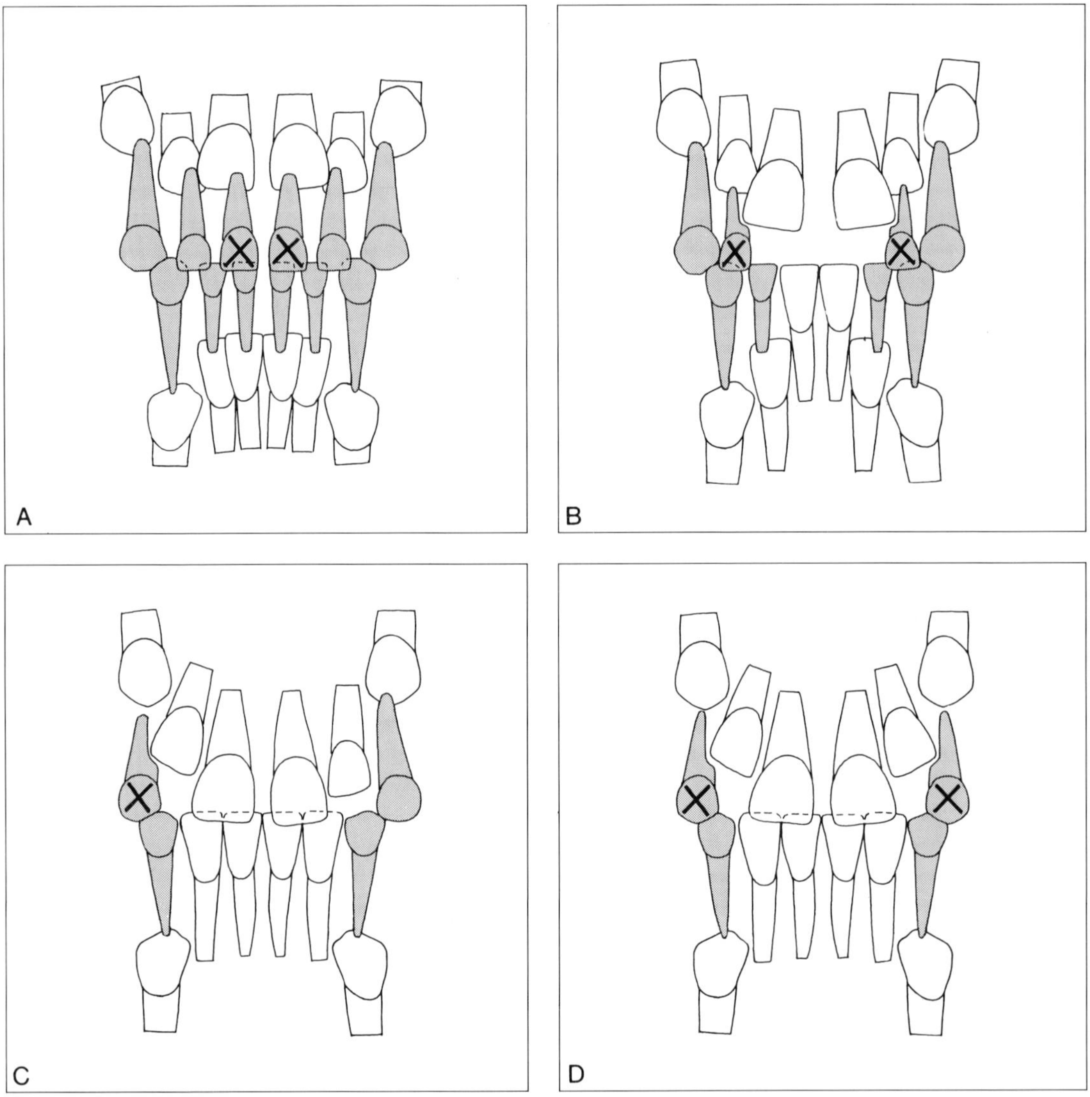

Fig. 5-5 Premature loss of deciduous incisors and canines in the maxilla due to trauma (A) or in association with the eruption of adjacent permanent teeth in a small anterior section of the apical area (C, D, E). (From Van der Linden.[223])

A Premature loss of one or two maxillary central deciduous incisors due to trauma will not disturb development of the dentition when the position and formation of the successors are not affected.

B Premature loss of both lateral deciduous incisors due to resorption associated with the eruption of the permanent incisors. The increase in intercanine width, which is normally associated with the eruption of the maxillary central permanent incisors and is based on the contact between the crowns of the central permanent incisors and roots of the adjacent lateral deciduous incisors, will not take place.

C Premature loss of the maxillary right deciduous canine associated with the eruption of a large lateral permanent incisor. The permanent incisors will subsequently migrate toward the open space.
D Premature loss of both maxillary deciduous canines associated with the eruption of the lateral permanent incisors.

example thumb-sucking. The maxillary central permanent incisors do not emerge lingual to the position originally occupied by their predecessors, as is the case in the mandible. By nature of their labial inclination they soon start to protrude labially beyond the places where previously the labial surfaces of their predecessors were located. Contact is then established with the upper lip, and under its influence the lateral inclination becomes reduced. Upon further eruption the incisors reach the lower lip and establish contact with the mandibular incisors (Fig. 5-6). The position attained upon complete eruption depends on the original position and orientation of these teeth within the jaw and the eruption path as it becomes influenced after emergence by the factors mentioned above. Local conditions within the dental arches also have an influence. Crowding will be demonstrated by rotation, overlapping, eversion, linguoversion, inversion, or a combination of these. A sagittal deviation in the relation between the dental arches will affect the vertical and sagittal positions of the mandibular and maxillary incisors. Eruption will continue until vertical support is established. Normally, this will be attained by the maxillary incisors contacting the mandibular ones and the lower lip. In a distorelation of the jaws, the maxillary and mandibular incisors will reach a position where there is an increased overjet and overbite. When the lower lip becomes positioned lingual to the maxillary incisors, the labial inclination of the usually already everted incisors will increase. The mandibular incisors may become tipped lingually.
As explained previously, the path of eruption of maxillary lateral permanent incisors has a more labial inclination than that of the central incisors. Normally, the upper lip and later the lower lip will exert the pressure required to bring the labial surface of the lateral crown in line with that of the central incisors. This happens mainly after the permanent canine emerges, unless more than adequate space is available in the dental arch.
If insufficient space is available in the dental arch for a maxillary lateral permanent incisor to move labially before its emergence, the tooth will change its path of eruption and become palatally positioned. Although frequently the transition of the mandibular posterior teeth provides extra space for the alignment of the anterior teeth, this seldom occurs in the maxilla. Therefore, the location of a palatally positioned maxillary lateral permanent incisor will not usually improve spontaneously. In addition, the occlusion with the mandibular incisors usually interferes with spontaneous improvement of a palatally positioned maxillary lateral permanent incisor, when a reversed overbite of that tooth exists. In this respect, the situation is also different from that of a lingually positioned mandibular lateral permanent incisor.
The final position of the maxillary permanent incisor is determined by a variety of factors as explained above. The variation in location is larger than that of the mandibular incisors. This disparity is partly due to the fact that the mandibular incisors precede the maxillary ones in the process of the transition. However, the differences in morphology of the tooth-bearing parts of the jaws and their adjacent structures are

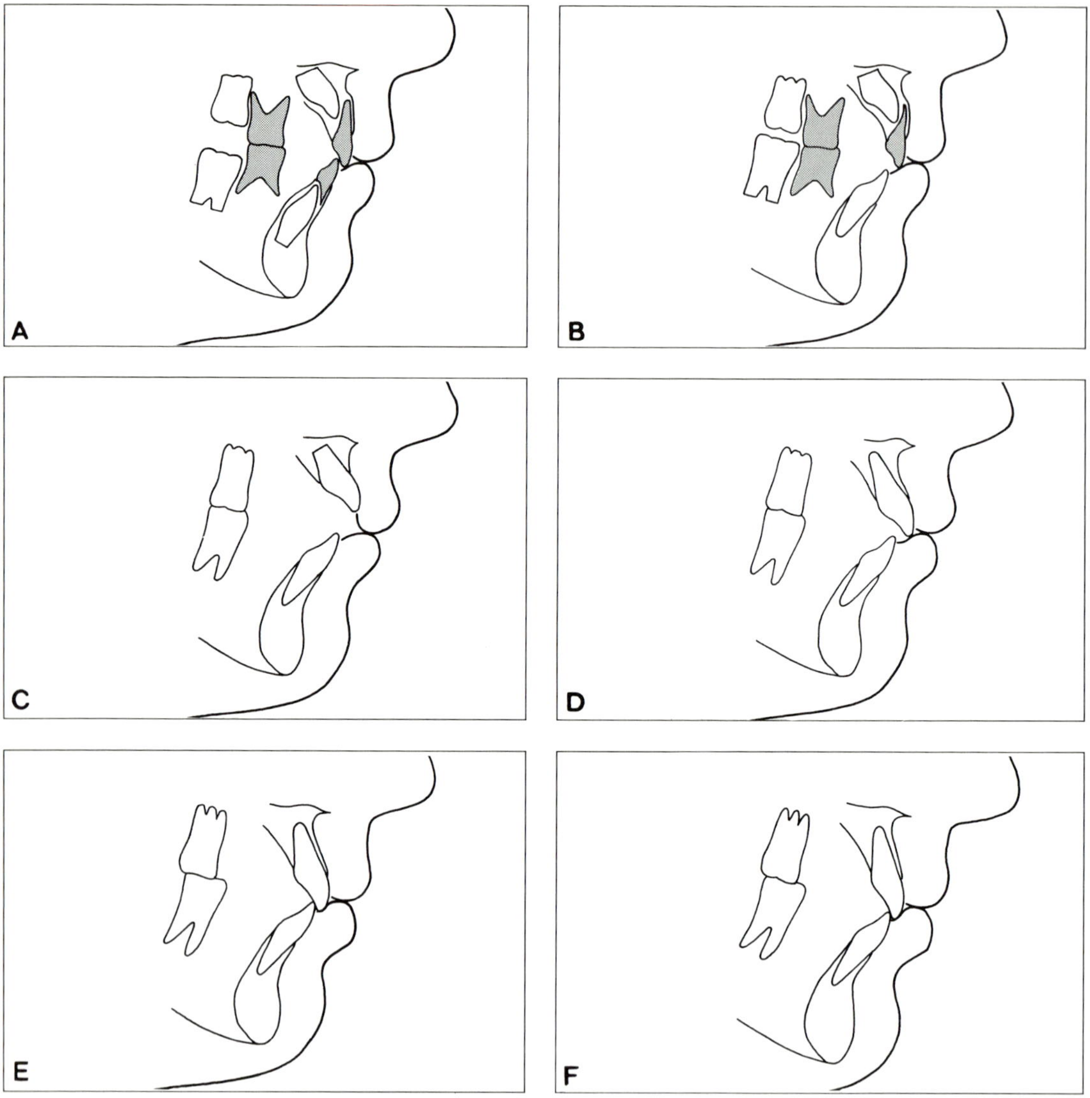

Fig. 5-6 Survey of the changes in vertical and sagittal direction in the central incisor region from the deciduous to the adult dentition. (From Van der Linden.[223])

A In the complete deciduous dentition the incisors are only slightly labially inclined. The permanent incisors are located lingually to their predecessors and are labially inclined. The pattern of resorption of the deciduous incisors is associated with the eruption of their successors.

B The mandibular central permanent incisor erupts after emergence in a direction corresponding to its original location within the jaw. The maxillary central permanent incisor has erupted further, and the resorption of its predecessor has proceeded.

C The mandibular central permanent incisor erupts further and the maxillary central permanent incisor emerged a few weeks or months after the loss of its predecessor.

D During eruption, the position of the mandibular incisor becomes influenced by the tongue and the lower lip. After emergence, the maxillary incisor establishes contact with the upper lip and its labial inclination reduces accordingly.

E The maxillary and mandibular incisors continue to erupt until vertical contact is reached and reciprocal vertical support between the incisors of both jaws is established. In addition, the lower lip plays an important role in the vertical support of the maxillary incisors. The upper and lower lips exert a lingual force in the maxillary incisor. Further, the lower lip is in contact with the mandibular incisors. The tongue provides support sagittally for the incisors of both jaws. This is also probably true for the vertical support, although to a lesser extent.

F After years, the maxillary and mandibular incisors have attained a steeper inclination in the adult situation. This change is associated with the continuation of jaw growth after the permanent teeth have established occlusion. The pressure exerted by the peri-oral musculature on the incisors also plays a role in the realization of this change in inclination.

more important in this respect. The same applies to the influences of normal and abnormal factors that in general affect the position of the maxillary incisors more than that of the mandibular ones.

5.5 Patterns in transition of maxillary incisors

The changes associated with the transition of maxillary incisors also are frequently not symmetrical. Differences between left and right sides are often encountered.

Five patterns are distinguished in the transition of the maxillary incisors. The guideline used to distinguish the varying patterns was, as for the mandible, the degree of rotation around the long axis of the incisors during emergence. The patterns will be presented by means of photographs of longitudinal series of dental casts and schematic drawings.

5.5.1 Maxillary Incisor Transition Pattern A

Emergence of the central and lateral permanent incisor in a nonrotated or slightly rotated position, with a normal labial inclination, and a normal mesiodistal angulation (Figs. 5-7 and 5-8). The central incisors emerge and erupt more labially than their predecessors. They are usually slightly distally angulated with a central diastema of about 3 mm between the mesial incisal corners. When sufficient space is available the lateral incisors will emerge without contacting the central incisors. Their labial inclination reduces during subsequent emergence and the incisal edges become aligned with those of the central incisors. The lateral incisors may be in contact with the mesial surfaces of the deciduous canine crowns; however, diastemata can also be present. Diastemata between the maxillary deciduous canines and first deciduous molars are usually closed before the emergence of the lateral incisors.

A lateral deciduous incisor will rarely be lost prematurely without any crowding or without a close proximity between the erupting central permanent crown and the root of the adjacent lateral incisor. When all four permanent incisors are fully erupted they will be located on an arch segment that is larger and more ventral than that of their

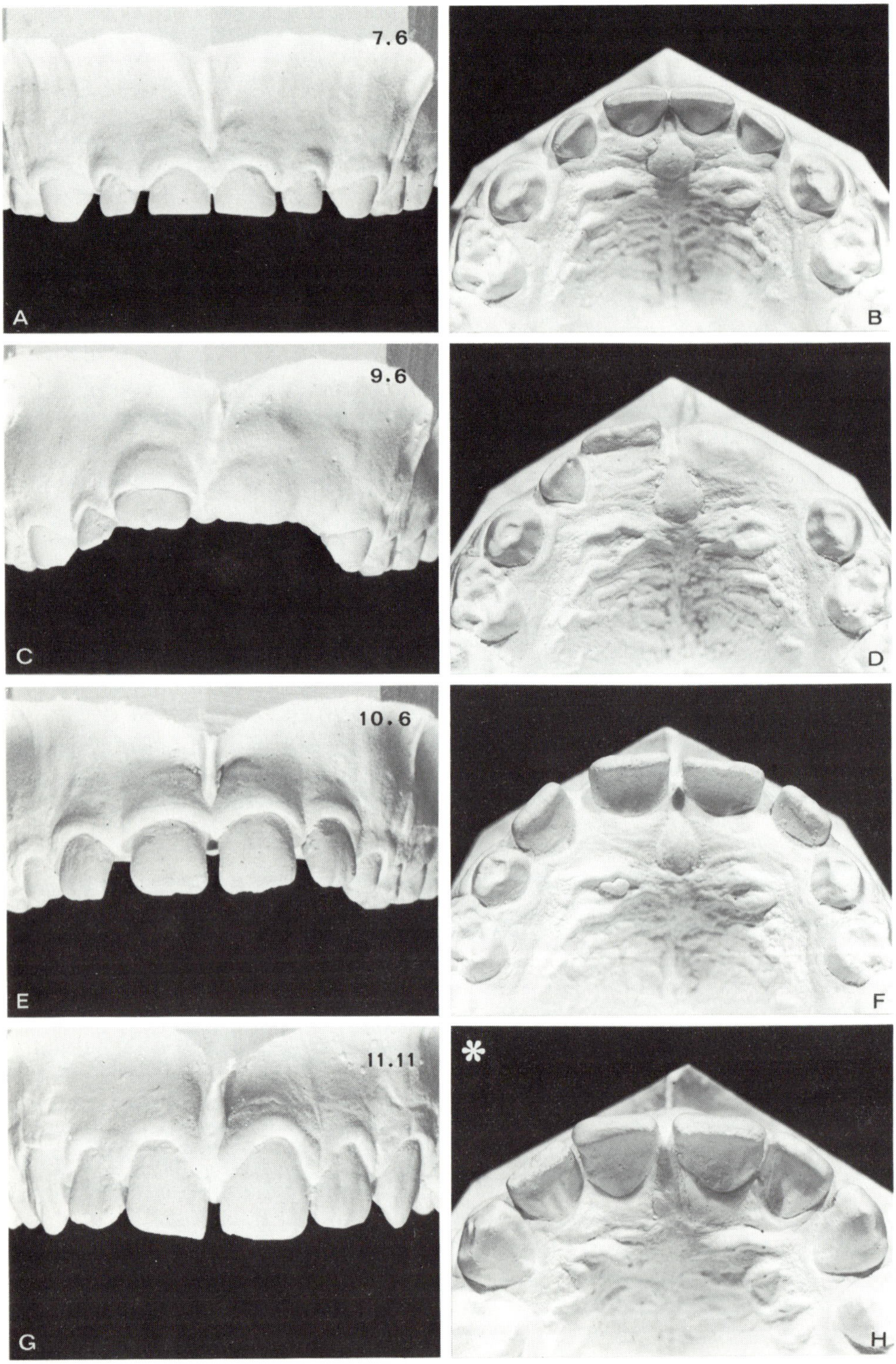

Figure 5-7

Fig. 5-7 Frontal and occlusal views of a longitudinal series of dental casts of a large anterior section of the apical area. This series demonstrates bilaterally the Maxillary Incisor Transition Pattern A, which is characterized by emergence of the central and lateral permanent incisors in a nonrotated or slightly rotated position, a normal labial inclination, and a normal mesiodistal angulation.

A, B Moderate diastemata are present in the anterior region between the deciduous teeth. The deciduous incisors form a harmonious arch with the other deciduous teeth.

C, D The maxillary right central permanent incisor has emerged in a more labial position than that occupied by its predecessor. The left permanent incisor will soon emerge in a similar position. Perforation of the overlying mucosal tissue will uncover the incisal edge, which is only slightly superior to that of the other central incisor. The right central permanent incisor has emerged without contacting the lateral deciduous incisor, which was, if at all, only slightly distally displaced. The maxillary left lateral deciduous incisor is prematurely lost without any crowding or close proximity with the crown of the central permanent incisor.

E, F The lateral incisors have emerged without making contact with the crowns of the central incisors. Diastemata are present between the four incisors. On the right side the lateral incisor contacts the crown of the deciduous canine. This is not the case on the left side where the lateral incisor occupies a more labial position. Both lateral incisors are distally angulated. Their apices are still close to those of the central incisors. The incisal edges of the four incisors extend labially beyond the position occupied by their predecessors. The distance between the deciduous canines increased only slightly during the transition of the incisors. A favourable aspect in the case demonstrated here is that the mesiodistal crown dimensions of the permanent incisors are not much larger than those of their predecessors.

G, H The permanent canines have emerged and the diastemata between the incisors have been reduced. The apices of the lateral incisors were able to move distally after the crowns of the permanent canines had descended. As a rule, the central diastema closes during or shortly after completion of the eruption of the permanent canines. (The dental casts presented in G and H are not from the same child as those in A to F. They serve as a substitute to demonstrate the changes that normally occur. See note at Fig. 2-7, page 40).

Fig. 5-8 (see page 116) Schematic drawing of the Maxillary Incisor Transition Pattern A, characterized by emergence of the central and lateral permanent incisors in a nonrotated or only slightly rotated position, a normal labial inclination, and a normal mesiodistal angulation, in a large anterior section of the apical area.

A There are large diastemata between the anterior deciduous teeth. The central permanent incisor crown has started to erupt, reducing the initially limited overlap of the crown of the lateral incisor. No contact exists between the crown of the central permanent incisor and the adjacent root of the lateral deciduous incisor. This contact may, however, be attained later, leading to a distal displacement of the lateral deciduous incisor. The central and lateral permanent incisors are located in the jaw in a nonrotated position; they erupt with that orientation.

B After complete eruption of the central permanent incisor, the lateral incisor will start to descend. The overlapping by the crown of the central incisor has been fully eliminated. The lateral incisor can erupt in accordance with its orientation within the jaw in a nonrotated and in a more labial direction than did the central incisor. The lateral deciduous incisor may

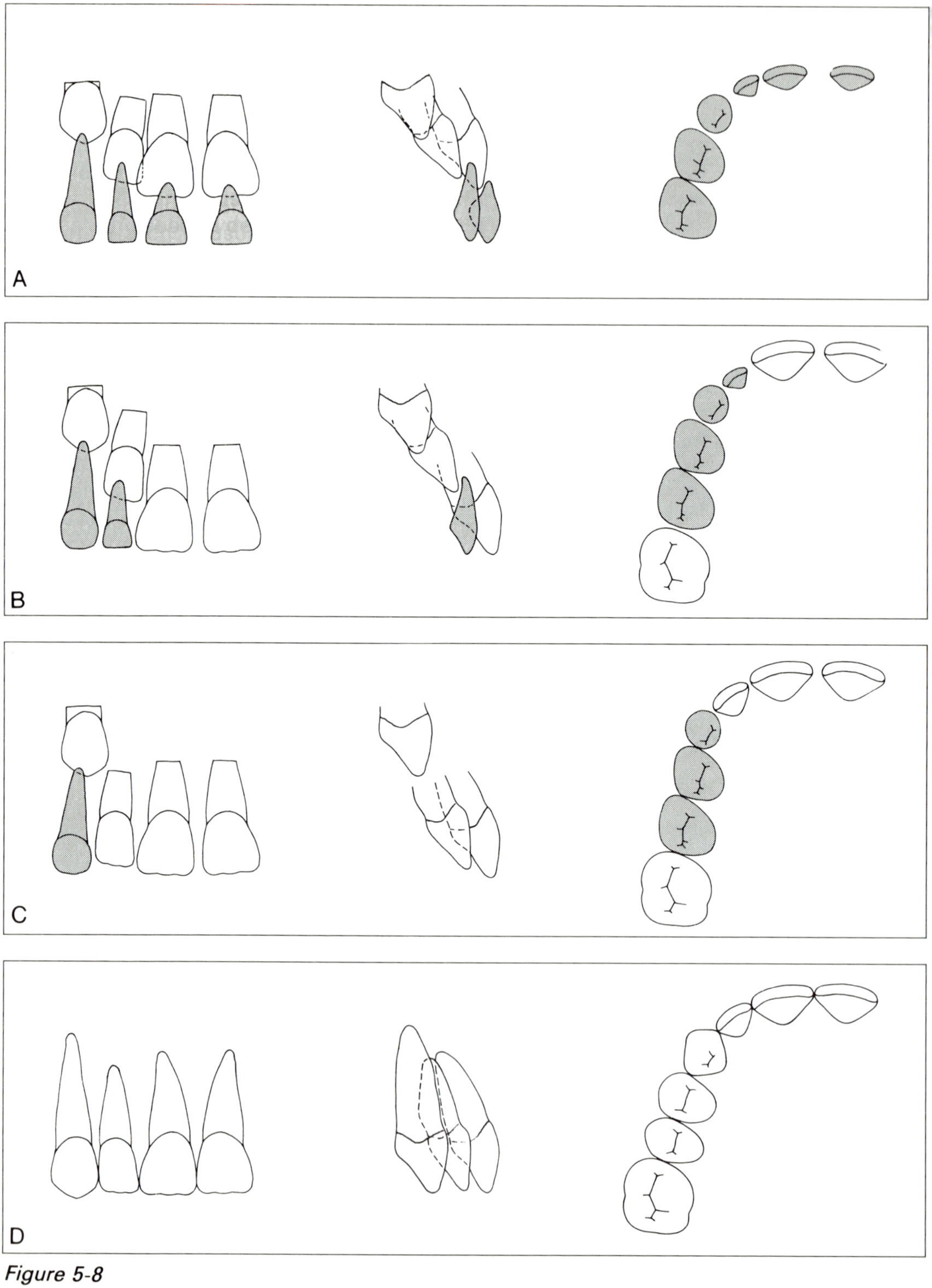

Figure 5-8

establish contact with the deciduous canine, and the intercanine distance may therefore increase. Diastemata are present between the incisor teeth.

C *After complete eruption of the lateral permanent incisor its mesiodistal angulation still is affected by the presence of the large permanent canine crown in close proximity to its root. The incisors are separated by diastemata and are located more labially than their predecessors were.*

D *In the adult dentition the incisors and canines are well aligned and in contact with each other. The apex of the lateral incisor is vertically approximately half way between the apices of the adjacent central incisor and canine. The lateral incisor is no longer distally but is now mesially angulated. This is also the case for the central incisors, although to a lesser degree.*

predecessors. The lateral permanent incisors extend labially beyond the buccal surfaces of the deciduous canines.

In a medium anterior section of the apical area the permanent lateral incisors usually erupt in contact with the central incisors and the central diastema will concomitantly be reduced. The lateral incisors will then also be in contact with the deciduous canine crowns. The apices of the central and lateral permanent incisors will be close together and the lateral incisors will be distally angulated. Some eversion of the incisors can also be present.

In a small anterior section of the apical area the lateral deciduous incisor is likely to be resorbed in association with the eruption of the central permanent incisor. The increase in intercanine width related to the eruption of the permanent central incisor in contact with the root of the deciduous lateral incisor does not take place. A deciduous canine can be prematurely lost in association with the eruption of the permanent lateral incisor. The space remaining in the dental arch for the permanent canine will be too small. If a deciduous canine does not resorb prematurely the fully erupted permanent incisors will be located labially and in eversion. The lateral incisors will be markedly distally angulated, and their distal incisal corners may overlap the labial surfaces of the deciduous canines.

5.5.2 Maxillary Incisor Transition Pattern B

Emergence of the central and lateral permanent incisors in mesiolabial rotation, with a rather upright labial inclination (Figs. 5-9 and 5-10). The deciduous incisors are normally aligned. Before emergence there is nothing to indicate that the permanent incisors are located in a rotated position within the jaw. The mesial incisal corner of the lateral permanent incisor crown is situated labial to the distal incisal corner of the central incisor. Usually, the permanent incisors are less labially inclined than normal. They will therefore erupt and emerge in a more upright position. In most instances the distal surface of the crown of the erupting central permanent incisor will make contact with the root of the deciduous lateral incisor, leading to a distal displacement of the latter. The permanent lateral incisor will emerge rotated mesiolabially and its distal incisal corner will become located not buccal to but palatal to the deciduous canine. The four incisors will attain an upright labiopalatal inclination and assume positions in the dental arch that are only slightly labial to those of their predecessors. The size of

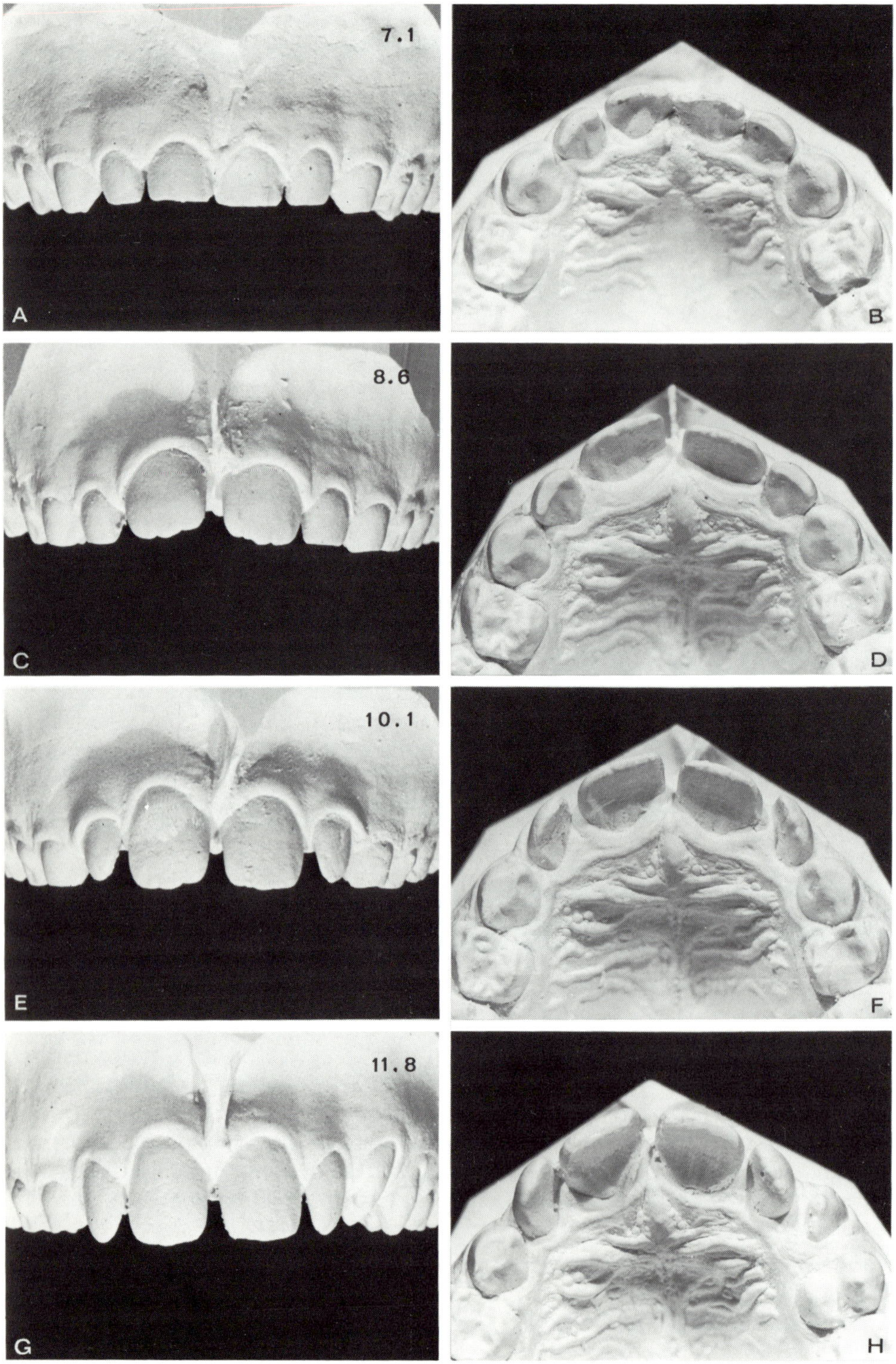

Figure 5-9

Fig. 5-9 Longitudinal series of dental casts of a medium anterior section of the apical area, showing bilaterally the Maxillary Incisor Transition Pattern B, which is characterized by emergence of the central and lateral permanent incisors in a mesiolabial rotation with an upright labial inclination.

A, B *Normally aligned deciduous dental arch with only a few small diastemata.*
C, D *The right central permanent incisor emerged mesiolabially rotated in a somewhat more labial position than its predecessor. The left central incisor emerged more in line with the original deciduous dental arch. A diastema is present between the two central incisors. The small diastemata on both sides of the deciduous canines are closed.*
E, F *The initial rotation of the right central permanent incisor is somewhat improved and the central diastema reduced. The lateral permanent incisors have emerged mesiolabially rotated without contacting the central incisors. Their mesial incisal corners extend labially beyond the distal incisal corners of the central incisors. The distal incisal corners of the lateral incisors do not extend buccally to the adjacent deciduous canines. The intercanine distance increased during the transition of the incisors.*
G, H *The maxillary right lateral incisor has moved palatally, probably under the influence of the erupting permanent canine crown. On the left side the permanent canine emerged and is located buccally to the lateral incisor, which has also moved palatally. The incisors are only slightly labially inclined; the diastemata between them have become reduced.*

Fig. 5-10 (see page 120) Schematic drawing of the Maxillary Incisor Transition Pattern B, characterized by emergence of the central and lateral permanent incisors in a mesiolabial rotation, with an upright labial inclination in a medium anterior section of the apical area.

A *The central and lateral permanent incisors are located in a mesiolabially rotated position and in an upright inclination within the jaw and do not overlap. The central incisor will pass the lateral incisor during its eruption. The distal corners of the central permanent incisors will not achieve contact with the roots of the adjacent lateral deciduous incisors.*
B *The central incisors are fully erupted and their rotation may improve slightly if circumstances are favourable. A central diastema is still present. The crowns of the lateral deciduous incisors may come in contact with those of the deciduous canines.*
C *The maxillary lateral permanent incisor has emerged in mesiolabial rotation. Its mesial incisal corner extends labially beyond the distal corner of the central incisor. Its distal incisal corner is more in line with the deciduous canine or it may be positioned palatally to it. The central diastema is reduced in size.*
D *In the adult situation the diastemata are closed and overlapping exists. The incisors are in an upright position and are still rotated. However, the rotation of the lateral incisor has been slightly corrected following the complete eruption of the canine. The mesial incisal corner of the canine lies buccal to the distal edge of the lateral incisor. The arch form has a tapered appearance.*

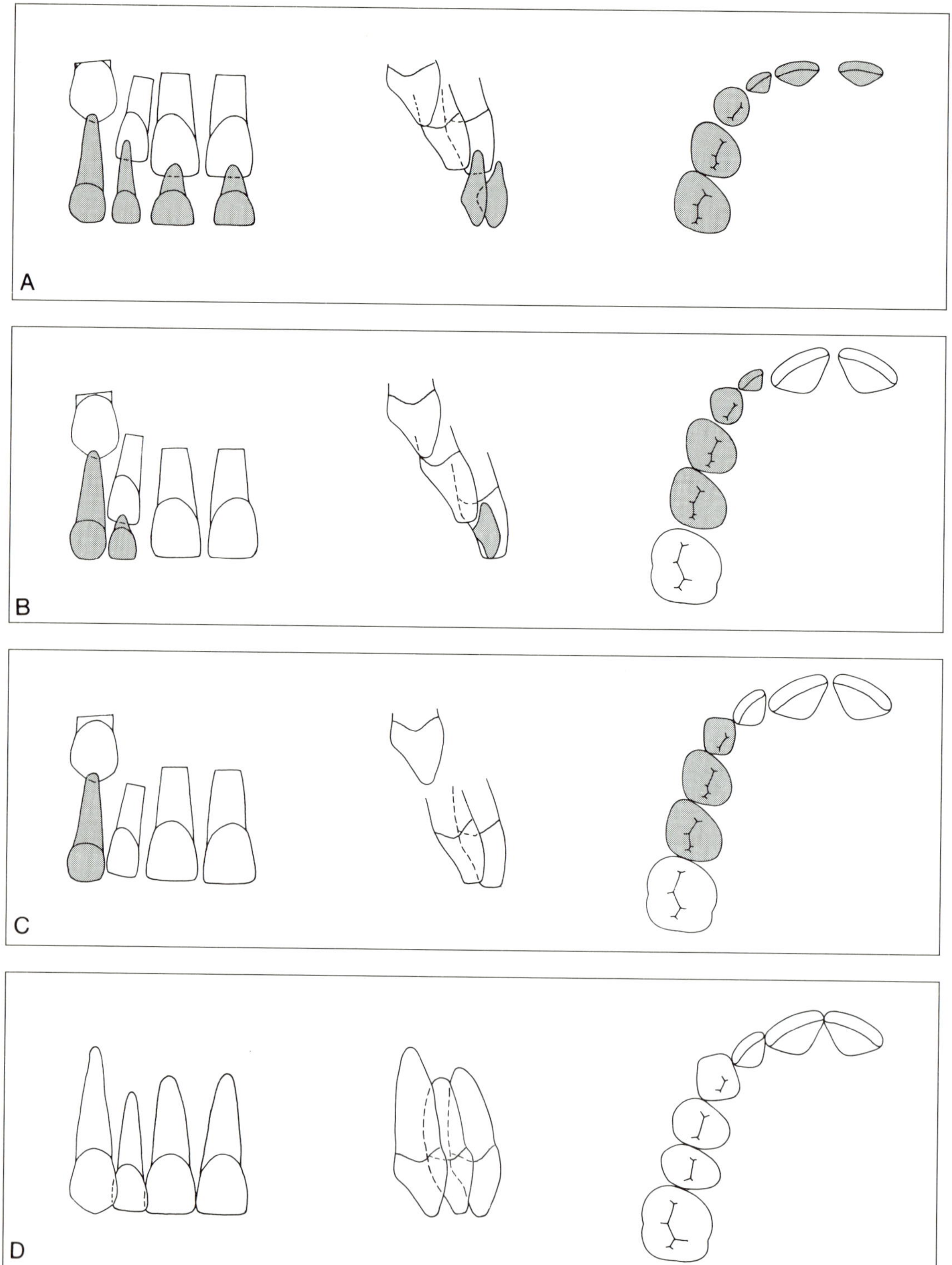

Figure 5-10

the anterior section of the apical area determines how far diastemata may remain. Occlusal forces may lead to a change in position of the incisors. The same holds true for the pressures exerted by the tongue and lips. However, maxillary incisors exhibit a considerably reduced tendency than do the mandibular ones to correct rotations that were initially present. This reduced tendency may be partly due to the less favourable spatial conditions within the maxillary dental arch than in the mandibular arch. Rotations of maxillary incisors seldom correct completely, even in cases of excess space. The crown of the permanent canine, during its eruption, may increase the rotation of the adjacent lateral incisor. After emergence of the canine, the rotation of the lateral incisor may subsequently improve, spatial conditions within the dental arch permitting.

In a large anterior section of the apical area the transition pattern with mesiolabially rotated central and lateral incisors will be associated with excess space and diastemata between the erupted permanent incisors. Rotations may then partially improve if the local conditions are favourable.

In a medium anterior section of the apical area more contacts will exist between the permanent and deciduous teeth during the transition, resulting in a relatively larger increase in intercanine distance.

In a small anterior section of the apical area, lateral deciduous incisors and canines are apt to be lost prematurely in accordance with the crowding and typical orientation of the permanent incisor crowns. Upon completed eruption, the incisors will usually be in contact and the arch form will be tapered. The incisor crowns may overlap each other considerably.

5.5.3 Maxillary Incisor Transition Pattern C

Emergence of the central permanent incisor in mesiolabial rotation and of the lateral incisor in distolabial rotation (Figs. 5-11 and 5-12). As in the previous patterns there are no visible indications of rotated permanent incisors in the dental arch before their emergence. The rotated positions are present from the beginning of formation and are maintained during eruption. The central incisors usually erupt in an upright labial inclination and a slight mesial angulation. Contact between the two central incisors is achieved soon after emergence. If this contact does not result in a reciprocal support, the two central incisors will start to overlap their mesial incisal corners. Sometimes the central incisors erupt more labially, are less mesially angulated, and the central diastema is not closed. During their eruption the permanent central incisors usually establish contact with the roots of the adjacent lateral deciduous incisors, leading to an increased intercanine distance. The lateral permanent incisors are rotated in the opposite direction to that of the central incisors. Their mesial incisal corners are palatally positioned and located close to the also palatally positioned distal incisal corners of the central incisors. The central incisors can erupt without being unfavourably influenced by the permanent lateral incisors. When eruption of the central incisor is complete, the lateral incisor can erupt in the labial direction because the overlapping of the permanent central incisor crown is eliminated. The rotation of the central incisors can be partially and sometimes totally corrected, mainly under the influence of the tongue and lip. However, most of these teeth maintain part of their rotation. This holds particularly true for the lateral incisors.

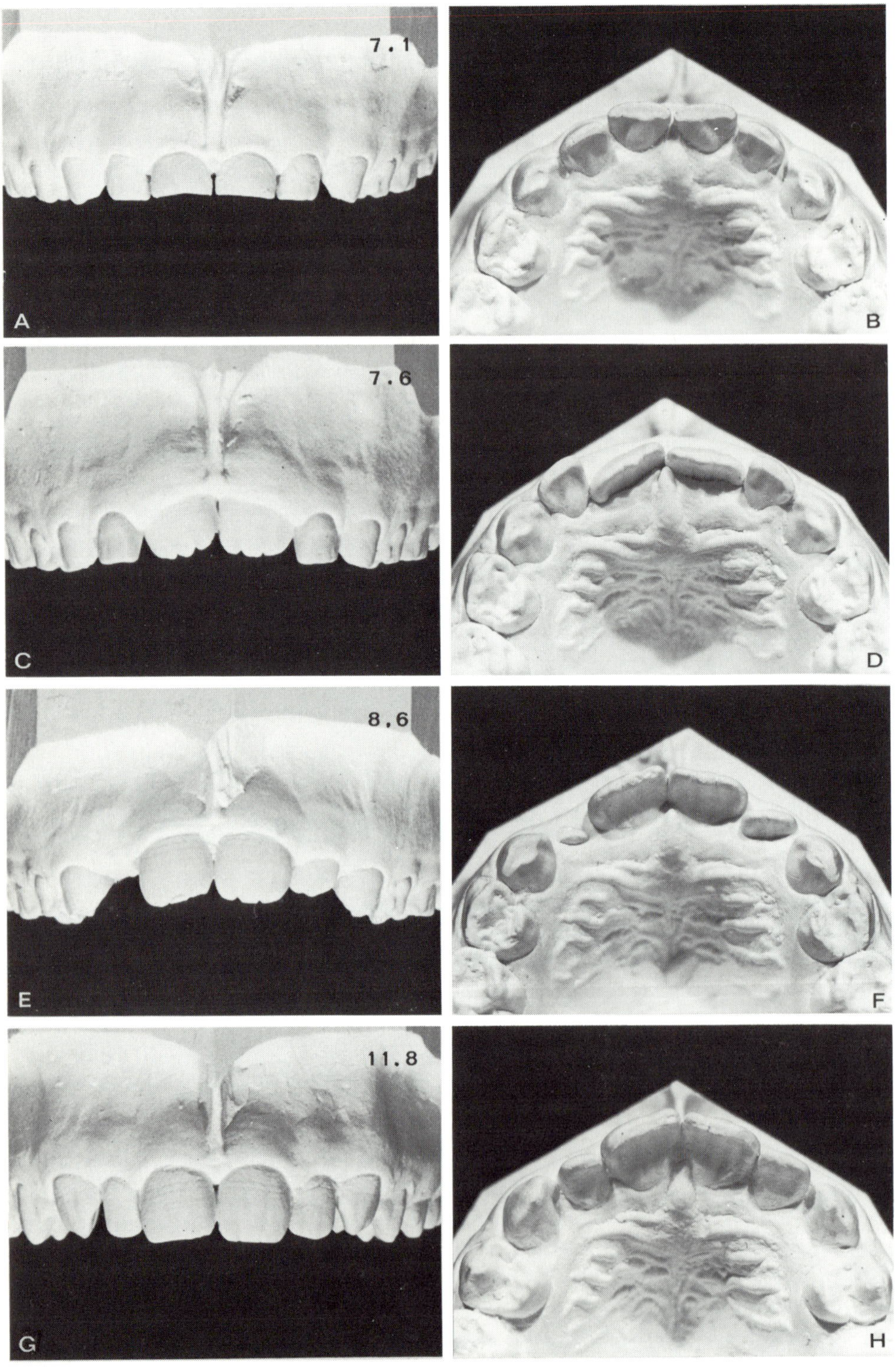

Figure 5-11

Fig. 5-11 Longitudinal series of dental casts of a medium anterior section of the apical area, showing bilaterally the Maxillary Incisor Transition Pattern C, characterized by emergence of the central permanent incisor in mesiolabial rotation and the lateral incisor in distolabial rotation.

A, B A few small diastemata are present between the deciduous anterior teeth.
C, D The central permanent incisors have emerged in an upright labial inclination and mesial angulation. They are initially positioned more palatally than their predecessors were. The central permanent incisors are in contact with each other and with the lateral deciduous incisors. The intercanine distance has increased substantially.
E, F Rotations of the central incisors are slightly reduced. The lateral permanent incisors have emerged distolabially rotated. They will be able to erupt in a labial direction because there will be no interference caused by overlapping of the central incisor crowns.
G, H The lateral incisors are fully erupted and more labially located than at emergence. The rotation of the left lateral incisor has been partly corrected. The lateral and the central incisors have become more labially inclined. The central incisors are less mesially angulated than previously. The permanent canines have emerged but are not yet completely erupted.

Fig. 5-12 (see page 124) Schematic drawing of the Maxillary Incisor Transition Pattern C, characterized by emergence of the central permanent incisor in a mesiolabial rotation and the lateral incisor in a distolabial rotation, in a medium anterior apical area.

A The central permanent incisors are orientated in the jaw in a mesiolabial rotation, the lateral incisors in a distolabial one. The overlapping of the lateral permanent incisor crown by that of the central incisor will be eliminated when the central incisor descends further.
B Soon after the central incisors emerge they will attain contact and support each other reciprocally. No overlapping in the median line will then occur. The rotation and mesial angulation of the central incisor are unfavourable for establishing contact between the distoincisal corners of the central incisors and the roots of the lateral deciduous incisors.
C The lateral permanent incisor is able to erupt in a labial direction because no overlapping remains. The mesial angulation and rotation of the central incisors may reduce. The contact between the lateral permanent incisor and the deciduous canine does not usually favour correction of rotation of the lateral incisor.
D In the adult situation some rotations are still present; the contacts leave something to be desired.

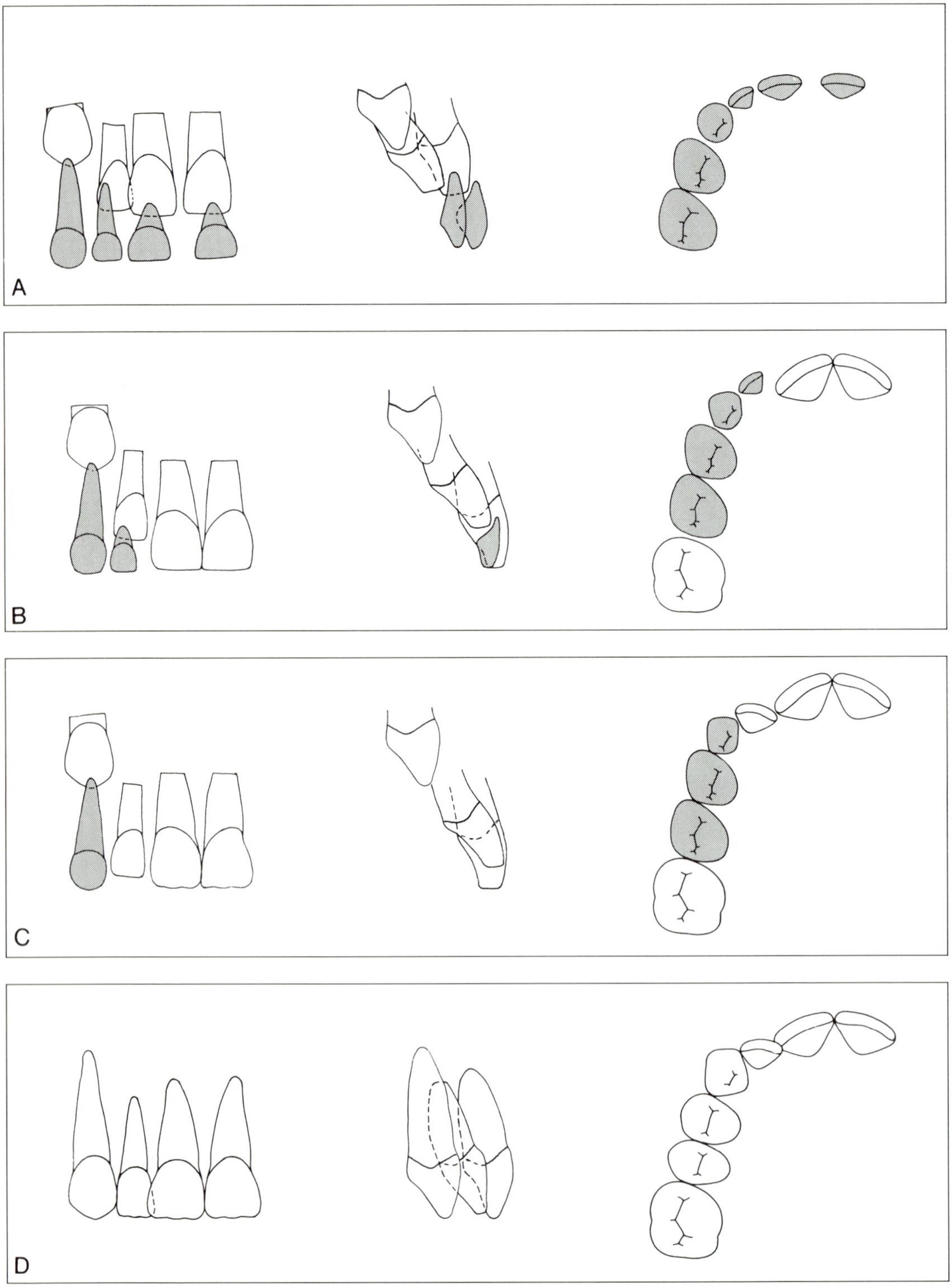

Figure 5-12

In a large anterior section of the apical area diastemata are present during the transition and rotations are more likely to be corrected.
In a medium anterior section of the apical area less diastemata will be found, the intercanine distance may increase more, and rotations and overlapping will be found in the adult situation.
In a small anterior section of the apical area deciduous teeth may be lost prematurely. Marked rotations and overlappings will be maintained.

5.5.4 Maxillary Incisor Transition Pattern D

Emergence of the central permanent incisor in a nonrotated position and of the lateral incisor in a mesiolabially rotated position (Figs. 5-13 and 5-14). The central permanent incisors usually erupt in an upright labial inclination and a slight distal angulation. A small central diastema is initially present. The permanent lateral incisor erupts in a mesiolabially rotated position and soon after emergence begins to protrude beyond the labial surface of the adjacent central incisor. When adequate space is available the lateral incisor may become less labially inclined and move back in the direction of the dental arch. The rotation may also become reduced. Before the crown of the permanent canine erupts it usually inhibits labial movement of the root of the lateral incisor. When the permanent canine descends and emerges, the inclination of the lateral incisor can change. After the permanent canine emerges buccal to the lateral incisor, thc inclination of the lateral incisor will change again and its distal corner will move palatally. As such the rotation that was initially present will increase. The pattern of transition of the incisors described here will often occur only unilaterally. The transition in the other quadrant then takes place differently.
In a large anterior section of the apical area diastemata will be present between the permanent incisors. The lateral incisor will improve in position, but slight rotation will usually remain.
In a medium anterior section of the apical area the lateral incisors may tip more labially, and this malposition will not be fully corrected. The same holds true for the rotation.
In a small anterior section of the apical area premature loss of deciduous teeth may take place and considerable crowding with exclusion of the permanent canines from the dental arch may result.

5.5.5 Maxillary Incisor Transition Pattern E

Emergence of the central permanent incisor in a normal position and of the lateral incisor in a palatal, nonrotated position (Figs. 5-15 and 5-16). This pattern of transition may occur in a small anterior section of the apical area. The process is comparable in essence to Pattern A (see 5.5.1) with, however, considerable crowding and unfavourable developmental conditions. Lateral deciduous incisors are often prematurely lost and the intercanine distance does not increase or does so only slightly.
A palatal position of the lateral permanent incisor may occur unilaterally or bilaterally. If it only occurs on one side it is usually an indication that only the lateral deciduous incisor on that side was lost prematurely and that the central permanent incisors drifted toward the resulting space. On the nonaffected side the position of the

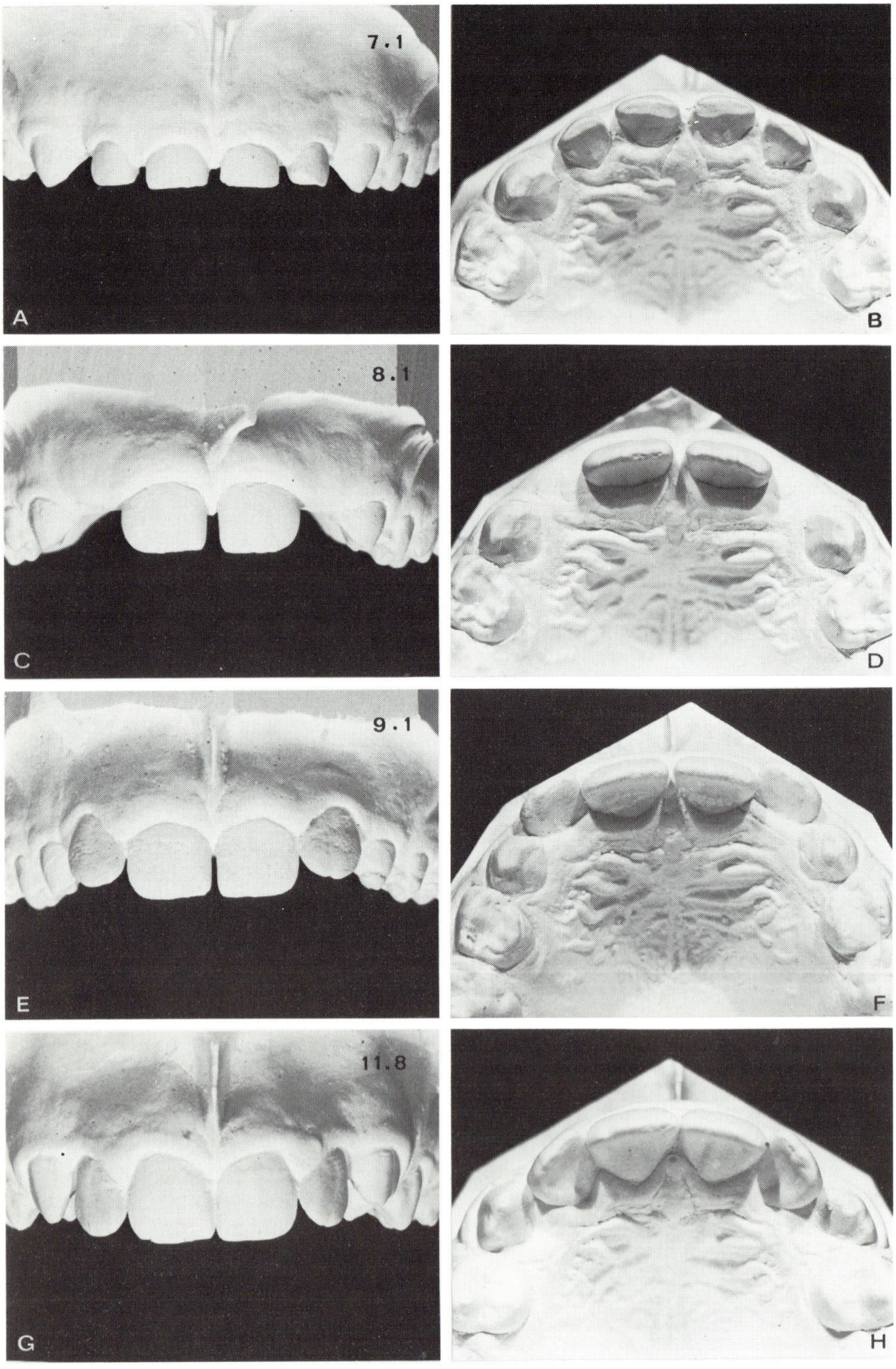

Figure 5-13

Fig. 5-13 Longitudinal series of dental casts of a medium anterior section of the apical area, showing bilaterally the Maxillary Incisor Transition Pattern D, characterized by emergence of the central permanent incisor in a nonrotated position and of the lateral incisor in a mesiolabially rotated position.

A, B *Diastemata are present between all deciduous anterior teeth.*

C, D *The central incisors erupt nonrotated with an upright labial inclination, without a mesiodistal angulation, and with a small central diastema. The lateral deciduous incisors were recently exfoliated and their successors will erupt shortly.*

E, F *Both lateral permanent incisors have emerged in a labial direction and passed the labial surfaces of the central incisors and deciduous canines. The central diastema is reduced.*

G, H *The left and right permanent canines emerge labially to the lateral incisors in contrast to the positions occupied by their predecessors. The rotation of the lateral incisors has changed accordingly. The distal edges have become displaced palatally. The central diastema is closed. All teeth are in contact. Some crowding exists.*

Fig. 5-14 (see page 128) Schematic drawing of the Maxillary Incisor Transition Pattern D, characterized by emergence of the central permanent incisor in a nonrotated position and of the lateral incisor in a mesiolabially rotated position, in a medium anterior section of the apical area.

A *Diastemata are present between the deciduous teeth in the anterior region. The lateral permanent incisor is located palatally to the central incisor and is slightly mesiolabially rotated.*

B *The central permanent incisor has erupted in a nonrotated position with a slight distal angulation. A central diastema is present. The crown of the lateral permanent incisor is no longer overlapped by that of the central incisor. It can erupt in a labial direction.*

C *The lateral incisor will be moved palatally by pressure of the lip and become more aligned with the central incisor. The lateral incisor may slightly overlap labially the distal incisal corner of the central incisor. The central diastema will be closed before the canines emerge.*

D *The permanent canine will emerge labial to the distal edge of the lateral incisor and move it more palatally. This rotation can be corrected when adequate space is available and the canine can move distally. The general arch form will have a slightly rectangular appearance.*

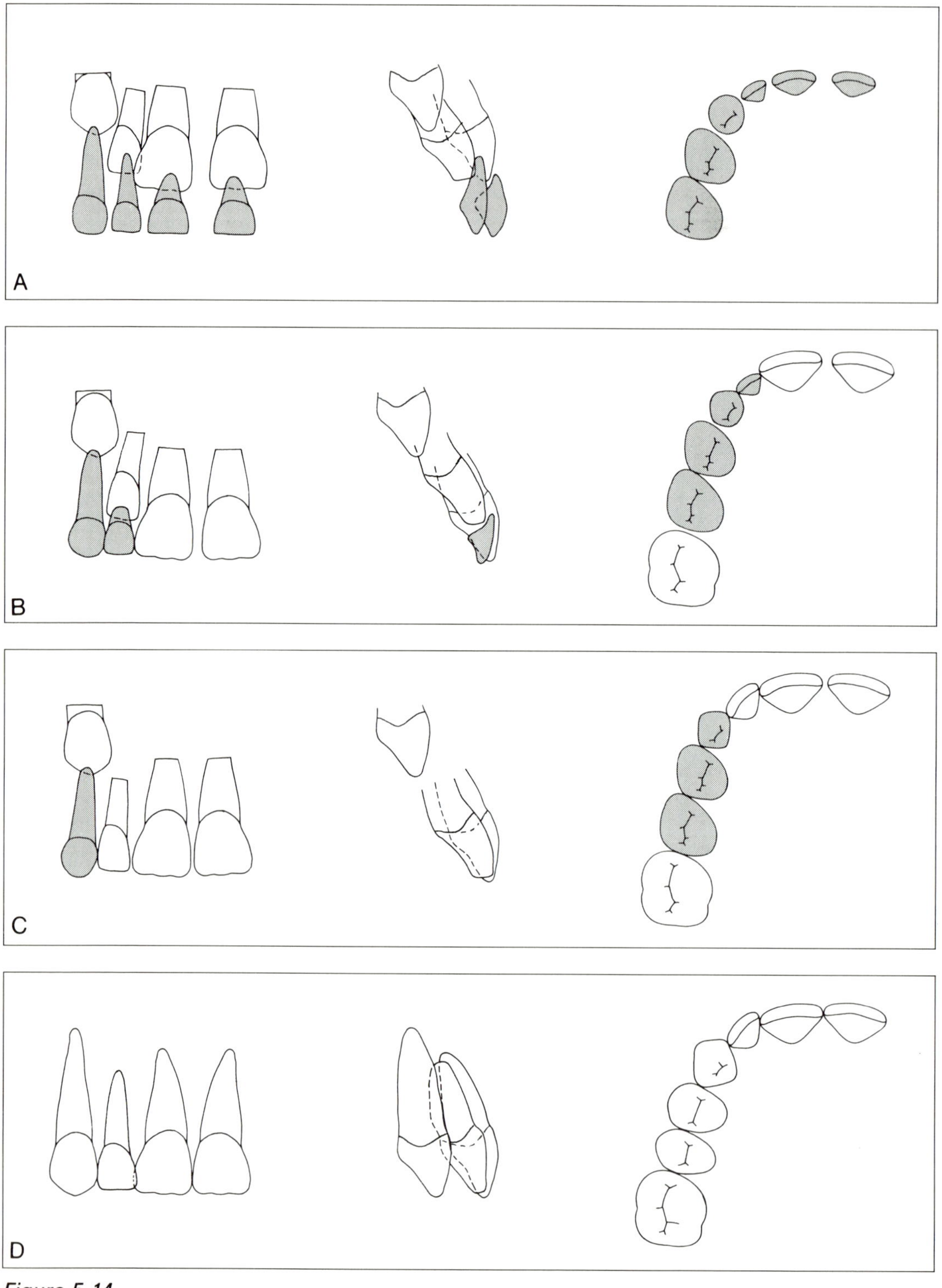

Figure 5-14

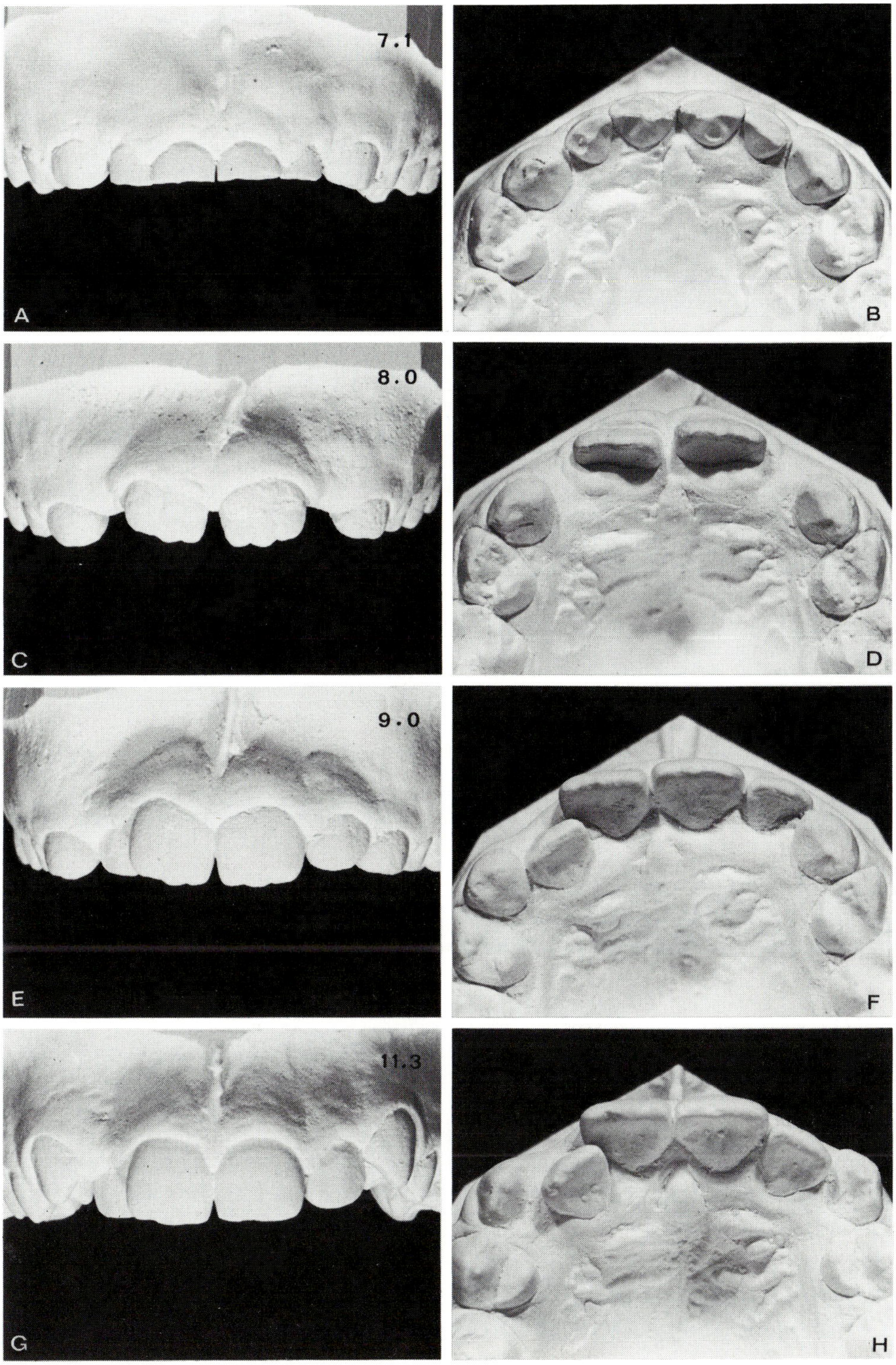

Figure 5-15

Fig. 5-15 (see page 129) Longitudinal series of dental casts of a small anterior section of the apical area, showing on the right side the Maxillary Incisor Transition Pattern E, characterized by emergence of the central permanent incisor in a normal position and of the lateral incisor in a palatal, nonrotated position.

A, B Small deciduous anterior teeth with no diastemata.
C, D The lateral deciduous incisors are prematurely exfoliated. The central permanent incisors have emerged with a distal angulation, hence a large central diastema. No increase in intercanine distance based on the contact between the central permanent incisor crowns and the adjacent lateral deciduous incisor can take place.
E, F The central incisors have moved toward the right side. The central diastema is closed and enough room has become available for the left lateral permanent incisor to erupt in a labial direction. Its distal incisal corner overlaps the deciduous canine labially. The right lateral permanent incisor is palatally placed in relation to the adjacent teeth. There is no room for it to move labially.
G, H Both permanent canines have emerged. The left one is buccally placed in relation to the adjacent lateral incisor, in contrast to the position occupied by its predecessor. The position of the left lateral incisor has changed accordingly. The right permanent canine is more buccally positioned than its predecessor. However, its larger labiopalatal and mesiodistal crown dimension does not allow the lateral incisor to move buccally.

Fig. 5-16 Schematic drawing of the Maxillary Incisor Transition Pattern E, characterized by emergence of the central permanent incisor in a normal position and of the lateral incisor in a palatal, nonrotated position, in a small anterior section of the apical area.

A No or only a few and small diastemata are present between the deciduous teeth in the anterior region. The central permanent incisor is angulated slightly distally; its crown overlaps half the lateral crown. Premature loss of the lateral deciduous incisor is likely to occur.
B Because of premature loss of the lateral deciduous incisor, the deciduous canine will not move laterally or only slightly so. Considerable shortage of space exists. The central incisor still overlaps the lateral incisor, preventing its eruption labially.
C The central diastema is closed prior to the emergence of the permanent canines. The lateral incisor has emerged in a palatal position. No diastemata are present.
D After the permanent canine emerges, the lateral incisor maintains its palatal position. The relation with the mandibular teeth will normally consolidate this palatal position because the mandibular anterior teeth will occlude labially to the maxillary lateral incisor and lingually to its adjacent teeth.

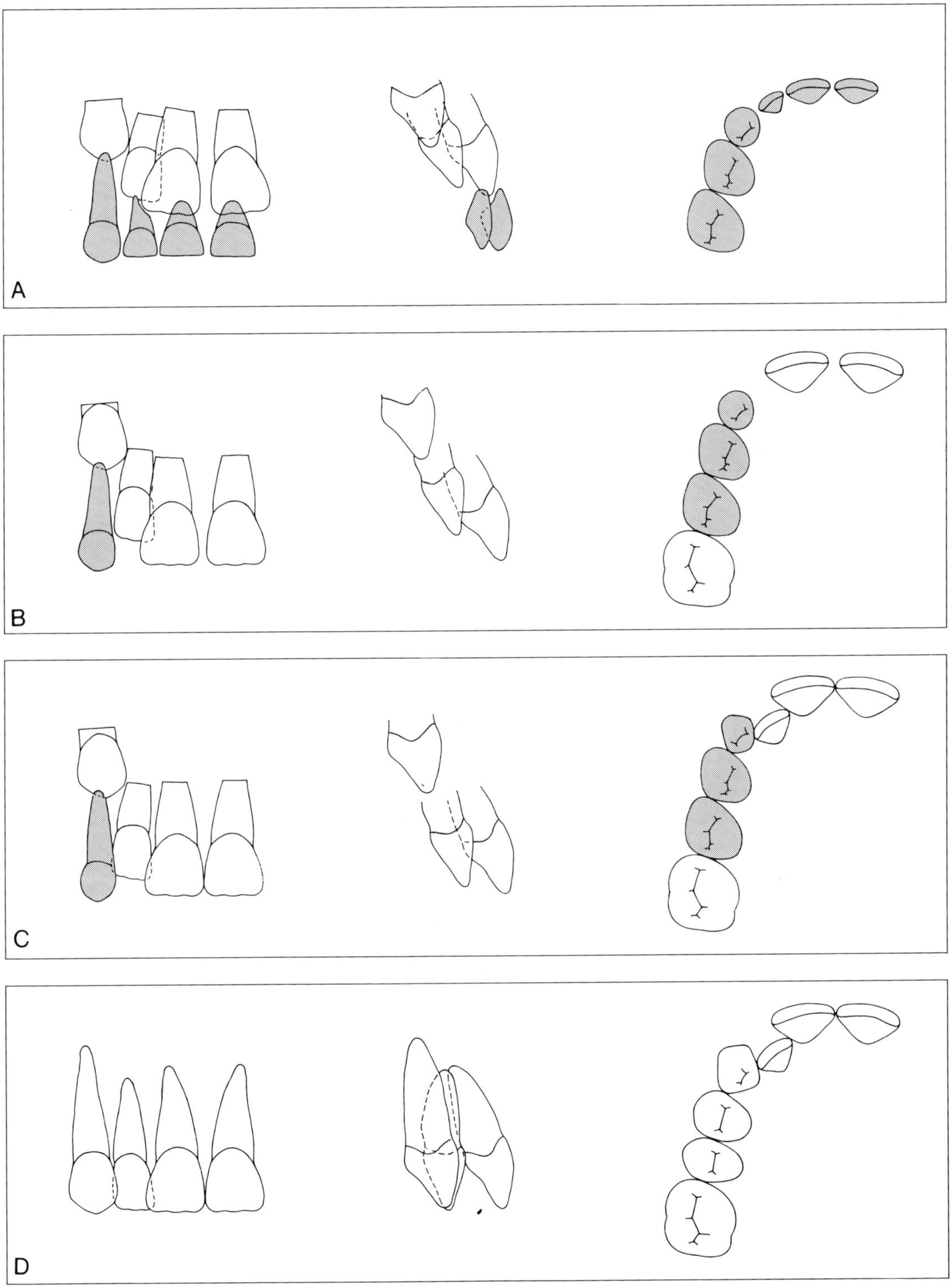

Figure 5-16

lateral permanent incisor and its relation with its adjacent permanent teeth may be normal. The palatal eruption of a lateral incisor usually occurs when overlapping of its crown by that of the central incisor is not eliminated. In a small anterior section of the apical area the crown of the central permanent incisor overlaps that of the lateral incisor by approximately half its width or more. The lateral incisor may not find the space required to erupt in labial direction upon the emergence and complete eruption palatally of the central permanent incisor. A palatally emerging and erupting lateral incisor will often lead to some labial movement of the adjacent central incisor.

5.6 Supplementary remarks

The five transition patterns of the maxillary incisors show a variation that is related to a number of different factors. The initial orientation of the permanent incisors at their morphogenesis determines the position in which they will form. It is questionable how far a rotated position of the permanent incisors has to be considered as a sign of crowding or as a phenomenon that is independent of the local spatial conditions both for the maxillary and mandibular incisor region. The inclination of the incisors before emergence probably depends on the size of the anterior section of the apical area. It is clear that a small anterior section is more likely to house the incisor teeth in a more labial inclination than a large anterior section. A comparable situation will exist in the transverse direction. A small anterior section of the apical area is usually associated with distally angulated central incisors that are formed with their mesial surfaces about parallel and close to the median suture.

Local circumstances within the dental arch partly determine what is going to happen during and after emergence of the teeth. Some of the variations observed are primarily due to these circumstances.

The role of the tongue and lips has been discussed only superficially. However, considerable importance must be attached to both, particularly in regard to the position the teeth will finally attain. The same comment applies to the occlusion. It may make quite a difference if a normal or abnormal sagittal relation exists in the anterior region.

A few remarks may be appropriate to compare the transition of the maxillary incisors to that of the mandibular ones. The functional forces that act on the mandibular dental arch tend to move the teeth lingually. The forces of the tongue act in the opposite direction. However, in the mandibular dental arch the contained arch principle plays a major role in preventing lingual collapse.[140] Adequate contacts between adjacent teeth prevent the lingual movement of individual mandibular teeth. A comparable mechanism does not exist for the maxillary arch because the occlusal and other forces work mostly in a buccal direction. In addition, maxillary incisors have a larger range for their position than mandibular incisors. This larger range in variation is also related to differences in morphology of the teeth, the surrounding alveolar bone and adjacent structures, normal functional forces, and abnormal influences.

Chapter 6

Variations in Transition of Maxillary Posterior Teeth*

6.1 Introduction

The space available in the dental arch for the transition of the maxillary posterior teeth is bounded as in the mandible by the distal surface of the crown of the lateral permanent incisor and by the mesial surface of the crown of the first permanent molar. The sum of the mesiodistal crown dimensions of the maxillary deciduous molars and canine is slightly larger than that of their successors. The first premolar has approximately the same mesiodistal crown dimension as its predecessor. The second premolar is usually smaller than the preceding deciduous molar; however, the difference between the two is less marked than between the corresponding mandibular teeth. The maxillary permanent canine has a considerably larger mesiodistal crown dimension than the deciduous one. This difference is larger for boys than for girls and more marked in the maxilla than in the mandible.[71] The excess in the sum of the mesiodistal crown dimensions of the deciduous molars and canine in relation to their successors is smaller in the maxilla than the mandible. Yet the average leeway space is larger in the maxillary dental arch. Seemingly a contradiction, it is related to the occurrence of more and larger diastemata between the teeth of the involved segment of the dental arch. The disparity in the transition of the maxillary posterior teeth and that of the mandibular teeth is related not only to the differences in mesiodistal crown dimensions and in the leeway space; size and shape of the middle section of the apical area and the sequences of emergence also play a role.
The transition of the maxillary posterior teeth is discussed in relation to the space available for the permanent canine and the premolars in the middle section of the apical area and in the dental arch. Variation in the location of the permanent teeth concerned, and their relation to each other, to their predecessors, and to the adjacent lateral permanent incisor and first molar are indicated. The differences in emergence sequence and associated preemergence and postemergence behaviour are discussed. Seven transition patterns are distinguished, five of which are presented in detail.

* Reproduced from: "Transition of the upper posterior teeth" by Hein J.W. Wassenberg, Paul J.M.R. Bakker and Frans P.G.M. van der Linden. In: *Transition of the human dentition.* Monograph No. 13. Craniofacial Growth Series., Pg 101-123. Ed. Frans P.G.M. van der Linden. Center for Human Growth and Development. The University of Michigan, Ann Arbor, U.S.A., 1982.

6.2 The middle section of the apical area and arrangement of the permanent canine and premolars before emergence

As has been described before, the anterior section of the apical area in the maxilla is bounded laterally by the permanent canines. Before their emergence, the large permanent canine crowns limit the space initially available for the forming permanent incisor crowns and subsequently for their roots. After complete eruption of the permanent canines their apices form the lateral boundaries of the anterior section of the apical area. The room then normally available is adequate to contain the relatively small roots of the permanent incisors. As explained previously, the anterior section of the apical area is initially too small to house the forming permanent crowns in an arrangement comparable to what they will occupy after their eruption is completed. A corresponding situation exists in the maxilla for the middle section of the apical area. In the sagittal direction the middle section of the apical area is too small to house the forming premolars and permanent canine at the same level. Further, the size of the transverse dimension and the presence of the deciduous teeth roots allow only a limited variation in buccopalatal direction. The first premolar and permanent canine are formed close together, and their crowns occupy positions of different levels prior to their eruption.

The size and shape of the middle section as well as of the anterior section depend upon the morphology and location of the piriform aperture. The permanent canines are formed lateral to the anterior section and are, of all teeth, at the greatest distance from the occlusal plane. The permanent canines will develop the longest roots of the entire dentition. In the preeruptive phase the premolars are distinctly closer to the occlusal plane than the permanent canine. The initial arrangement of the premolars and permanent canine in the maxilla resembles that in the mandible. However, there are marked differences. The maxillary canine is not usually situated mesial to the first premolar crown but superiorly, and it overlaps it vertically. The distal corner of the permanent canine crown develops almost in contact with the mesial cementoenamel junction of the first premolar. The mesial concavity of the first premolar can be thought to result from this relation.

In accordance with the situation in the mandible the crown tip of the maxillary permanent canine is located palatally to the apex of its predecessor. The mesial part of the crown is in close proximity to the root of the fully erupted lateral permanent incisor and frequently overlaps the root buccally. The premolars are located between the roots of their predecessors. The first premolar is more to the buccal and closer to the occlusal plane than the second premolar. Compared to the mandible, the space between the mesial surface of the first premolar crown and the distal surface of the root of the lateral permanent incisor is smaller.

The middle section of the apical area in the maxilla shows a large individual variation in size and shape. The differences appear primarily in the location of the canine and first premolar. Considerable variation, more than in the mandible, is encountered in the sagittal and transverse locations of these teeth. As in corresponding previous chapters, prepared human skulls serve to demonstrate the variation in size and shape of the middle section of the apical area and the associated arrangement of the forming permanent teeth (Figs. 6-1 to 6-3).

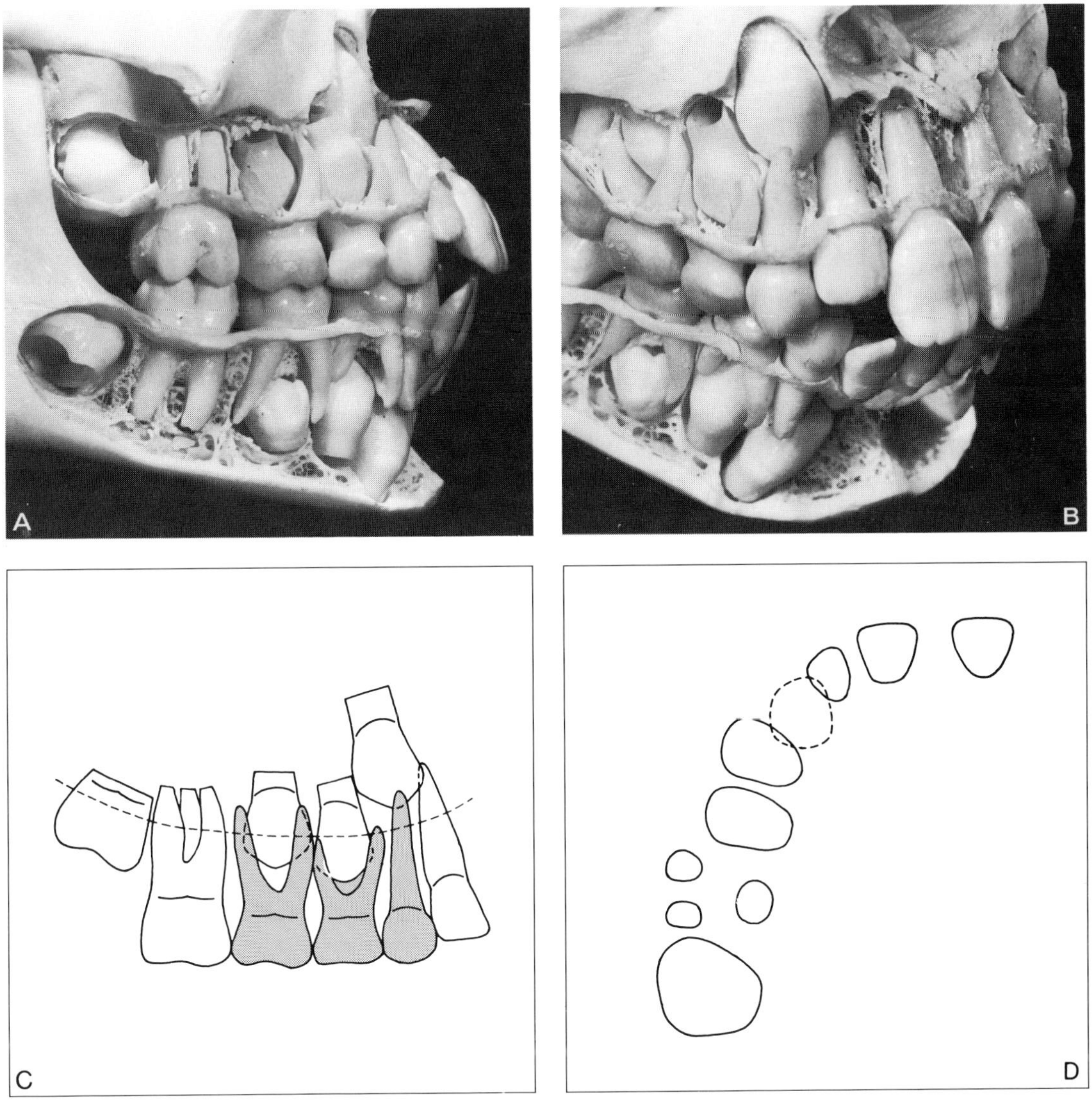

Fig. 6-1 *Large middle section of the apical area in the maxilla. The relation between the mesiodistal crown dimensions of the maxillary permanent canine and the premolars and the size and shape of the middle section of the apical area is favourable. However, no diastemata are present in the dental arch.*

A *The permanent canine is located more superiorly and palatally than the premolars and is mesially angulated. This is in accordance with the morphology of the adjacent structures. Both maxillary premolars are closer to the occlusal plane and at about the same level. The second deciduous molar has a larger mesiodistal crown width than its successor.*

B *The permanent canine crown slightly overlaps the root of the lateral incisor. Its cusp tip is palatal and slightly mesial of the apex of its predecessor. The canine partly overlaps the first premolar in a mesiodistal direction. Its distal corner is in close proximity to the first premolar.*

The deciduous canine crown is smaller than the permanent one.

C *Schematic drawing with a dotted line indicating the section presented in D. Both premolar crowns are about the same level and in a comparable relation with the roots of their predecessors. Some space exists between the mesial surface of the first permanent molar root and the second premolar crown. The first premolar crown is mesially inclined and close to the second premolar, which is normally oriented perpendicular to the occlusal plane.*

D *The premolar crowns are not in contact with each other and do not overlap. Both are harmoniously positioned in a buccopalatal direction. The distance between the first premolar crown and the lateral incisor root is relatively large. At this stage of development the permanent canine crown overlaps both adjacent teeth slightly. However, later on there will be sufficient room in the alveolar process to house the root of the permanent canine with its smaller circumference.*

(Legend 6-2 continued)

B *The permanent canine is medially situated above the first premolar, almost totally overlapping it in the vertical plane. Both teeth are mesially angulated, particularly the canine. In addition, the first premolar is mesiopalatally rotated, extends buccally, and is situated closer to the occlusal plane than the second premolar. The mesial surface of the canine crown extends anteriorly to the line that can be constructed as the continuation of the mesial surface of the lateral incisor root.*

C *The differences in vertical position of the crowns of the premolars and permanent canine are associated with the overlapping of these teeth. The distance in the dental arch between the mesial surface of the first permanent molar and the distal surface of the lateral incisor is small.*

D *The second premolar is located more palatally and the first premolar more buccally than normal. The space available between the mesial surface of the first premolar and the distal surface of the lateral incisor is limited.*

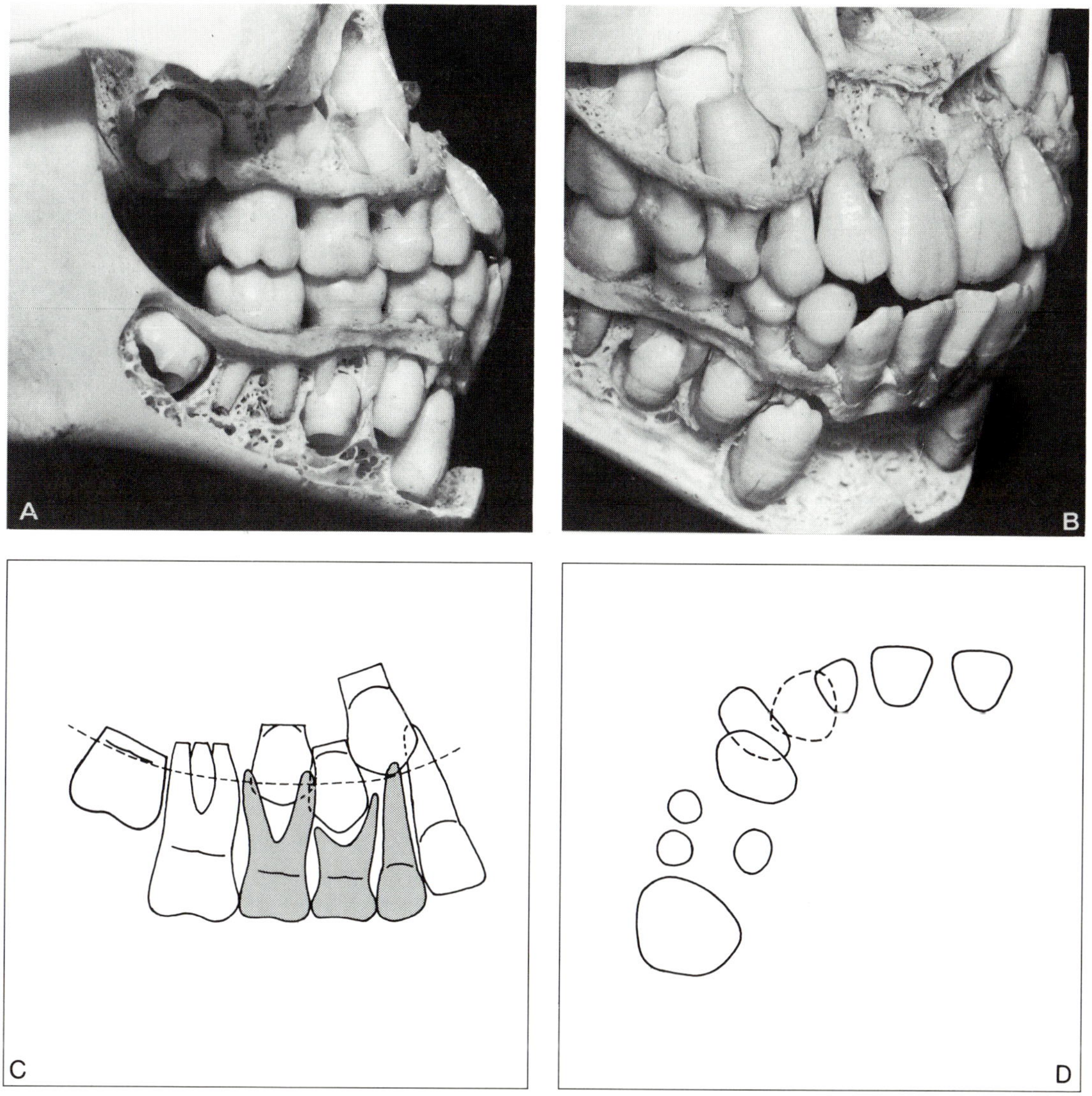

Fig. 6-2 Medium middle section of the apical area in the maxilla. The position of the permanent canine crown, its proximity to the lateral permanent incisor root and first premolar crown, and the differences in the mesiodistal crown dimensions of the corresponding deciduous and permanent teeth are critical.

A Both premolars are close together. The second premolar is situated close to the first permanent molar. The mesiodistal crown dimensions of the deciduous canine and molars are small in relation to those of their successors.
(Legend continues on page 136)

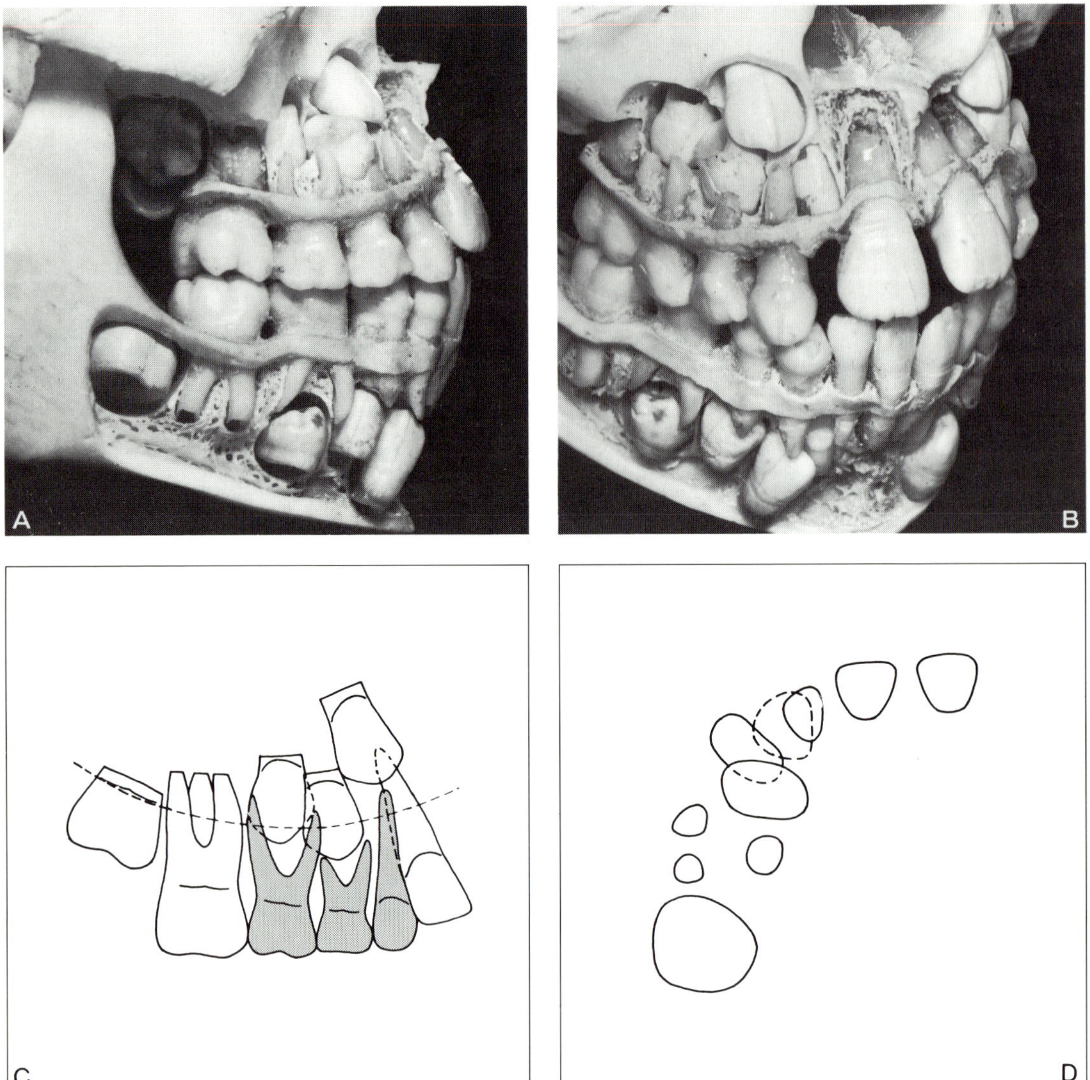

Fig. 6-3 Small middle section of the apical area in the maxilla in an instance where the lateral deciduous incisor was lost prematurely and its successor has not yet emerged.

A The permanent canine crown is in a superior position and markedly mesially angulated. The forming part of the first premolar is located buccal to the canine crown. The canine crown is in close proximity to the second premolar crown. Little room is available for the second premolar, which is close to the root of the first permanent molar.

B The permanent canine crown is close to the piriform aperture, which has a small transverse width. The crown of the canine is distobuccally rotated and overlaps the crown of the permanent lateral incisor to a large extent. The first premolar crown is only partially situated between the roots of its predecessor. The same holds true for the second premolar crown.

C The differences in vertical position of the crowns of the premolars and of the canine, their overlapping, the close proximity with the first permanent molar root, and the overlapping of the lateral incisor are expressions of an extremely crowded condition.
D The remark made under C also applies to the palatal position of the second premolar crown and the buccal position and rotation of the first premolar crown. The space available between the lateral incisor and the first premolar is very small.

As was the case for other groups of corresponding deciduous and permanent teeth discussed in prededing chapters, a moderate correlation also exists between the sum of the mesiodistal crown dimensions of the maxillary deciduous molars and canines and that of their successors. Correlations for corresponding individual teeth have low values, particularly for the canines.[142, 144]
Compared to the mandible, a larger variation exists in the size and shape of the middle section of the apical area and in the arrangement of the teeth, prior to emergence. Further, the middle section of the apical area is smaller in the maxilla than in the mandible. This difference between both jaws is related to the fact that the structures that determine the size and shape of the middle section of the apical area in the maxilla are placed on a smaller arch segment than those in the mandible. As such the mean perimeter of the middle section of the apical area of the maxilla is shorter than the combined mesiodistal dimension of the involved permanent tooth crowns concerned. In the mandible the situation is reversed. These differences between both jaws partly explain why the transition of maxillary posterior teeth proceeds in a manner different from that of mandibular teeth and usually encounters other complications.

6.3 Eruption before emergence

As in the mandible, no uniformity exists in the eruption sequence of the maxillary premolars and permanent canine. However, as explained above, the spatial conditions are initially less favourable for the maxilla than for the mandible. The maxillary teeth are usually housed in a smaller compartment than that required to accommodate the crowns adjacent to each other without vertical overlapping. Consequently, the tooth that is closest to the occlusal plane must begin eruption before the one that is situated at a higher level can start to descend. In most cases the maxillary first premolar must erupt before the permanent canine can do so. Only in a large middle section of the apical area and with spatial conditions that allow the canine to pass the first premolar in its eruption process can the canine emerge first.
The most common sequence of emergence is: first premolar, second premolar, canine. Occasionally, the last two will emerge simultaneously. Sometimes the canine emerges prior to the second premolar. For more details regarding the transitional process in the most frequently observed emergence sequence refer to Fig. 3-4 (page 59). For some variations in the sequence of emergence of the posterior teeth, including the second permanent molar, see Fig. 3-5 (page 60).
The direction of eruption will depend primarily on the orientation of the teeth within the jaw as determined to a large extent by the spatial conditions. When adequate space is available the premolars and canines can erupt and emerge without restrictions.

However, with a medium and small middle section of the apical area the initial positions of the premolars and canine will be less favourable, as explained above. The direction of eruption of the premolars will vary accordingly (Fig. 6-4). A small middle section of the apical area will be associated with mesially angulated eruption of the first premolar and canine. Depending upon the relation between the first premolar, canine, lateral incisor, and the spatial conditions in the dental arch, the canine will emerge more buccally or more palatally than normal. Abnormal eruption of the canine can be accompanied by rotation in mesiobuccal or mesiopalatal directions. An overlapping of the lateral incisor root by the canine crown will lead to a mesiobuccal rotation of the latter.

In general there will be a shortage of space in the middle section of the apical area in the canine-first premolar region. The second premolar is usually less affected because its predecessor has a larger mesiodistal crown dimension. However, an exception has to be made for cases of a mesially angulated erupting first permanent molar in which the distal surface of the second deciduous molar can resorb, leading eventually to a premature loss of that tooth (see Chapter 16). The transition of the posterior teeth that takes place some years later will then encounter special difficulties. This is also the case for premature loss of the second deciduous molar due to caries or extraction. The same holds true for the first deciduous molar, though to a lesser extent (see Chapter 14).

In a small middle section of the apical area the second premolar will be more distally located in relation to its predecessor without any deviation in its mesiodistal orientation. The mesially angulated first premolar and canine will erupt more mesially than normal.

Frequently, the space available between the first premolar and the root of the lateral incisor for eruption of the canine is limited. The first premolar will move distally when space in the dental arch and occlusion allow this migration to occur. Further, the position of the lateral incisor will change because the large canine crown will descend in close proximity to its root, which increases in circumference from the apex to the cementoenamel junction. Before emergence of the canine, the root of the lateral permanent incisor will be displaced mesially and palatally and its crown tipped distally and laterally. The extent of this movement of the lateral incisor is related to the lack of space encountered by the erupting canine and the presence or absence of the deciduous canine.

In exceptional instances the crown of the canine will be located not labially but palatally to the root of the lateral incisor. When adequate space is available the eruption path of the canine will then be slightly different and the tooth will usually emerge less buccally in the dental arch but in the appropriate transverse relation with the mandibular teeth. In the postemergence phase the canine will erupt further, move buccally, and gradually adopt the appropriate position. However, in conditions of insufficient space a canine crown initially positioned palatal of the root of the lateral incisor will erupt in a deviating direction and not attain a normal position within the dental arch. The canine cannot move buccally, either before emerging or in the postemergence eruption phase. The canine will emerge palatally or not emerge at all and becomes impacted.

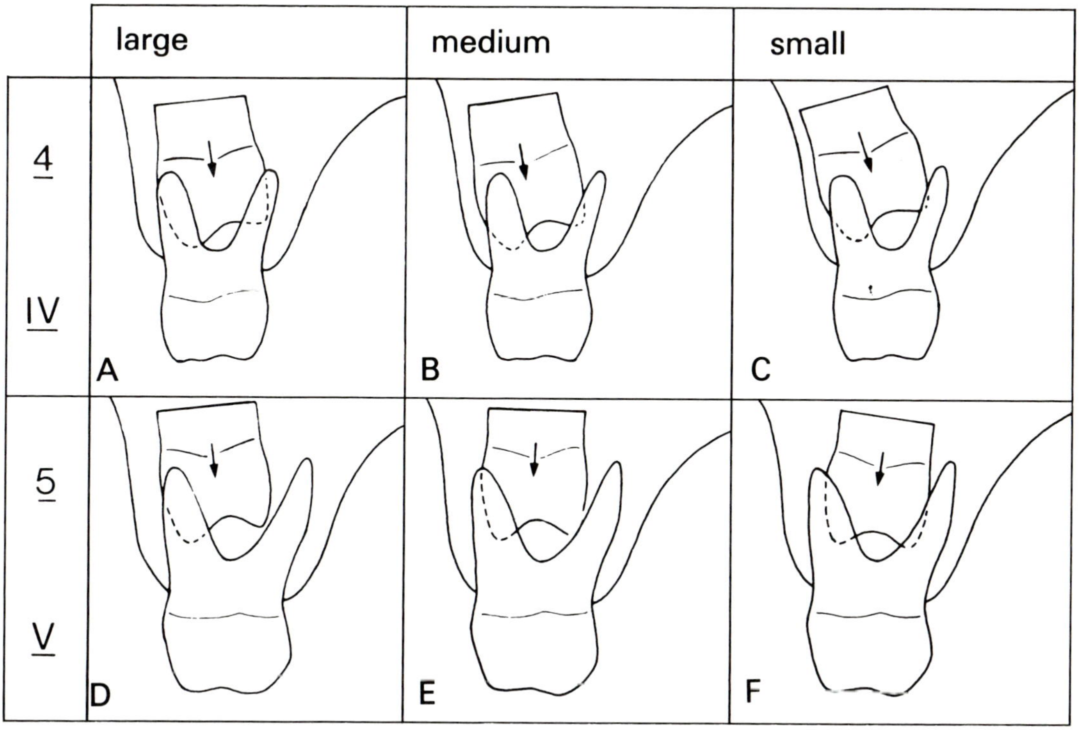

Fig. 6-4 Variations in the transverse position and direction of eruption of the maxillary first and second premolars related to the size of the middle section of the apical area. A shortage of space in the middle section of the apical area will affect the position and direction of eruption of the first premolar more than that of the second premolar.

A In a large middle section of the apical area the first premolar will be positioned superior to the first deciduous molar and its path of eruption will be slightly palatally directed.

B In a medium middle section of the apical area the first premolar will be more buccally placed and erupt in a more palatal direction.

C In a small middle section of the apical area the crowded conditions lead to excessive buccal displacement and a palatal direction of eruption.

D In a large middle section of the apical area the second premolar is located superior to its predecessor and more buccally. It will erupt in a slightly palatal direction.

E In a medium middle section of the apical area the second premolar is situated more central and superior to its predecessor. Its direction of eruption is about perpendicular to the occlusal plane.

F In a small middle section of the apical area the second premolar is more palatally located and erupts in a slightly buccal direction.

6.4 Eruption after emergence and subsequent change in orientation

As in the mandible, with a large middle section of the apical area the maxillary premolars emerge within the contour of the crown of their predecessor in accordance with both the position occupied before and the direction of the eruption movement (Fig. 6-4, page 141). In a medium middle section and particularly with a small middle section of the apical area, the first premolar is more buccally positioned and its path of eruption more palatally directed. A different situation exists for the second premolar. In a small middle section of the apical area the second premolar will be more palatally positioned and erupt in a buccal direction. In a medium middle section of the apical area the second premolar is approximately centred above its predecessor and erupts perpendicularly. In a large middle section of the apical area the second premolar will be more buccally positioned and will erupt in a more palatal direction. The sites of emergence of the first and second premolars depend on their direction of eruption. In situations with a small middle section of the apical area, first premolars tend to emerge more buccally and second premolars more palatally in the dental arch.

Simultaneous emergence of both premolars results in a situation different from that following sequential emergence. This aspect will be dealt with in detail in the discussion of the different transition patterns.

Depending on the local conditions in the dental arch and on the size of the middle section of the apical area the canine will emerge more or less buccal to the lateral incisor. When the largest circumference of the canine crown approaches the cementoenamel junction of the lateral incisor, the labial inclination of the lateral incisor will become reduced.

The erupting canine causes a palatal movement of the crown of the lateral incisor if both teeth are in close proximity. In accordance with the change in relation between the permanent canine and the lateral incisor, the latter will become distopalatally rotated. The movement of the root of the lateral incisor is no longer restricted by the presence of the large canine crown within the alveolar process. The more the canine with its tapering root descends, the more space will become availabe for a change in position of the root of the lateral incisor. The ultimate position of the lateral incisor will also depend on the space available within the dental arch and its contact with the mandibular teeth. Likewise, the changes associated with the preemergence and postemergence eruption of the maxillary permanent canine depend on the size of the middle section of the apical area and the space available in the dental arch for displacement of the first premolar and lateral incisor.

As in the mandible, emergence of the second permanent molar before the second deciduous molar is exfoliated will lead to more mesial migration of the first permanent molar than when the second permanent molar emerges after completion of the transition of the premolars and the canine. In contrast to the situation in the mandible, the incisor region will not usually profit from the leeway space. In general, maxillary permanent canines do not occupy a more distal position within the dental arch than their predecessors, as is the case in the mandible.[222]

As already indicated previously, premature loss of a deciduous canine or deciduous molars presents special problems. Particularly the loss of the maxillary second deciduous molar results in undesirable, often irreversible changes. The first perma-

nent molar will rotate mesiopalatally and the space for the second premolar will become reduced. The rotational movement of the first permanent molar will cause the remaining space to be trapezoidal in shape with its largest side palatal. The erupting second premolar, in unfavourable situations already palatally positioned to start with (Fig. 6-4, page 141), will erupt and emerge palatally in the dental arch.[223] The lost space is not regained (see Chapter 14).
The postemergence eruption and the subsequent location of the maxillary premolars are determined mainly by the initial contacts that develop between the opposing teeth and by the final occlusion. In this respect the mandibular teeth serve more as a guide for the maxillary teeth than vice versa. The mandibular premolars usually precede the maxillary premolars in their emergence. The morphology of the mandible allows a smaller range of variation in transverse location of the premolars than that of the maxilla. The final position of the maxillary permanent canine is also more determined by the occlusal contacts of the teeth of the mandible rather than the other way round.
Some of the comments made above can be summarized in the statement that an overall larger variation in transverse direction is found in the maxilla than in the mandible. This applies to the initial location of the deciduous teeth and the sites of formation of their successors, the transition of the posterior teeth, and the transverse location of the canines, premolars, and permanent molars after occlusion is attained.

6.5 Patterns in transition of maxillary posterior teeth

The categorisation of the transition of the maxillary posterior teeth into patterns is based, as for the mandible, on differences in emergence sequence and in the leeway space. Table 6-1 presents a survey of nine theoretically distinguishable patterns. Five of them will be illustrated by means of photographs and schematic drawings. Two will be discussed briefly in connection with the others. Special attention will be given to the changes in the position of the lateral incisor in the different transition patterns.
The sequence of emergence and the differences in mesiodistal crown dimensions of corresponding deciduous and permanent teeth play an essential role in the transition of the posterior teeth. These factors seem to be next in importance after consideration of the space available in the dental arch and the size of the middle section of the apical area.
The size and shape of the middle section of the apical area on the left and the right side are usually about the same. That does not hold true for the sequence and time of emergence of the premolars and permanent canine. Changes associated with the transition of the maxillary posterior teeth frequently do not take place symmetrically. The influence of the emergence of the second permanent molar is only occasionally mentioned in the presentation of the patterns.

TABLE 6-1
*Survey of nine combinations in the transition of the maxillary posterior teeth based on three emergence sequences. Combinations based on other emergence sequences are not incorporated in order to reduce the complexity of the presentation. Five patterns are illustrated (Figs. 6-5 to 6-14).**

leeway space / sequence of emergence	large > +2.1 mm	medium +2.1 to +0.7 mm	small < +0.7 mm
(3,4,5)	A	—	—
4(5,3)	X	B	C
4,5,3	X	D	E

* Numbers in parentheses indicate simultaneous emergence; "—" = pattern cannot occur for reasons explained in the text; "X" = pattern is discussed briefly in combination with the patterns demonstrated.

6.5.1 Maxillary Posterior Teeth Transition Pattern A

Pattern A is characterized by the emergence sequence (3,4,5) (more or less simultaneous emergence of all three teeth) and a large leeway space (Figs. 6-5 and 6-6). Simultaneous eruption of the permanent canine and both premolars usually only takes place when a large leeway space is accompanied by a large middle section of the apical area. Then the three crowns can be situated at the same level before and during emergence. The relation between the permanent canine crown and the lateral incisor root depends on the situation in the anterior section of the apical area. A large middle section of the apical area is not necessarily associated with a large anterior section. The canine crown may be situated at some distance from the root of the lateral incisor. However, overlapping in different degrees can also be found, and the position and inclination of the lateral incisor will vary accordingly.
Simultaneous emergence of the three teeth is usually not encountered in instances of a small or medium leeway space, because the first premolar then emerges before the canine, as discussed earlier.

6.5.2 Maxillary Posterior Teeth Transition Pattern B

Pattern B is characterized by the emergence sequence 4 (5, 3) and a medium leeway space (Figs. 6-7 and 6-8). The first premolar emerges first. It can take up a proper position within the dental arch because spatial conditions are favourable. The mesiodistal dimension of the first deciduous molar crown is usually larger than that of its successor in situations with a medium leeway space. The subsequently erupting canine can move the first premolar distally if necessary. The simultaneous emergence of the canine and second premolar offers the possibility that the extra space that becomes available in the second premolar region can be utilised for improving the relation between the canine and lateral incisor. This will not be necessary if the anterior section of the apical area is also large. However, when that is not the case, the initial overlapping of the lateral incisor by the canine can disappear by distal movement of the latter.

The emergence sequence 4 (5, 3) combined with a large leeway space will usually result in a harmonious permanent dental arch. Enough space will be available for the canine to move distally if required.

6.5.3 Maxillary Posterior Teeth Transition Pattern C

Pattern C is characterized by the emergence sequence 4 (5, 3) and a small leeway space (Figs. 6-9 and 6-10). In a small middle section of the apical area, frequently associated with a small leeway space, the maxillary first premolar is buccally and the second premolar palatally positioned before eruption starts. The canine and both premolars are crowded and the first premolar is the first tooth to emerge as it forms an obstacle to the descent of the crowns of the two adjacent permanent teeth. The simultaneous emergence of the second premolar and the permanent canine allows the first premolar to move distally after exfoliation of the second deciduous molar. The somewhat palatally positioned second premolar is likely to emerge accordingly. This can particularly be the case if the first permanent molar migrates mesially because of an early emergence of the second permanent molar. However, in by far the majority of cases, the second premolar may find enough space in the dental arch and attain a proper position.

When the first premolar does not move distally the emerging canine will not find enough space in the dental arch and will end up in a buccal position, usually overlapping the lateral incisor labially. Existing crowding in the incisor region can increase. However, in the emergence sequence 4 (5, 3) the crowding generally tends to show up more in the second premolar region than in the canine-incisor region in comparison with the sequence 4, 5, 3 (see 6.5.5).

6.5.4 Maxillary Posterior Teeth Transition Pattern D

Pattern D is characterized by the emergence sequence 4,5,3 and a medium leeway space (Figs. 6-11 and 6-12). That the transition is more critical in instances of a medium leeway space than of a large leeway space also applies here. The most favourable sequence of emergence is the one discussed here. The first premolar can move distally and occupy some of the extra space that becomes available after loss of the second

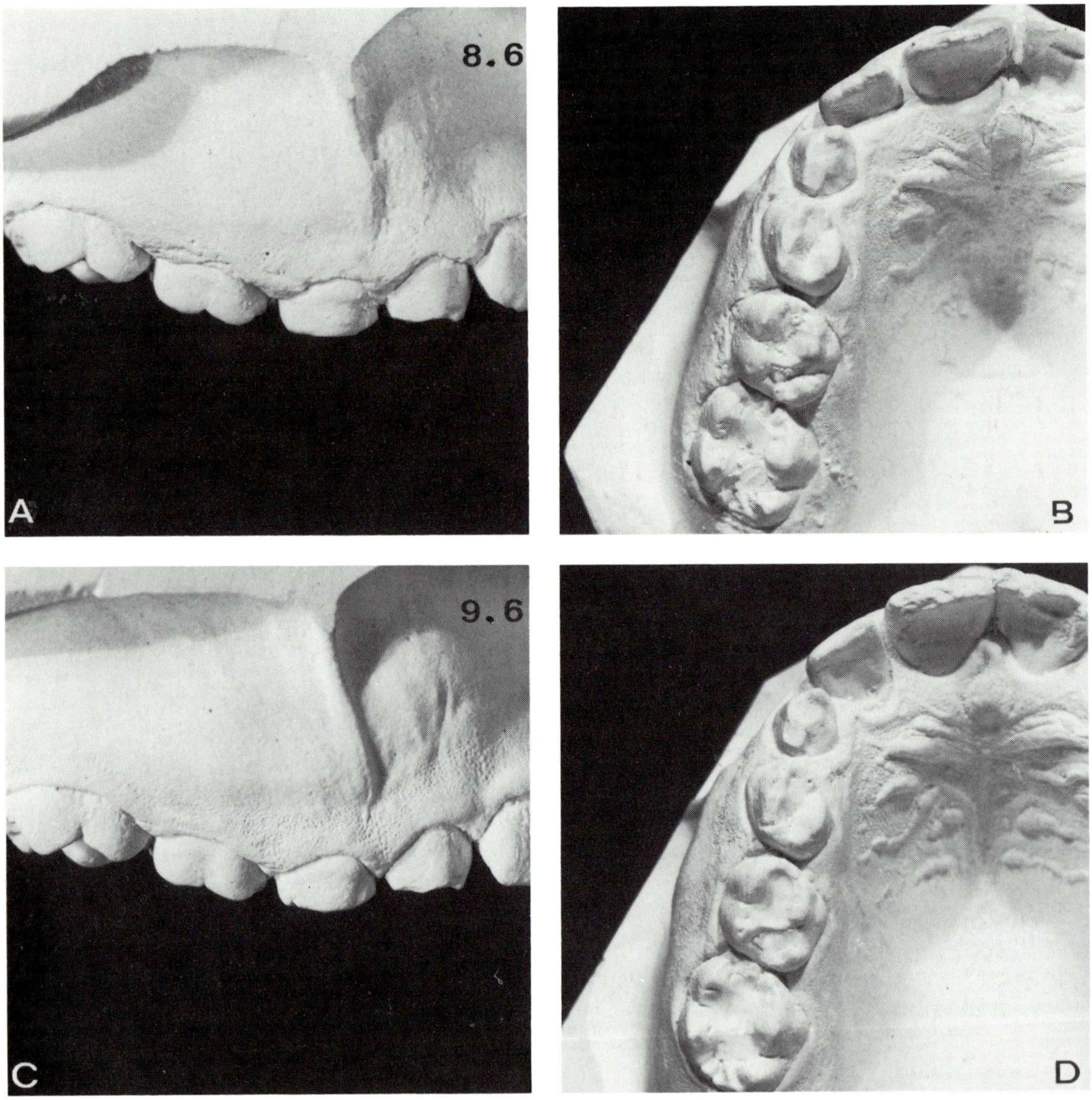

Fig. 6-5 Lateral and occlusal views of a longitudinal series of dental casts of the Maxillary Posterior Teeth Transition Pattern A, characterized by simultaneous emergence (3, 4, 5) and a large leeway space.

A, B *Diastemata are present in the dental arch. The position, angulation, and inclination of the lateral incisor are indicative of a medium anterior section of the apical area.*

C, D *Space exists between the deciduous canine and the first and second deciduous molars. The diastema between the lateral and central incisor is reduced in size.*

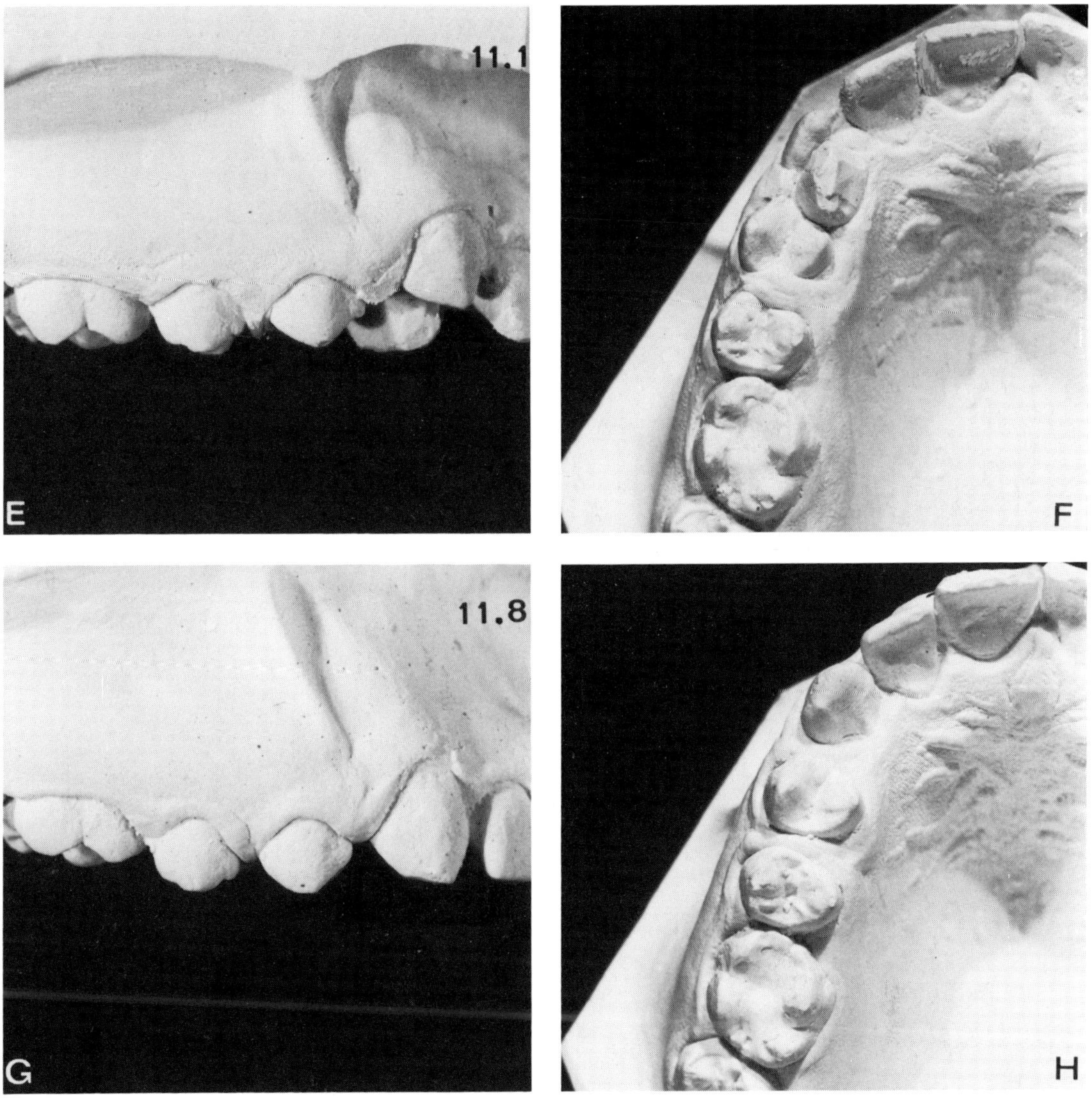

E, F *The premolars and the permanent canine have recently emerged. The latter erupts buccal to its predecessor, which had become palatally displaced. The permanent canine has emerged in contact with the lateral incisor and overlaps it slightly. The diastema between the lateral and central incisors is closed. A diastema is present between both premolars. The second premolar has emerged in contact with the first permanent molar and is buccally positioned.*

G, H *The premolars and canine have erupted further. A good contact exists between the canine and the lateral incisor, which is not rotated. Also, the canine did not rotate. The second premolar has attained a better position. Note the large diastemata on both sides of the first premolar and the relatively small canine crown.*

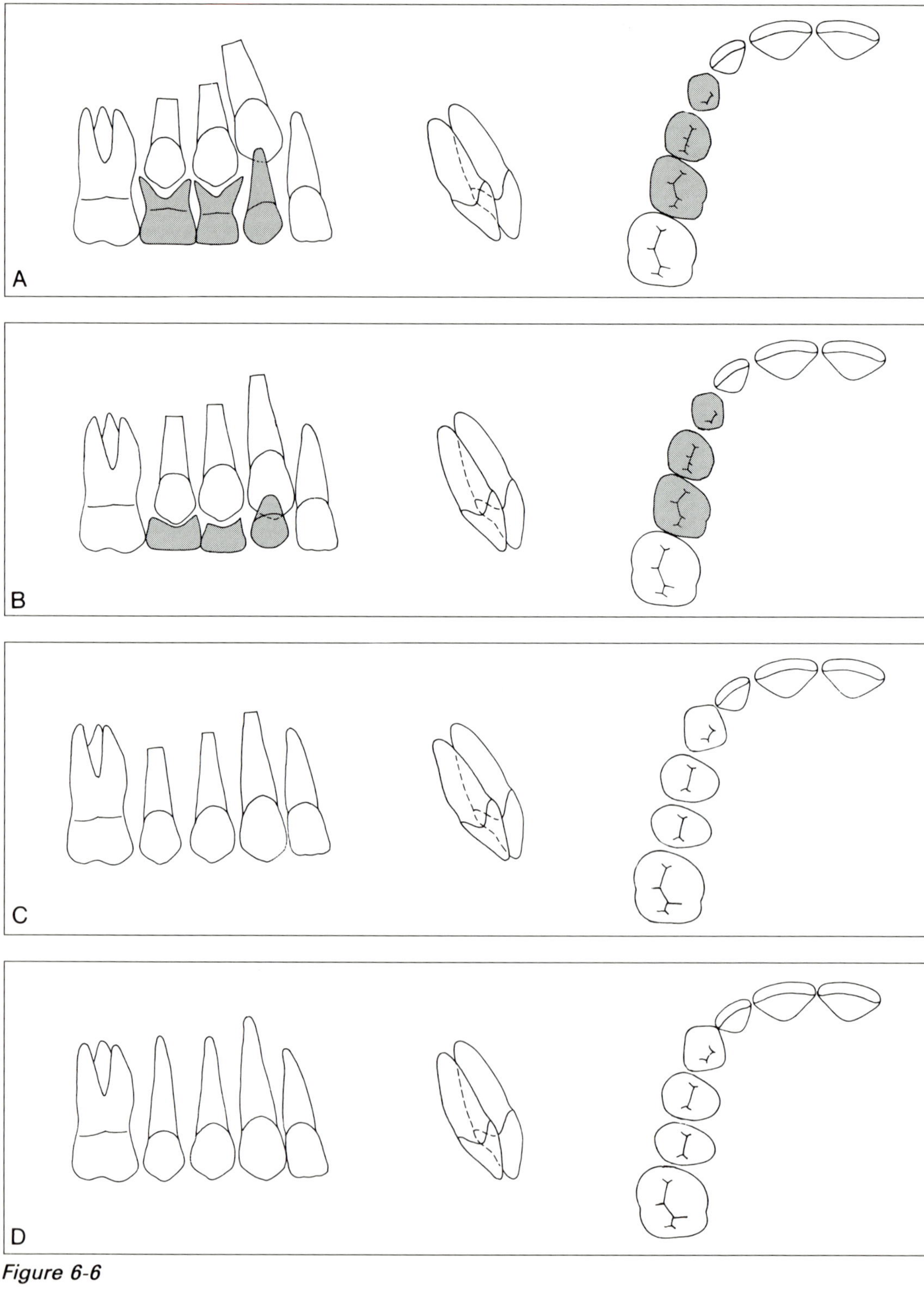

Figure 6-6

Fig. 6-6 Schematic lateral and occlusal views of the Maxillary Posterior Teeth Transition Pattern A, characterized by simultaneous emergence (3, 4, 5) and a large leeway space.

A Diastemata are present between the teeth and also in the anterior region when a large anterior section of the apical area exists. Both premolars and permanent canine are approximately at the same level with spaces between them. The canine crown does not vertically overlap the crown of the first premolar.
B The three teeth involved can descend and emerge simultaneously. The canine erupts more quickly than the first premolar. No overlapping of the lateral incisor will take place if a large anterior section of the apical area is also present, allowing the lateral incisor to move labially.
C More than enough space is available in the dental arch for the three teeth involved.
D After complete eruption the posterior teeth are harmoniously placed in the dental arch if the occlusion with the opposing mandibular teeth is favourable. Diastemata usually exist for some time after the transition is completed.

deciduous molar concomitantly with the emergence and eruption of the canine. However, the extra space may also be consumed primarily by mesial migration of the first permanent molar. Differences in the timing of emergence of the teeth involved influence the course of events. If a relatively long period elapses between emergence of the second premolar and emergence of the permanent canine, it is less likely that the canine can benefit from the extra space associated with the transition of the second deciduous molar than when the interval is small. The relation between the canine and the lateral incisor determines how much distal migration of the canine is desirable for improvement in the anterior region of the dental arch.
The emergence sequence 4, 5, 3 combined with a large leeway space offers favourable conditions. The transition will take place without problems. The excess space initially present will gradually become reduced. A harmonious alignment of the teeth can be attained.

6.5.5 Maxillary Posterior Teeth Transition Pattern E

Pattern E is characterized by the emergence sequence 4, 5, 3 and a small leeway space (Figs. 6-13 and 6-14). In general, cases of pattern E have a small middle section of the apical area and a small anterior area. No excess space is present in the arch and the incisors are frequently crowded. The premolars are not located centrally between the roots of their predecessors but are transversally displaced, the first one buccally, the second one palatally. However, after emergence, the first premolar usually attains a good position within the dental arch, particularly when the second deciduous molar is lost shortly thereafter. The second premolar will emerge palatally and subsequently move buccally. When a good occlusion exists between the mandibular and maxillary first permanent molars, the maxillary molar will not migrate too far mesially. The crowded condition will show up in the canine region when the deciduous canine is replaced by the permanent canine. The larger the difference in mesiodistal crown dimension between these two teeth, the greater the deficiency. The emergence and eruption of the permanent canine can lead to increased crowding of the incisors. Already existing overlap will usually increase. Good contact relations may become disturbed.

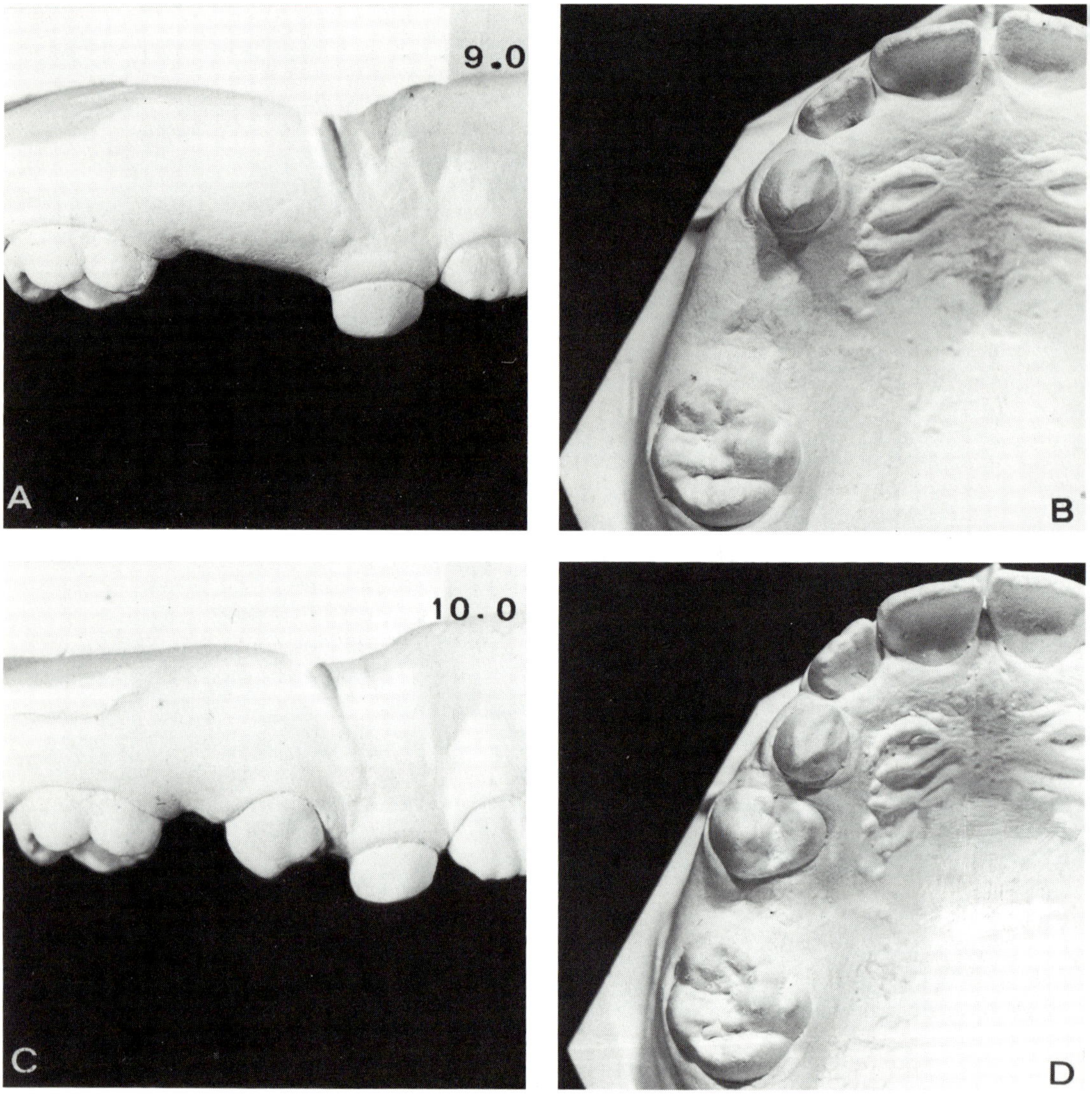

Fig. 6-7 Longitudinal series of dental casts showing the Maxillary Posterior Teeth Transition Pattern B, characterized by the emergence sequence 4 (5, 3) and a medium leeway space. The case demonstrated here is complicated by premature loss of the second deciduous molar.

A, B *Diastemata are present between the anterior teeth. The second deciduous molar was lost just before the stage shown here.*

C, D *The first permanent molar rotated mesially. The first premolar has emerged slightly buccally. The crown of the lateral incisor moved labially and its root palatally under influence of the erupting canine. The central diastema was reduced.*

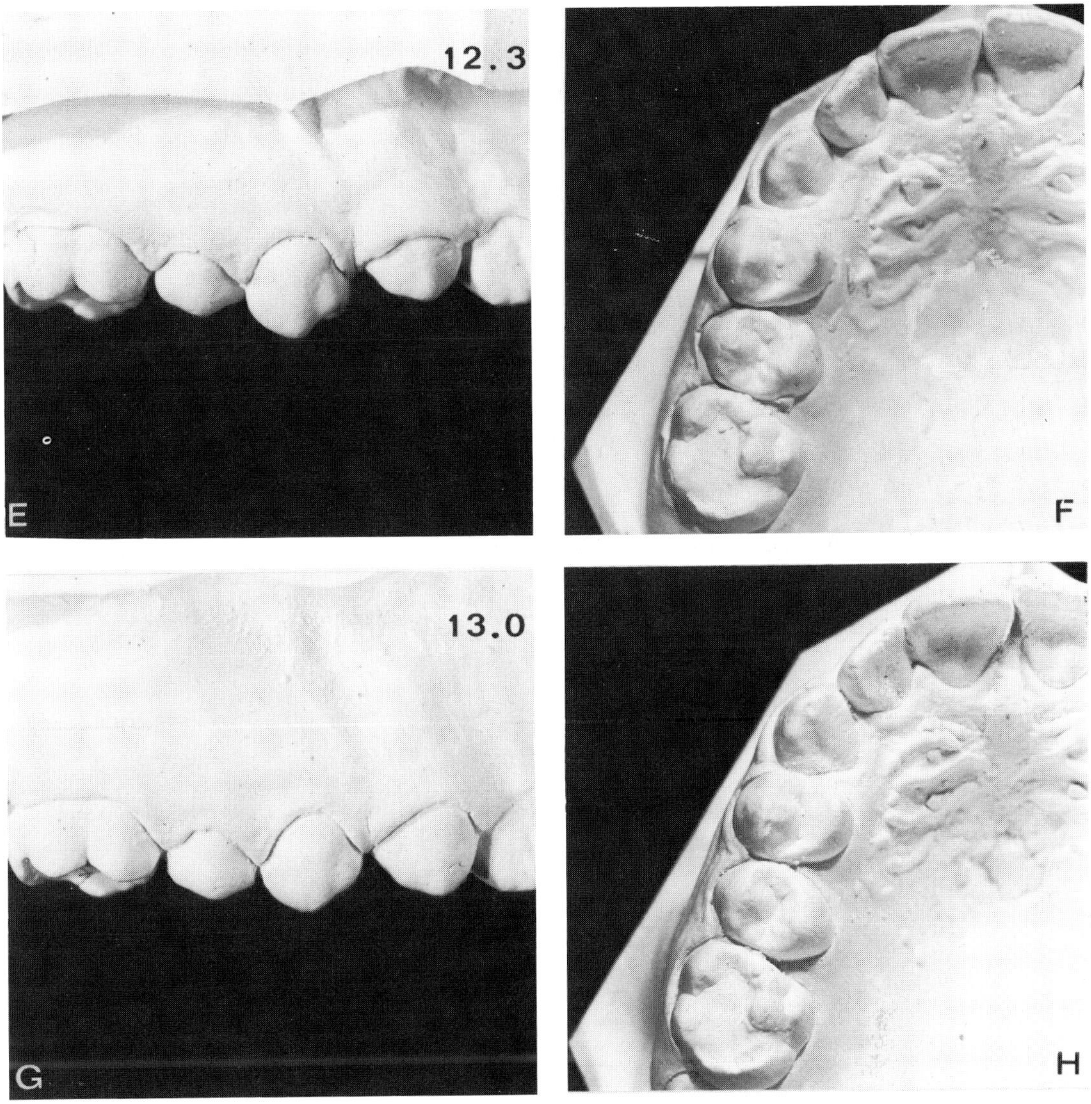

E, F *The permanent canine has emerged in contact with the lateral incisor and overlaps it slightly. The distal corner of the latter moved palatally. Some space still exists distal to the canine. The second premolar emerged slightly palatally.*

G, H *The lateral incisor rotated back toward its original position. The canine can still move distally and the contact with the lateral incisor can improve further. The premolars occupy a good position in the dental arch.*

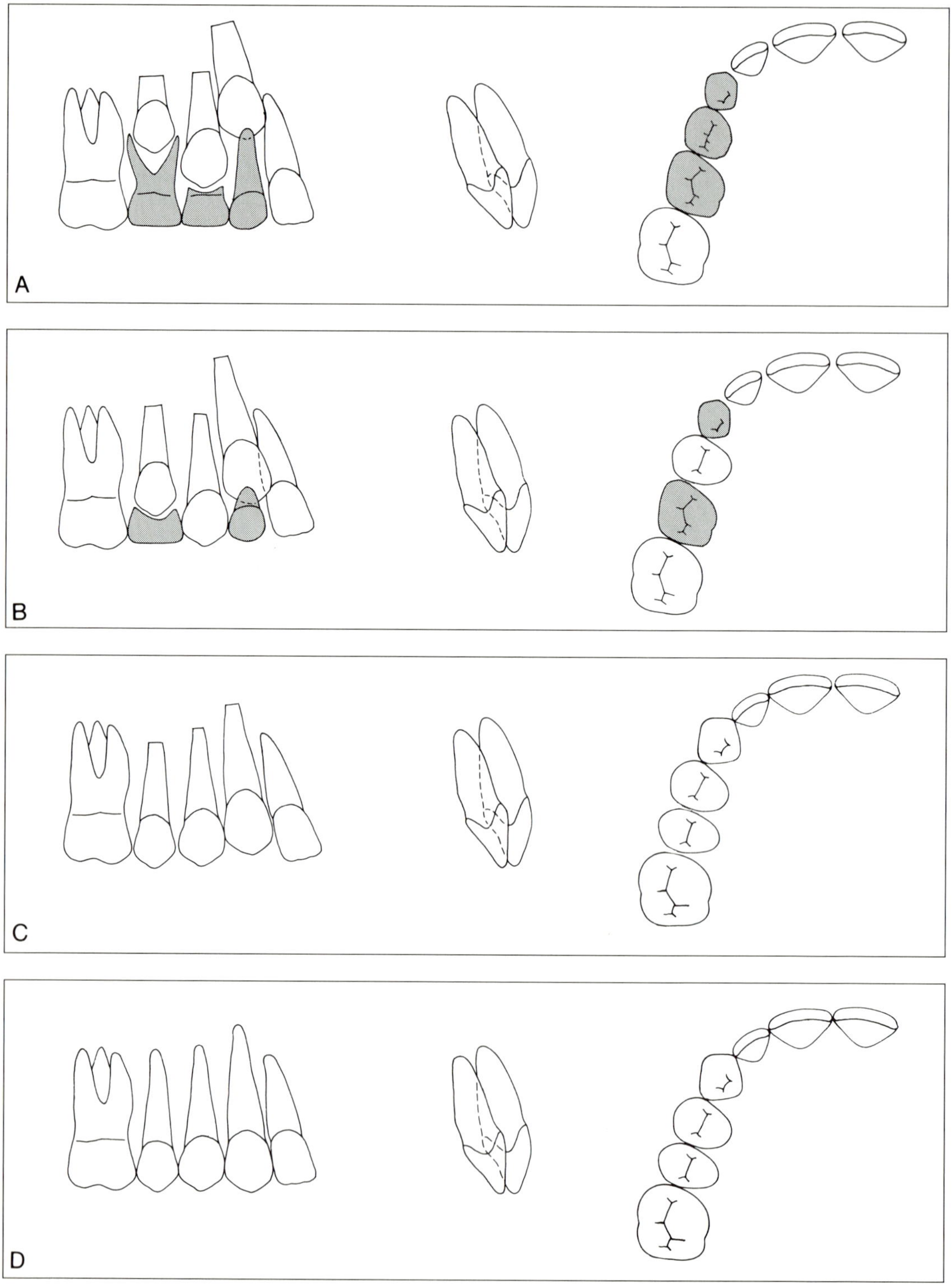

Figure 6-8

Fig. 6-8 Schematic drawing of the Maxillary Posterior Teeth Transition Pattern B, characterized by the emergence sequence 4 (5, 3) and a medium leeway space.

A Diastemata are present in the dental arch. The first premolar is closer to the occlusal plane than the two adjacent permanent teeth. The canine crown vertically overlaps the crown of the first premolar only slightly.
B The first premolar emerged without interferences and adequate space is available for the two other teeth to emerge.
C The second premolar and canine have emerged simultaneously. If necessary for the improvement of the canine-lateral incisor relationship, the first premolar can move distally. The diastemata in the incisal segment reduce with the eruption and emergence of the canine. Depending on the relation between the canine and lateral incisor the latter will experience a change in position and inclination with the eruption of the former.
D The situation upon completion of the transition will be harmonious if no unfavourable contacts with the mandibular teeth exist.

6.6 Supplementary remarks

The transition of the maxillary posterior teeth will encounter few difficulties in instances of a large leeway space. The sequence of emergence is then not important. A harmonious dental arch and good contacts between all permanent teeth can be realized.
The sequence of emergence plays an essential role in instances of a medium leeway space. That also holds true for differences in mesiodistal crown dimensions of corresponding deciduous and permanent teeth and for the location of the excess space in the form of diastemata. If the excess is centred in the canine region and a diastema is present between the permanent lateral incisor and the deciduous canine, the emergence sequence (4, 5) 3 is favourable. That also holds true when the permanent canine has only a slightly larger mesiodistal crown dimension than its predecessor. However, when in this respect a relatively large difference exists between the second premolar and its predecessor, then the emergence sequence 4 (5, 3) is more favourable.
In a small leeway space it is less likely that a harmonious dental arch will ultimately result. The difference between the sums of mesiodistal crown dimensions of the corresponding deciduous and permanent teeth is small and sometimes negative and diastemata are missing. As a rule, only the second deciduous molar then has a larger mesiodistal crown dimension than its successor. Crowding in the canine-premolar segment can develop when the first permanent molar migrates mesially in association with an early emergence of the second permanent molar. When the leeway space is small then only with the emergence sequence 4 (5, 3) and a favourable combination of the other variables involved will a reasonable dental arch be realized.
Characteristic for the transition of the maxillary posterior teeth are the changes in position and inclination of the lateral permanent incisor associated with eruption of the

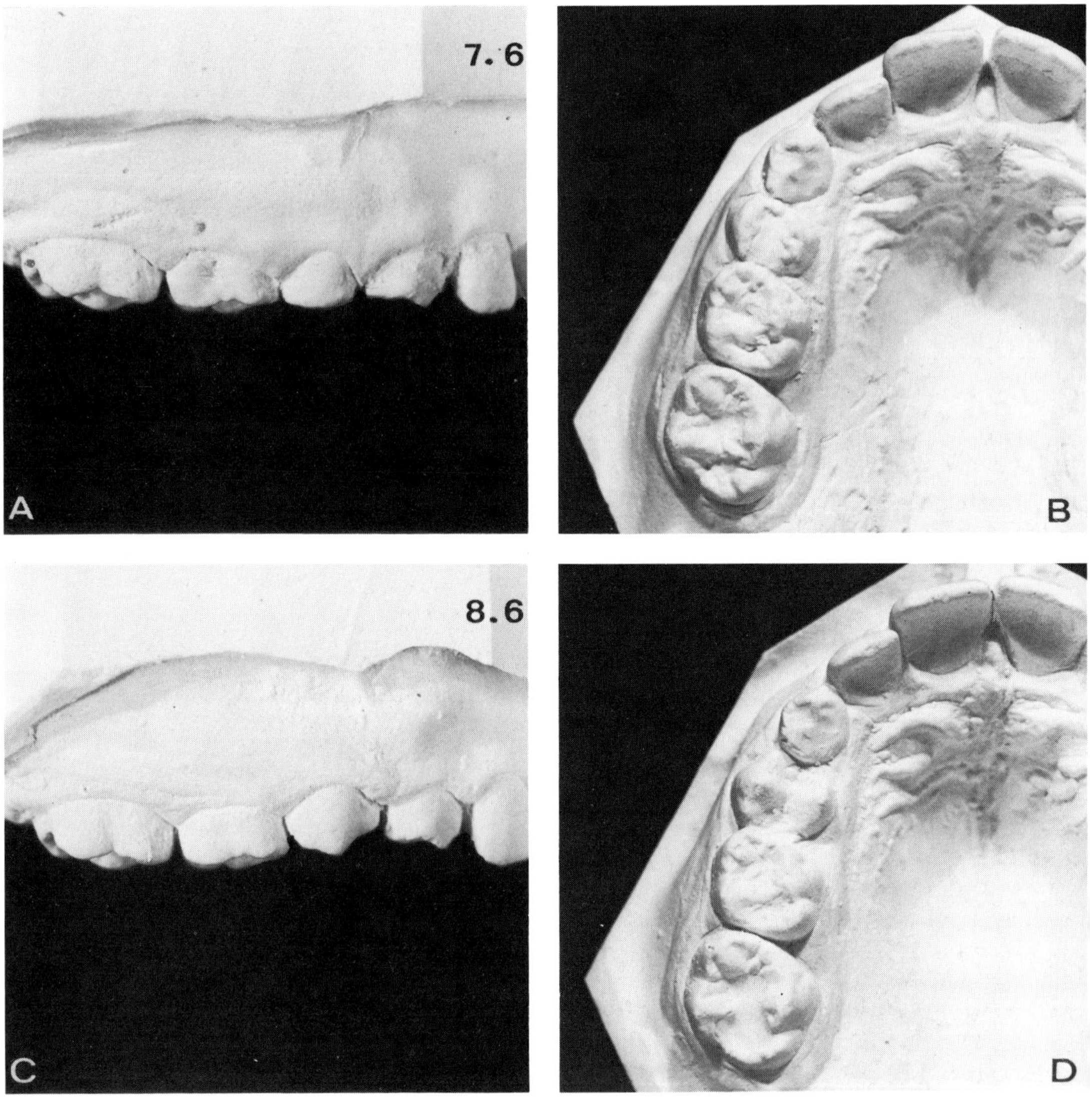

Fig. 6-9 Longitudinal series of dental casts showing the Maxillary Posterior Teeth Transition Pattern C, characterized by the emergence sequence 4(5,3) and a small leeway space.

A, B *Crowding exists in the incisal region. The central diastema is small. The lateral incisor is located palatally.*

C, D *The first premolar has emerged and assumed a position mainly affected by the restricted available space between the deciduous canine and second molar. The latter has a relatively large mesiodistal crown dimension compared to its successor. The central diastema is closed.*

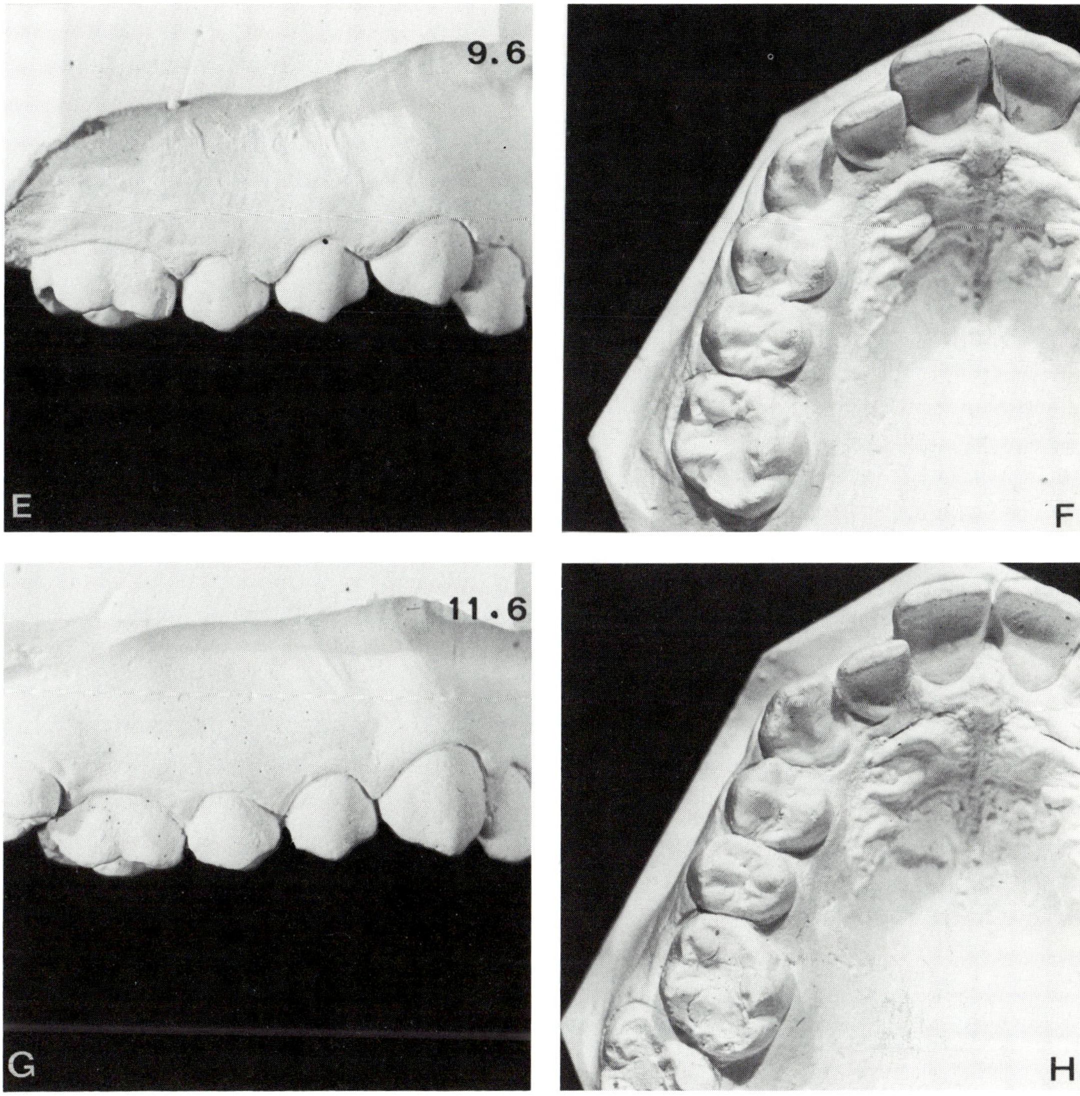

E, F The second premolar and permanent canine have emerged. The latter is in contact with the first premolar that has been moved distally. The second permanent molar has not yet emerged. The canine overlaps the lateral incisor and has moved it palatally.

G, H The canine is located buccally, the lateral incisor more palatally. Insufficient space is available for the second premolar, which is positioned excessively buccally and not palatally, as is usual in these cases.

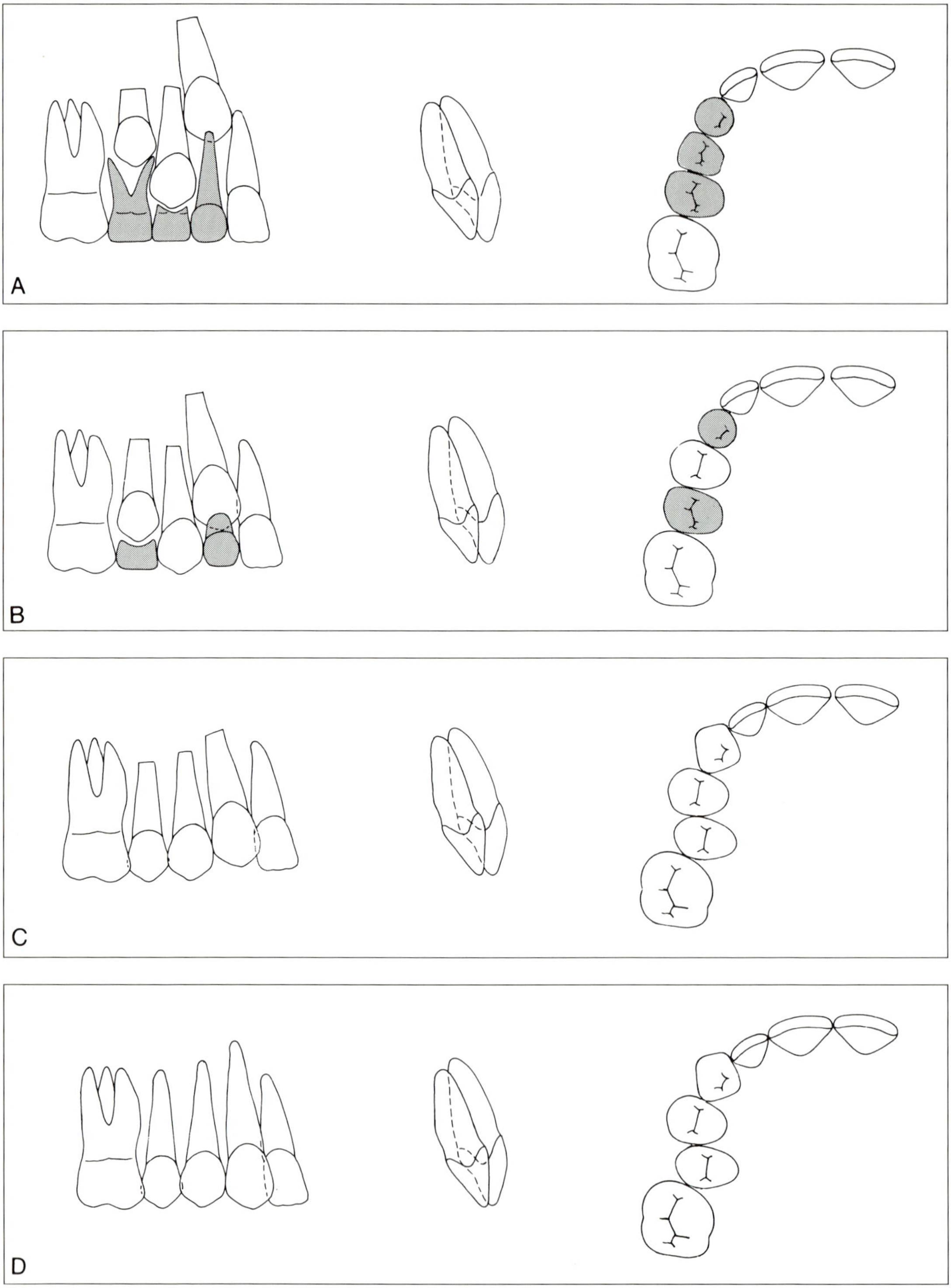

Figure 6-10

Fig. 6-10 Schematic drawing of the Maxillary Posterior Teeth Transition Pattern C, characterized by the emergence sequence 4 (5, 3) and a small leeway space.

A Both premolars overlap each other in a transverse and vertical direction. The canine overlaps the first premolar vertically. No diastemata are present distal to the lateral permanent incisor.
B The first premolar has emerged and may move distally after the second deciduous molar exfoliates.
C The permanent canine and second premolar emerged simultaneously. Insufficient space may remain for the second premolar, particularly if the first permanent molar migrates mesially. The permanent canine overlaps the lateral incisor labially.
D In a crowded situation the first premolar will be positioned buccally, the second premolar palatally. The permanent canine is placed buccally. If crowding exists in the incisor segment it can increase.

permanent canine, as explained in this chapter. Depending on the spatial relationship between these two teeth the crown of the lateral incisor will be more or less labially displaced initially. This displacement in a labial direction can increase in the early phase of canine eruption. As the canine crown descends further the inclination of the lateral incisor will change in the other direction and the crown will then become palatally displaced. The latter movement can be associated with a distopalatal rotation of the lateral incisor crown. Depending on the spatial conditions, the displacement of the lateral incisor can subsequently be restored and result in a harmonious alignment. Compared with the mandible, the transition of the maxillary posterior teeth in a small leeway space seems to result less frequently in crowding in the canine-premolar region. It may be that the larger range in variation in location of the premolars and permanent canine in transverse direction in the maxilla than in the mandible is associated with this difference. Further, it appears that relief of space deficiency in the posterior region by the increase in incisor crowding occurs more readily in the maxilla than in the mandible.

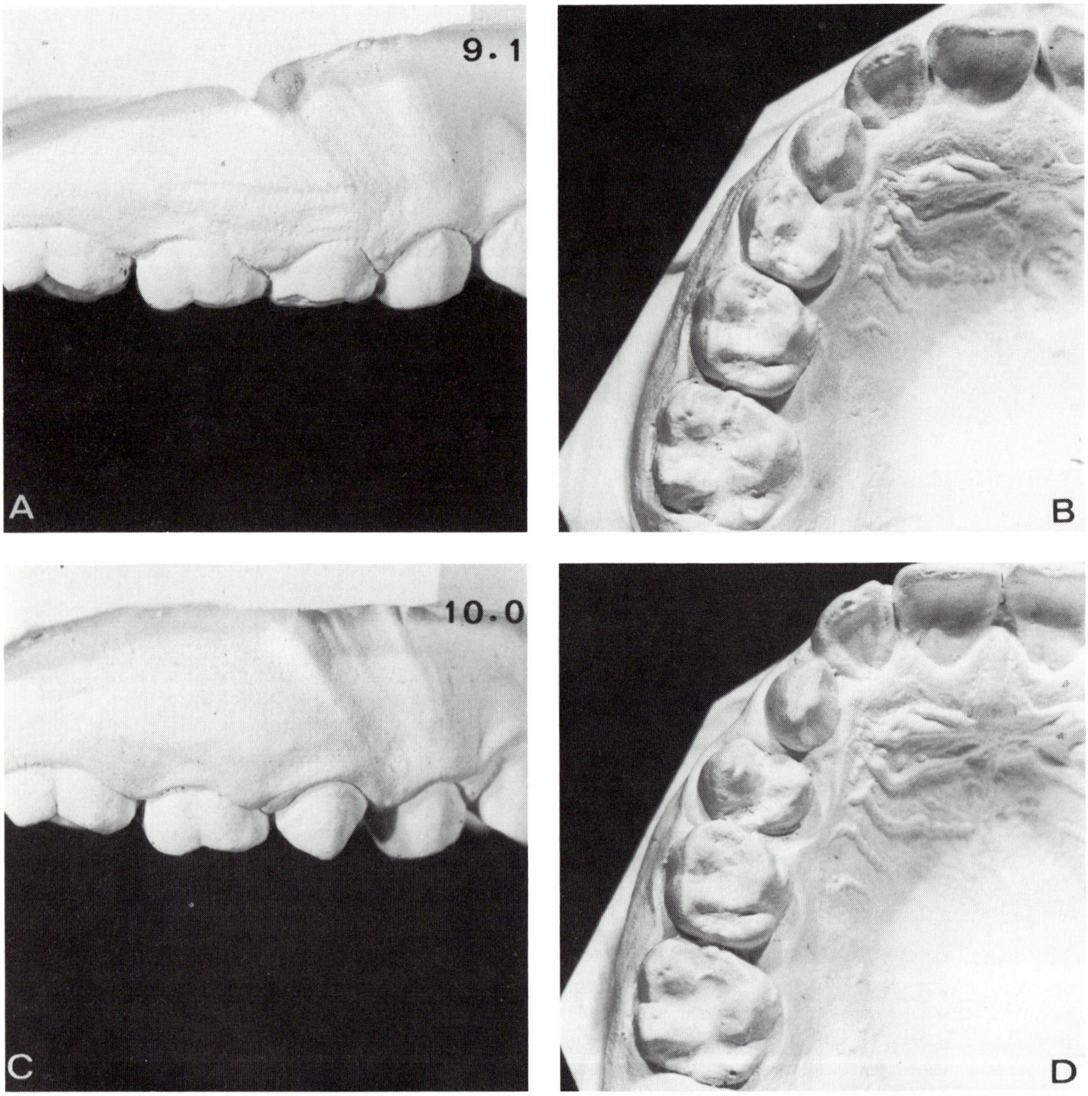

Fig. 6-11 Longitudinal series of dental casts showing the Maxillary Posterior Teeth Transition Pattern D, characterized by the emergence sequence 4, 5, 3 and a medium leeway space.

A, B A central diastema is present. Both permanent incisors are in eversion.
C, D The first premolar has emerged first. The lateral incisor moved labially under influence of the eruption of the permanent canine.

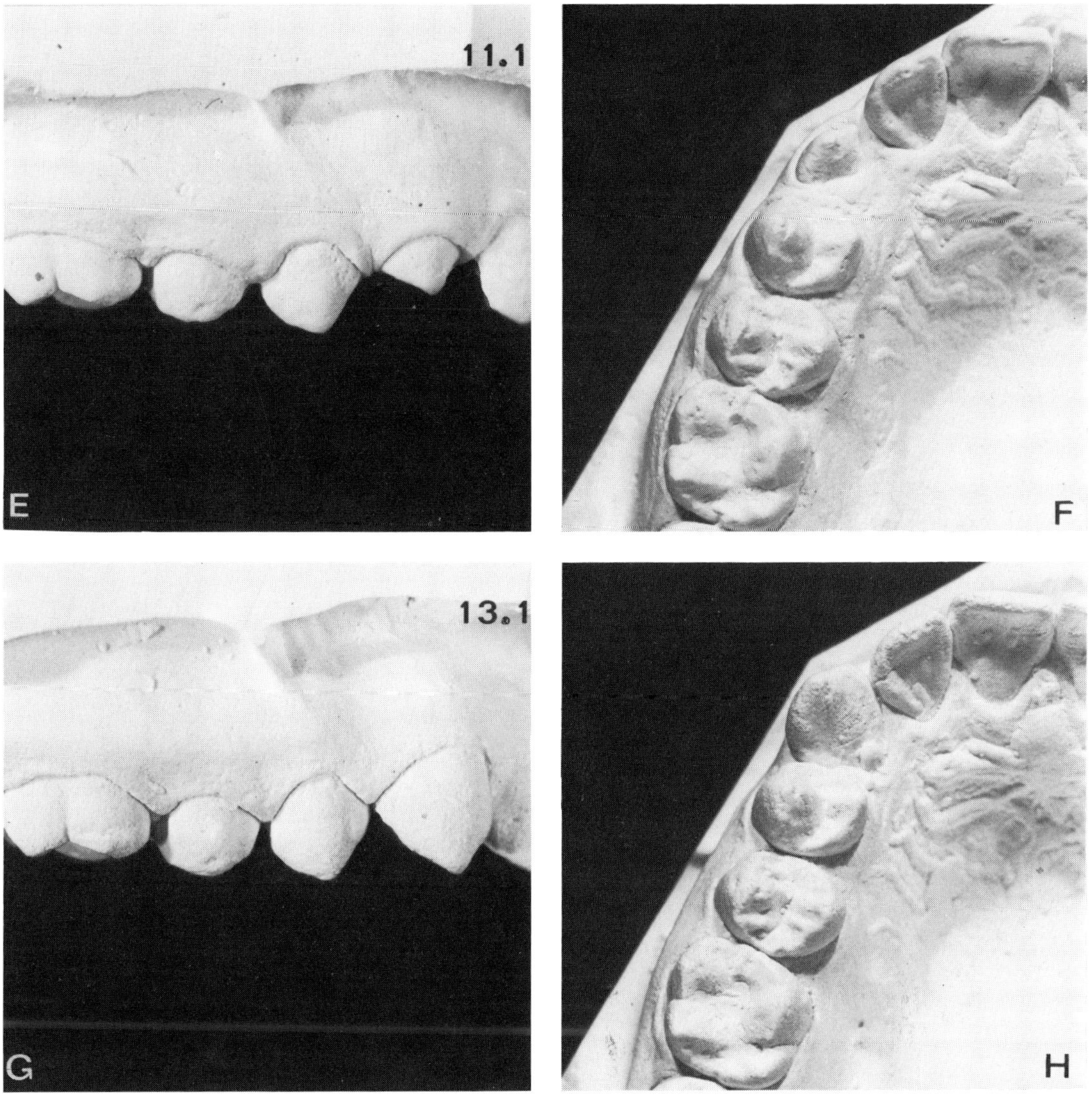

E, F *The second premolar has emerged before the permanent canine. The latter erupts in contact with the lateral incisor, which has already moved palatally. The lateral incisor did not experience a rotational movement in association with the eruption and emergence of the permanent canine. The first premolar migrated distally after exfoliation of the second deciduous molar. Extra space became available for the canine.*

G, H *After the full eruption of all teeth no diastemata are present in the dental arch. Slight crowding exists in the incisor-canine region. The canine is somewhat buccally positioned, the lateral incisor palatally positioned.*

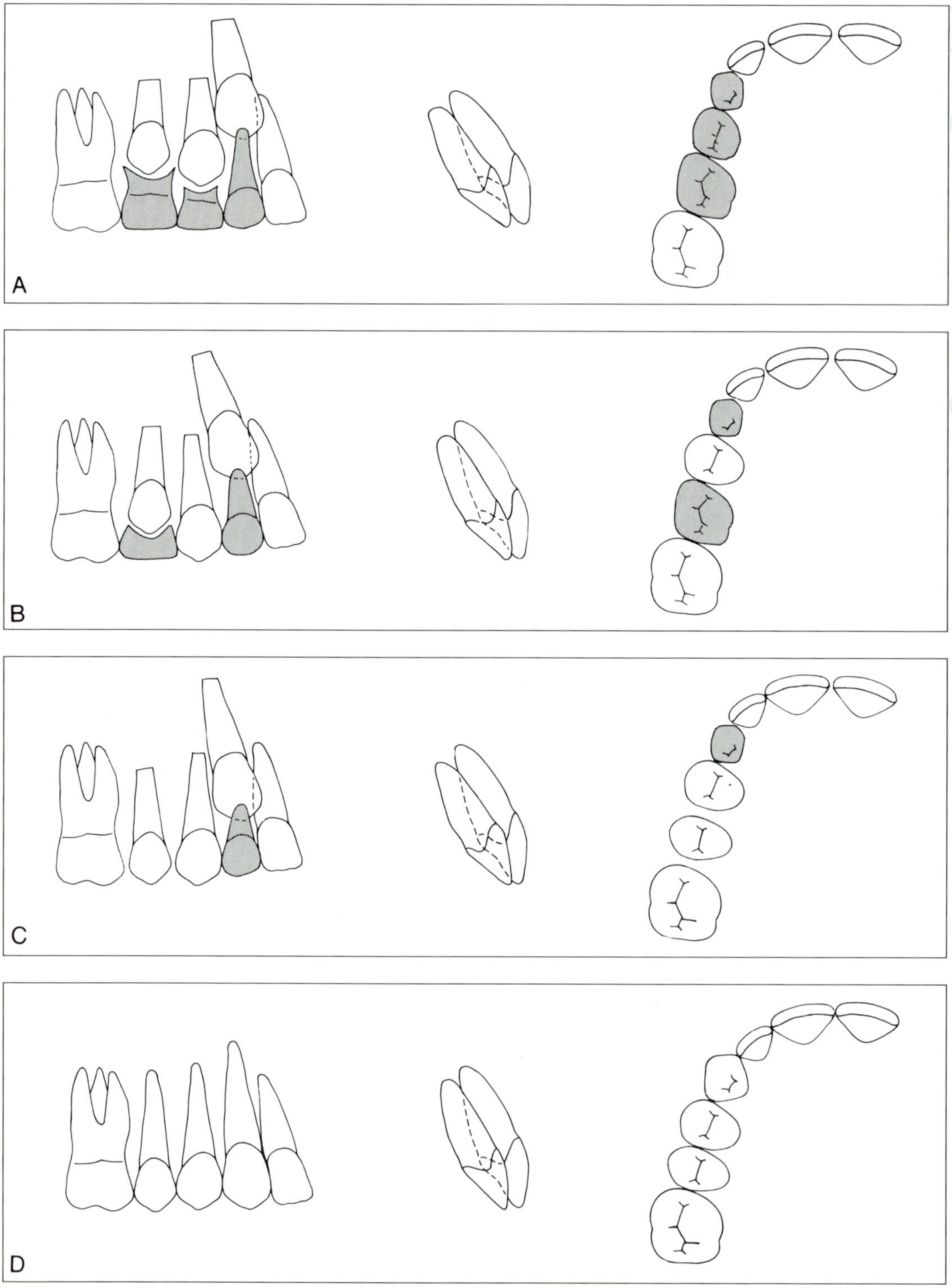

Figure 6-12

Fig. 6-12 Schematic drawing of the Maxillary Posterior Teeth Transition Pattern D, characterized by the emergence sequence 4, 5, 3 and a medium leeway space.

- *A Less space is available than with a large leeway space. The permanent canine vertically overlaps the first premolar. The relation between the permanent canine and the lateral incisor depends mainly upon the size of the anterior section of the apical area.*
- *B The first premolar emerges first. The crown of its predecessor has maintained sufficient space for the premolar.*
- *C The second premolar emerges with excess space. The premolars may become well aligned transversally before the canine emerges. The canine can, in its eruption, displace the first premolar distally, leading to more favourable conditions for the canine-lateral incisor relation.*
- *D Upon complete transition a harmonious dental arch or one with only slight crowding in the incisor-canine region will be found. The mesial migration of the first permanent molar, which is influenced by the time of emergence of the second permanent molar, will also affect the end result.*

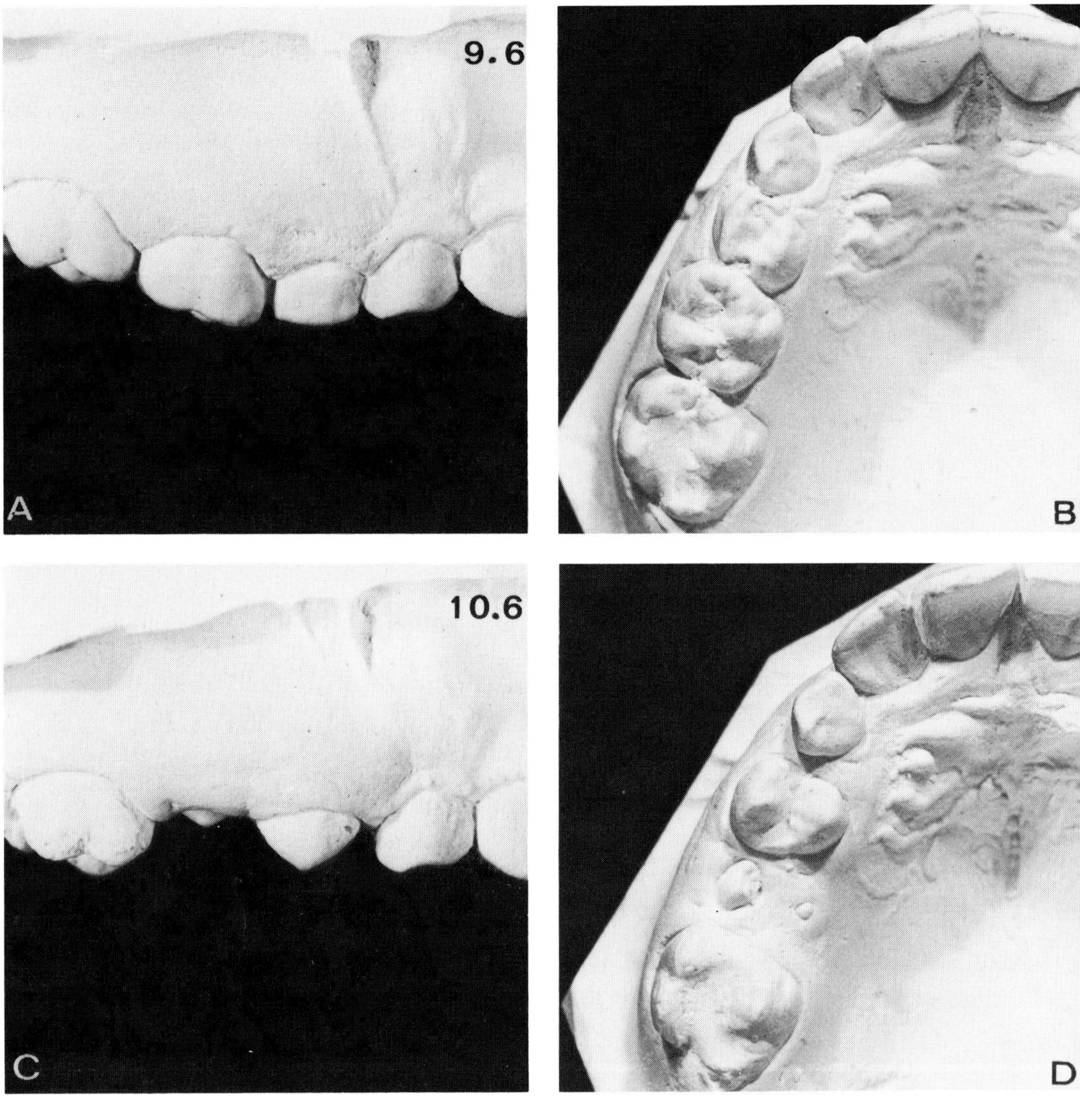

Fig. 6-13 Longitudinal series of dental casts showing the Maxillary Posterior Teeth Transition Pattern E, characterized by emergence sequence 4, 5, 3 and a small leeway space.

A, B Crowding exists in the incisal region. The lateral incisor is in eversion. No central diastema is present.

C, D The first premolar has emerged and has already moved distally, occupying some of the space that became available after the second deciduous molar was exfoliated. The second premolar has emerged soon after the first premolar and slightly palatally. Note the space between the deciduous canine and first premolar.

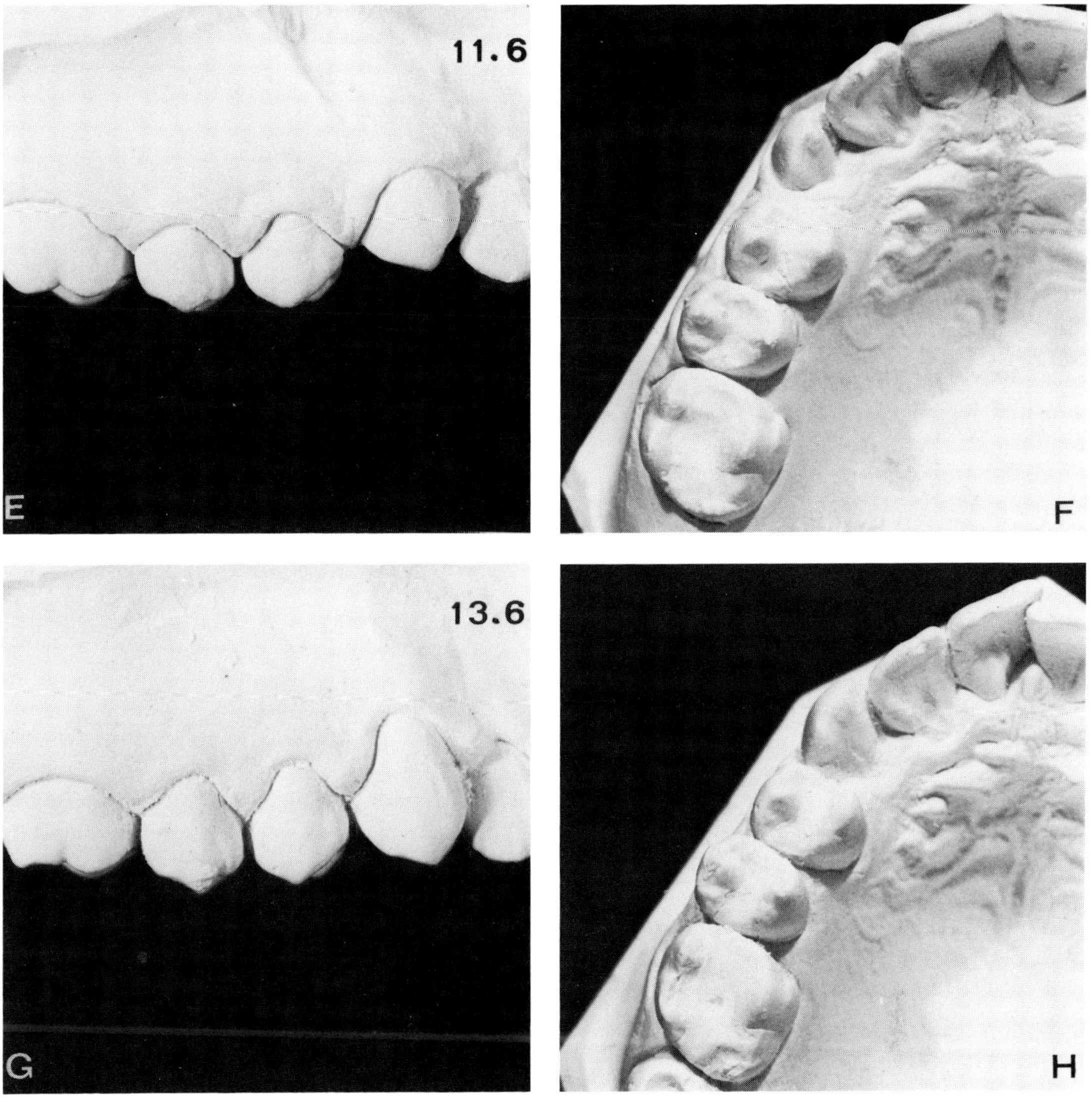

E, F *The second premolar has moved buccally. The permanent canine has emerged in contact with the lateral incisor and overlaps it. However, the short time interval between emergence of the first and second premolars and the fact that the second permanent molar did not emerge before the transition was complete did not prevent the considerable mesial migration of the first permanent molar, as can be concluded from the relationships between the posterior teeth and the lateral rugae points.*[222]

G, H *Further eruption of the canine is associated with its mesiobuccal rotation, palatal movement of the lateral incisor, and increased crowding of the incisors. Note the overlapping of the central incisors and the considerably larger mesiodistal dimension of the permanent canine compared with that of its predecessor.*

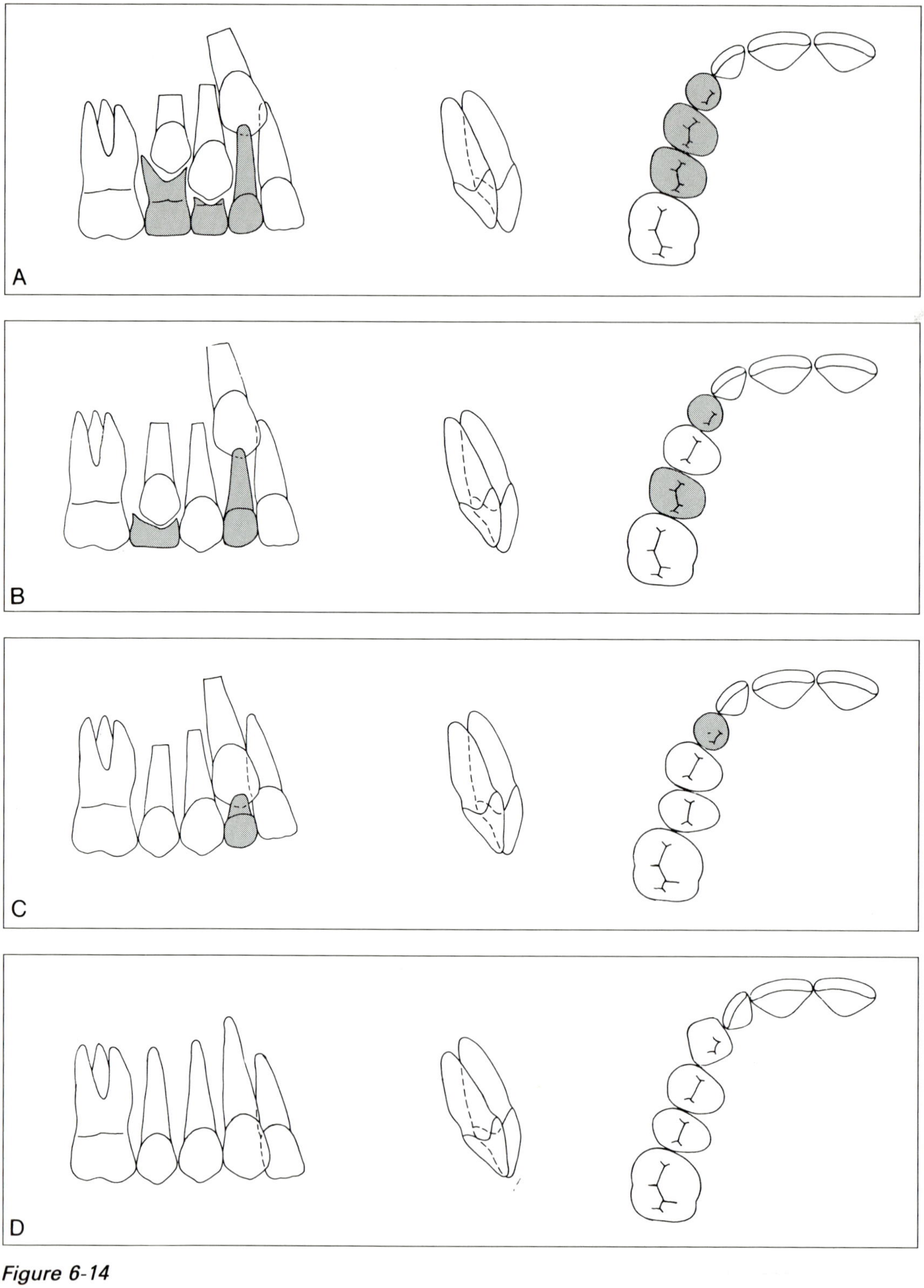

Figure 6-14

Fig. 6-14 Schematic drawing of the Maxillary Posterior Teeth Transition Pattern E, characterized by the emergence sequence 4,5,3 and a small leeway space.

A The two premolars overlap vertically and transversally. The canine overlaps the first premolar vertically and the root of the lateral incisor buccally. No or small diastemata are present in the arch. Crowding frequently exists.

B The first premolar has emerged first and can migrate distally when the second deciduous molar is exfoliated.

C The second premolar has emerged. The first premolar is initially situated buccally, the second premolar palatally. Both can attain a better position subsequently, if the first permanent molar does not migrate too much mesially. The permanent canine will erupt more or less in contact with the first premolar and the lateral incisor. The latter will demonstrate the typical rotational and labiopalatal movement associated with eruption of an overlapping canine.

D The permanent canine will rotate mesiobuccally and the lateral incisor will become palatally displaced and distopalatally rotated. The canine will attain a crowded and buccally positioned location. The crowding of the incisors can increase, depending on the situation in the anterior region, allowing the canine to attain a less buccal position.

Chapter 7

Changes in the Maxillary Incisor Region Associated With the Transition of Maxillary Posterior Teeth*

7.1 Introduction

As has been explained in the preceding chapters, a marked difference exists between the two jaws in the size and shape of the anterior and middle sections of the apical areas. The differences in tooth sizes, tooth positions before eruption, emergence sequences, and directions of eruption are also reflected in the changes in the maxillary incisor region associated with the transition of the maxillary posterior teeth. The combination of differences between the two jaws results in, among other things, the fact that in general the maxillary canine and incisors do not move distally in the dental arch and do not occupy some of the leeway space that becomes available, as is frequently seen in the mandible.
The relation between the size and shape of the anterior and middle sections of the apical area is discussed. The orientation of and the relations between the teeth involved before and after transition of the posterior teeth are described. Three patterns of changes in the incisor region associated with the transition of the posterior teeth are differentiated on the basis of the spatial conditions in the anterior region before the transition of the posterior teeth. In addition, the changes are related to the conditions in the canine-premolar region.

7.2 Relation between the size and shape of the anterior and middle sections of the apical area

The combined anterior and middle sections of the apical area in the maxilla are considerably smaller than those for the mandible. This is understandable because both the anterior and middle sections of the apical areas are each smaller in the maxilla than

* Reproduced from: "Changes in the upper incisor region, associated with the transition of the upper posterior teeth" by Hein J.W. Wassenberg, Paul J.M.R. Bakker and Frans P.G.M. van der Linden. In: *Transition of the human dentition.* Monograph No. 13. Craniofacial Growth Series., Pg 125-135. Ed. Frans P.G.M. van der Linden. Center for Human Growth and Development. The University of Michigan, Ann Arbor, U.S.A., 1982.

in the mandible. The relatively larger maxillary permanent incisor and canine crowns lead temporarily to closer packing in the maxillary anterior section of the apical area before emergence than in the mandible. Later, the relatively small anterior section of the apical area in the maxilla will be sufficiently large to house the apices of the incisors. Further, the latter teeth are more labially inclined than mandibular incisors. As in the mandible, the permanent canine occupies a key position in the demarcation between the anterior and middle sections of the apical area. Its initial location lateral and adjacent to the piriform aperture is later reflected by the location of its apex. The distance by which the apex descends in the direction of the occlusal plane will depend on the amount of vertical growth of the face. As in the mandible, a large anterior section of the apical area is not always associated with a large middle section. The same holds true for a small section.

The variation in size of the anterior section of the apical area is restricted mainly in the transverse direction, and that of the middle section in the sagittal direction. The demarcation between the two (i.e., where the permanent canine crown is in close proximity to the lateral incisor root) is the region most susceptible to variations. The close proximity of the permanent canine and first premolar crowns before eruption complicates matters further. Both aspects play a special role in the changes in its position, inclination, and angulation that the lateral incisor undergoes when the canine erupts.

The size and anteroposterior position of the anterior segment of the dental arch as it is reflected by the perimeter of the incisal edges of the incisors and canines are affected less by the size and shape of the anterior and middle sections of the apical area in the maxilla than is the case in the mandible. As such the dental arch parameters play a more important role in the maxilla than in the mandible in relation to the changes in the incisor region associated with the transition of the posterior teeth.

7.3 Orientations of and relations between incisors, canine, and premolars before transition of the posterior teeth

The position of the maxillary incisors can vary markedly depending on the size of the anterior section of the apical area, local conditions in the dental arch, and influence of internal and external factors. The space available between their crowns can be considerable. However, contact can also exist and crowding can be present in different degrees. A comparable variation exists in the space available for the incisor roots; they can be far apart or close together. The permanent canine can overlap the root of the lateral incisor to a large extent or only slightly or not at all. In most instances the canine buccally overlaps the first premolar crown. Depending on the size of the middle section of the apical area this overlapping can be larger, smaller, or absent altogether. The second premolar crown does not contact the first premolar and is usually at some distance from the surface of the mesial root of the first permanent molar.

7.4 Conditions in the dental arch after transition of the posterior teeth

The changes experienced by the maxillary lateral permanent incisor in association with the eruption and emergence of the permanent canine have been discussed mainly in the previous chapter. The changes in position of the lateral incisor involve not only rotations and labiolingual movements, but also a mesial migration that will lead to establishing contact between the lateral and central incisor if that contact does not yet exist. The central diastema will become reduced and ultimately the central incisors will contact each other.

When diastemata are small there is only limited space available for the mesial migration of the lateral incisor. Particularly when diastemata are lacking, the lateral incisor may rotate and overlap the central incisor. When the displacement of the lateral incisor is limited the canine will tend to erupt more buccally. The abnormal buccal emergence of the maxillary permanent canine occurs usually when the space between the first premolar and lateral incisor is too small. The possibility of displacement of the two adjacent teeth is mostly limited and a canine that is excluded from the arch will result.

In general, the maxillary canine will emerge after the two premolars have replaced their predecessors. Some distal migration of the premolars may take place when not enough space exists for the erupting canine. Extra space will not usually be provided by the development of crowding in the premolar region; instead, the incisors will be moved closer together and crowding may occur or increase in this region. This difference between the premolar and the incisor region is probably related to three factors. First, the morphology of the incisor crowns, unlike the premolar crowns, facilitates the occurrence of overlapping and crowding. Second, the morphology of the incisor roots and their location within the jaw allow rotations to occur more readily. Third, occlusal interferences are less rigid for the maxillary incisors than for the premolars. It would appear that in critical conditions the incisor alignment will be the first to be sacrificed. Only in extreme conditions will the posterior region have to adapt. The latter is less likely to be the case in the mandible, probably because the limited transverse range of variation between the cortical plates does restrict the amount of possible variation.

7.5 Patterns in changes in the maxillary incisor region associated with transition of the posterior teeth

Symmetry in the size and shape of the middle section of the apical area usually exists in the mandible and maxilla. However, the position of the permanent canine crown can vary. The maxillary canine is the tooth that is most frequently displaced. This displacement usually involves a palatal position and abnormal inclination. It can occur unilaterally or bilaterally. This abnormality is not discussed here because it exceeds the range of normal variation; it is treated in Chapter 13.

Changes taking place in one side of the dental arch will affect the position of the teeth of the other side less than similar changes in the mandible. The central diastema, usually present, limits the transmission from one side to the other. Further, the

intermaxillary suture separates the roots of the two quadrants. These roots do not cross this suture. When the teeth on one side influence those on the other side, the displacement of the crowns and roots occurs within the limitations indicated here. However, it may still involve marked changes in mesiodistal angulation and the passing of the midline by the mesial surface of a central incisor crown.
Three patterns of change can be distinguished based on differences in the space available in the incisor region. Thereafter, the changes will be discussed in reference to the conditions in the canine-premolar region.

7.5.1 Maxillary Incisor Region Changes Pattern A

Pattern A is characterized by excess available space in the anterior segment of the dental arch (Figs. 7-1 and 7-2). The maxillary incisor crowns do not contact each other. There is not only a central diastema, but there are also diastemata between the central incisors and the lateral incisors. The four incisors are well aligned and not rotated. No contact exists between the lateral permanent incisor and the deciduous canine.
The permanent canine crown does not overlap the root of the lateral incisor or does so only slightly. Depending on this relation and the eruption pattern of the canine, the position and inclination of the lateral incisor will change. In instances of extremely excessive space, the erupting and emerging canine does not have a direct effect on the position of the lateral incisor. As a rule, the diastemata reduce after the transition is completed. The mesiodistal angulation of the incisors changes accordingly.

7.5.2 Maxillary Incisor Region Changes Pattern B

Pattern B is characterized by a balance between the required and available dental arch length for the incisors (Figs. 7-3 and 7-4). The incisors are positioned in good alignment

Fig. 7-1 Lateral and occlusal views of a longitudinal series of dental casts of the Maxillary Incisor Region Changes Pattern A, characterized by excess available space in the anterior segment of the dental arch.

A, B Diastemata between the central incisors and between the central and the lateral incisors. The incisors have a normal position and angulation for this stage of development. The first premolar has emerged buccally while its predecessor is still present.

C, D The second premolar, which had only a slightly smaller mesiodistal crown dimension than its predecessor, has emerged. Contact between the second premolar and first permanent molar is established. The permanent canine has emerged at the palatal cervical border of its predecessor. This occasionally happens when the permanent canine occupies a palatal position in relation to the deciduous one. It will then also be less palpable on the buccal side.

E, F The permanent canine is completely erupted without contacting the adjacent teeth. The diastemata between the incisors are reduced but not yet fully closed. The lateral incisor contacts the central incisor. The central diastema is still present. Note that upon completion of the transition, the maxillary second permanent molar has emerged distobuccally directed.

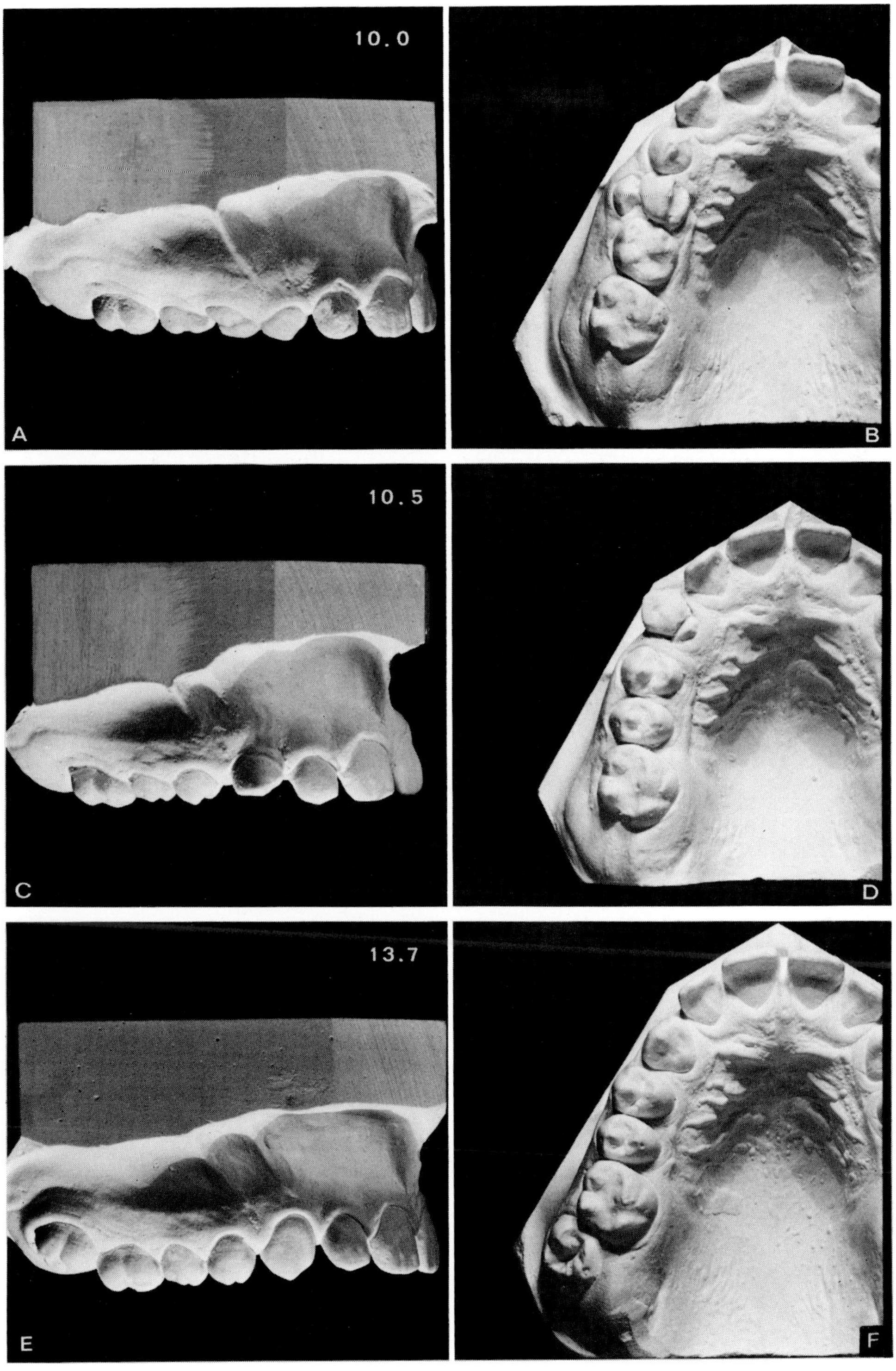

Figure 7-1

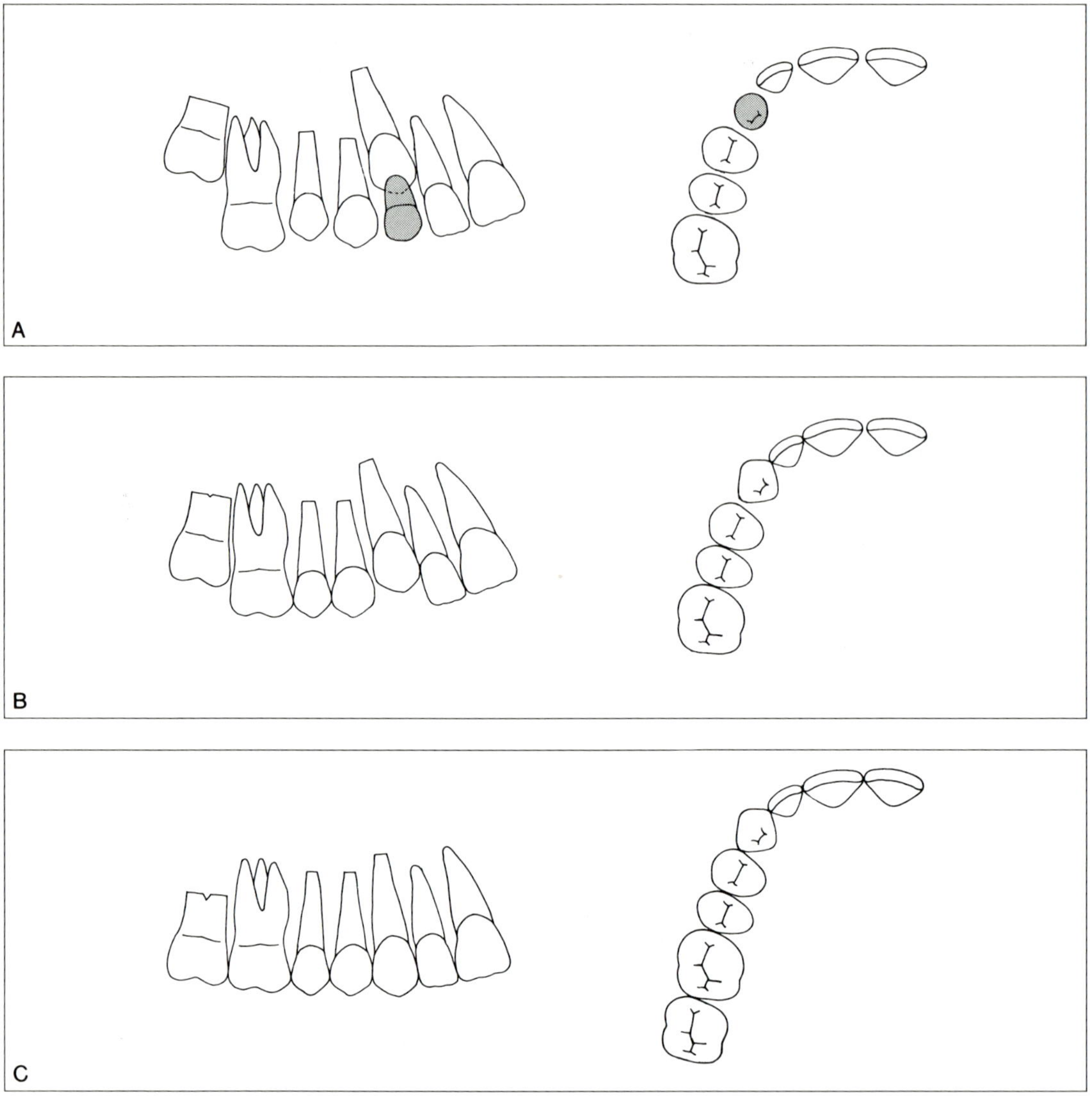

Fig. 7-2 Schematic lateral and occlusal views of the Maxillary Incisor Region Changes Pattern A, characterized by excess available space in the anterior segment of the dental arch.

- *A* *Diastemata exist between the incisors. The permanent canine is at some distance from the lateral incisor and will erupt and emerge without influencing the position of the lateral incisor. There is a diastema between the premolars and one mesial of the first permanent molar.*
- *B* *The permanent canine contacts the lateral incisor crown and moves it mesially. Diastemata in the incisor region become reduced. The lateral incisor contacts the central incisor. The first permanent molar migrated mesially and the diastemata between the premolars are closed.*
- *C* *All teeth are harmoniously aligned. Diastemata have disappeared.*

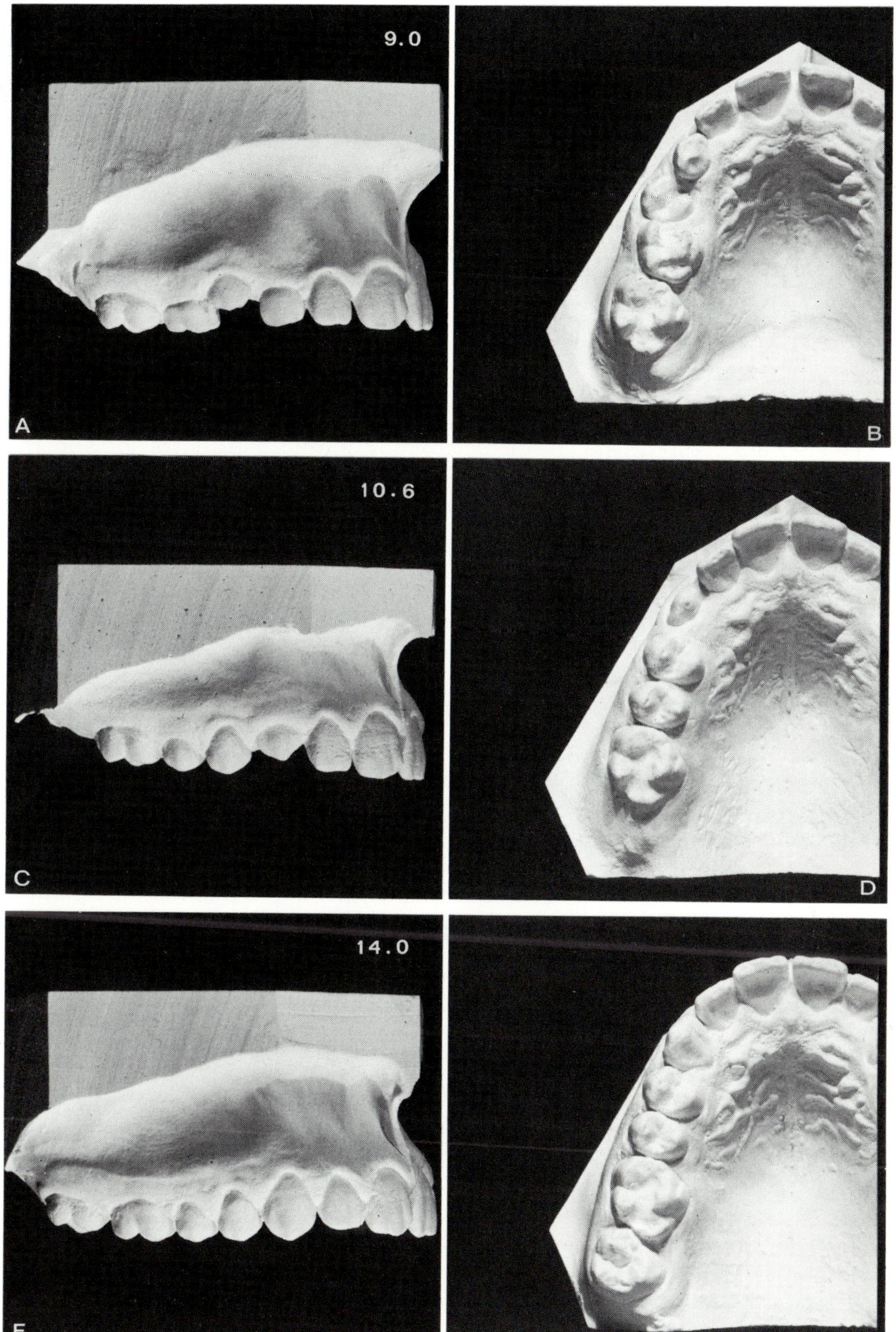

Figure 7-3

Fig. 7-3 (see page 173) Lateral and occlusal views of a longitudinal series of dental casts of the Maxillary Incisor Region Changes Pattern B, characterized by a balance between the required and available dental arch length for the incisors.

A, B The four incisors are positioned normally for this stage of development with a central diastema and contact between the lateral incisor and deciduous canine crown. The first premolar has emerged without excess space.

C, D The second premolar has emerged and is properly positioned within the dental arch. Good contacts exist in the premolar-molar region. The permanent canine has emerged in contact with the lateral incisor. The central diastema is reduced and will close when the canine erupts further.

E, F The canine is harmoniously placed between the adjacent teeth. All teeth are properly positioned.

with some diastemata present. The lateral incisor may contact the central incisor. The canine will erupt in close proximity to the root of the lateral incisor, resulting in the changes in position, inclination, and angulation of the lateral incisor as described in Chapter 6. The emergence and further eruption of the canine will lead to closure of the diastema and contact between the central incisors. Premolars will erupt undisturbed and attain a correct position within the dental arch. No diastemata remain after the transition is completed. The dental arch usually flattens in the anterior region.

7.5.3 Maxillary Incisor Region Changes Pattern C

Pattern C is characterized by a shortage of available space in the anterior segment of the dental arch (Figs. 7-5 and 7-6). Crowding exists in the incisor region. Diastemata are usually absent, and deviant contact points between the incisors reflect the crowded conditions. Prior to emergence the permanent canine is mesially angulated, buccally positioned, and overlaps the lateral incisor root considerably. The canine erupts close to the lateral incisor and will cause changes in the position, inclination, and angulation of the latter in accordance with the relation between the two during the descent of the canine crown. The premolars will usually not move distally and the lack of space will result in increased crowding of the incisors and a buccally positioned canine when it is fully erupted. The premolars may attain a more buccal position.

7.6 Influence of conditions in the canine-premolar segment on the maxillary incisor region during transition of the posterior teeth

As in the mandible, the same three main factors associated with the transition of the posterior teeth play a role in the changes that take place in the incisor region, namely the size of the middle section of the apical area, the size of the leeway space, and the emergence sequence of the premolars and canine. In the maxilla the early or late emergence of the second permanent molar is an additional factor.

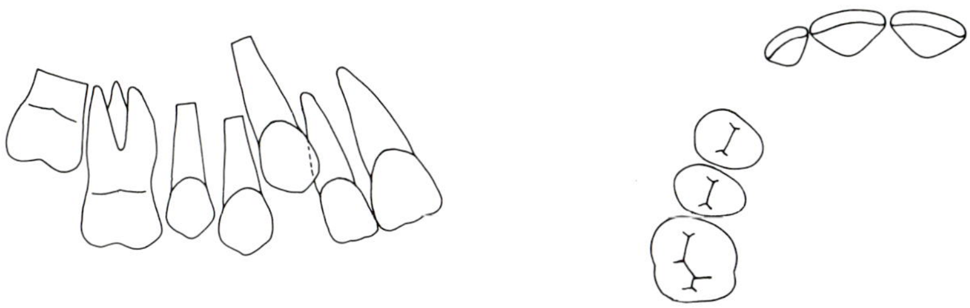

A

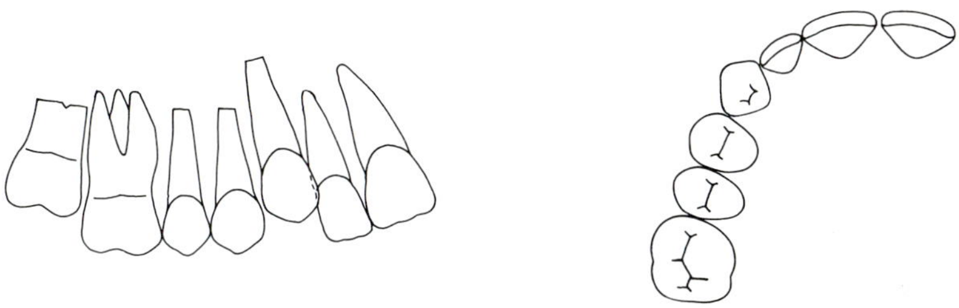

B

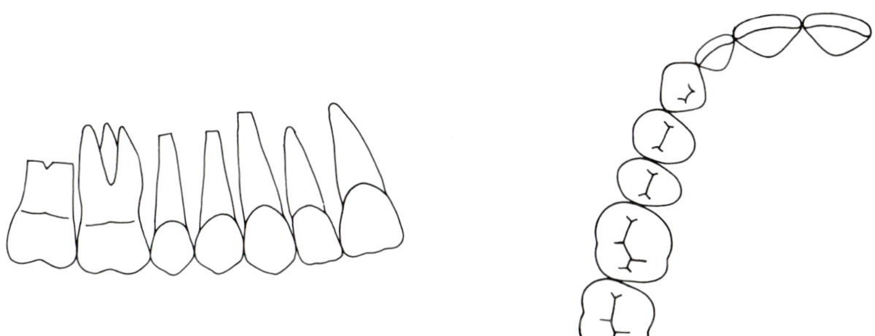

C

Fig. 7-4 Schematic lateral and occlusal views of the Maxillary Incisor Region Changes Pattern B, characterized by a balance between the required and available dental arch length for the incisors.

A The incisors are properly positioned. A central diastema exists. The lateral incisor may be in contact with or slightly separated from the central incisor. The erupting canine overlaps the lateral incisor. The diastemata between the incisors will become reduced.

B The diastemata between the premolars are closed because of the mesial migration of the first permanent molar. The canine has emerged properly positioned within the dental arch.

C The roots of the permanent teeth are about equally distributed over the space available within the alveolar bone. The dental arch usually flattens in the anterior region.

In cases of excess available space in the incisor region the four factors mentioned above are not important and do not affect the end result. The extra space required for the permanent canine crown, which is larger in size compared to its predecessor, is available in excess.

Cases of a balance between the required and available dental arch length for the incisors will depend on a favourable combination of the four factors involved. A small middle section of the apical area can lead to an undesirable development when an unfavourable sequence of emergence occurs (see Chapter 6). The relation between the permanent canine and lateral incisor is also critical. Considerable variation can exist in this respect (e.g., a mesially angulated, buccally placed permanent canine results in undesirable changes). Early emergence of the second permanent molar may lead to more mesial migration of the first permanent molar, with, as a consequence, a loss of leeway space otherwise utilised by the canine. The emergence sequence of the permanent canine, second molar, and finally both premolars is critical in this regard. Slight differences in timing may have a relatively large effect.

Cases of a shortage of available space in the anterior segment of the dental arch are even more dependent on a favourable combination of the four factors described. Incisors can demonstrate a marked increase in crowding and canines can assume positions completely outside the dental arch. In contrast to comparable situations in the mandible, only a little can be gained from the leeway space. Further, it would appear that maxillary permanent molars migrate mesially more readily than mandibular permanent molars[155] and are unlikely to spontaneously move distally later.

7.7 Supplementary remarks

The role played by the occlusion in the changes in position of the maxillary teeth is comparable to that for the mandibular teeth, which has been explained in Chapter 4. However, it would appear that the changes in position of the maxillary incisors depend

Fig. 7-5 Lateral and occlusal views of a longitudinal series of dental casts of the Maxillary Incisor Region Changes Pattern C, characterized by a shortage of available space in the anterior segment of the dental arch.

A, B Crowding in the incisor region with slight overlapping and abnormal contacts. No diastemata are present between the incisors and between the deciduous canine and the lateral incisor. The first premolar is almost fully erupted and the second premolar has recently emerged.

C, D The premolars attained a good position within the dental arch. The permanent canine emerged buccally and partly overlaps the lateral incisor crown. The diastema mesial to the second premolar reflects the mesially directed path of eruption of the canine.

E, F The canine is fully erupted and the incisor crowding has increased considerably. The canine is not in an extreme buccal position, which would have been the case had incisor crowding not been aggravated.

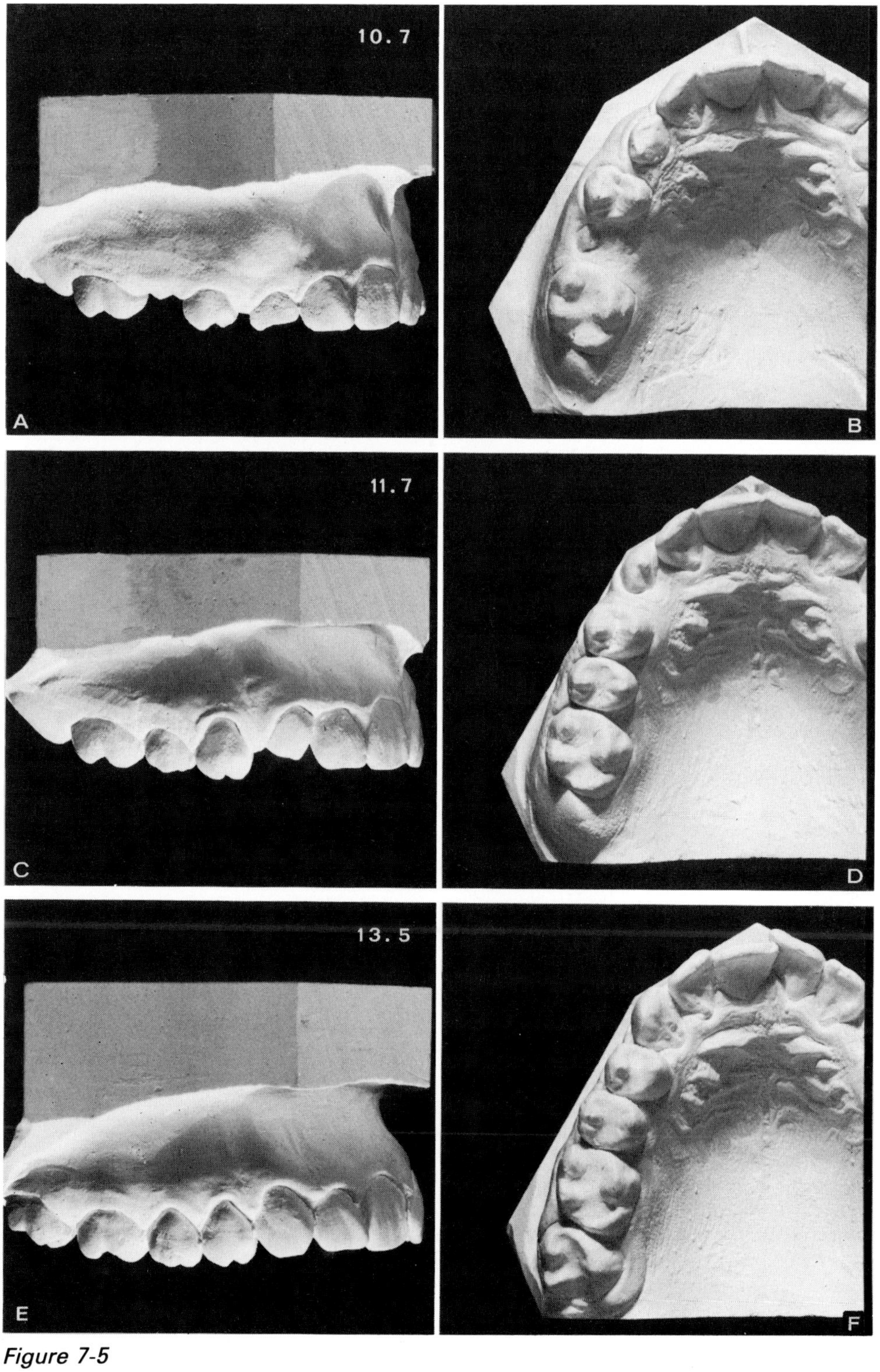

Figure 7-5

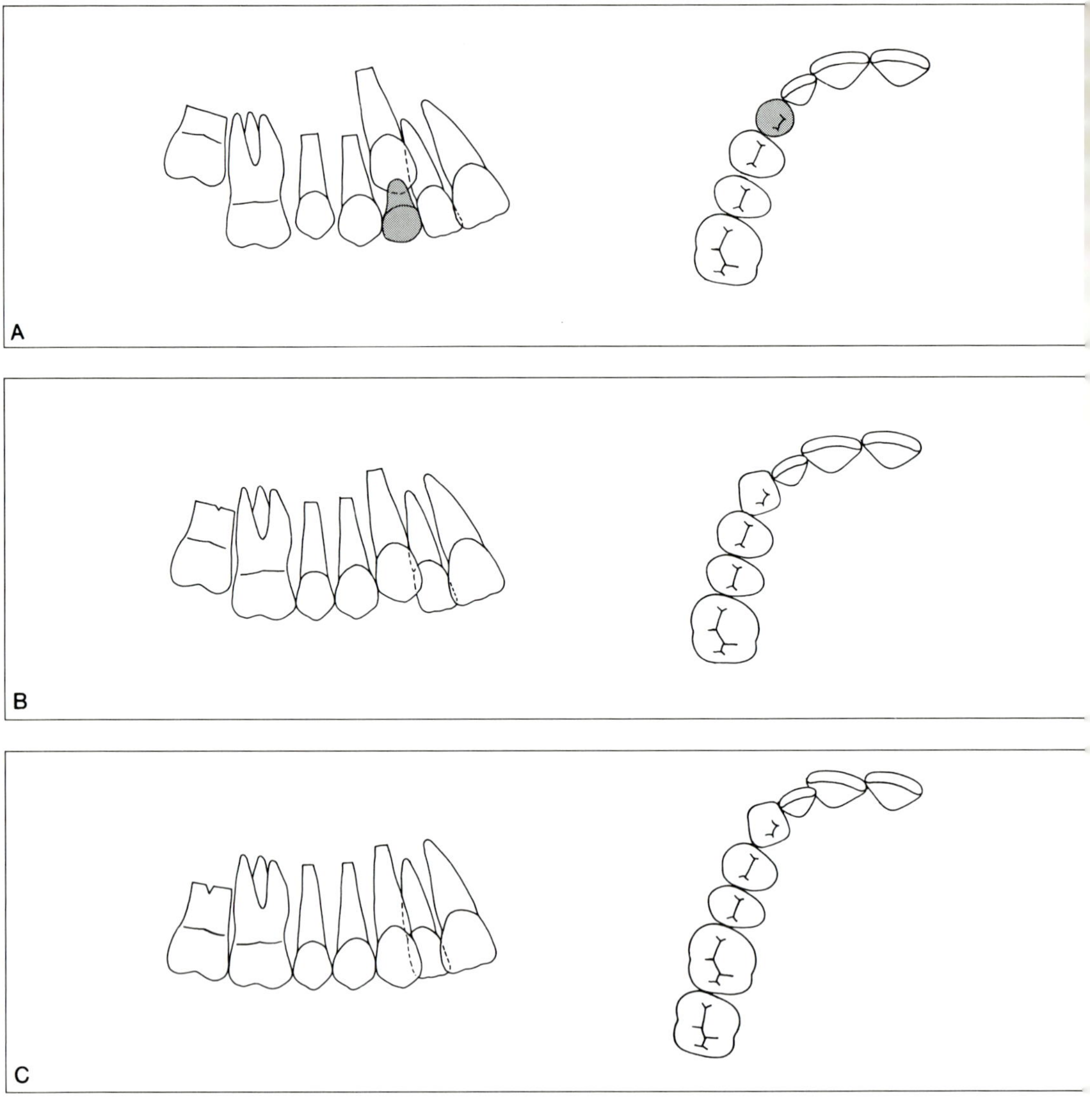

Fig. 7-6 *Schematic lateral and occlusal views of the Maxillary Incisor Region Changes Pattern C, characterized by a shortage of available space in the anterior segment of the dental arch.*

A *The crowded condition in the anterior region eliminates the possibility of normal mesial migration of the lateral incisor in association with the eruption of the permanent canine. The overlapping of the incisors will increase when the lateral incisor moves mesially.*

B *The permanent canine has emerged in mesiolabial rotation. It displaces the lateral incisor mesially but with an associated increase in crowding.*

C *The canine is not in an extreme buccal position. The incisors overlap. In cases where crowding of the incisors does not increase, the canine will become more buccally located.*

more on the development of the mandibular incisors than vice versa. In cases of good incisal occlusion in the anterior region, the location of the maxillary incisors and canines is partly determined by the position of the mandibular incisors and canines. The changes in the incisor region associated with the transition of the posterior teeth cannot take place independently in the mandibular or maxillary arch. The occlusion in the posterior and anterior regions plays an essential role in this respect.

The most sensitive and vulnerable area in the maxilla is the lateral incisor-canine-first premolar region. However, the latter tooth will seldom be abnormally placed because it usually emerges before the canine and its position does not readily change. That does not hold true for the lateral incisor, which will have to pay a portion of the debt in cases of lack of space. However, it is more frequently the canine that becomes displaced and excluded from the dental arch.

Chapter 8

Problems in the Transition of Mandibular and Maxillary Incisors

8.1 Introduction

Most children experience loosening of the central deciduous incisors as the first sign of the imminent transition from the deciduous to permanent dentition. The preceding increase in spacing between the deciduous incisors is scarcely noticed. It is commonly thought that deciduous teeth of a 5- or 6-year-old child are diminutive and that the successors, especially the maxillary central permanent incisors, are extraordinarily large. Both views are understandable and fit in with the picture of a continuously growing face in which the mesiodistal sizes of the crowns of the teeth do not increase. A maxillary central permanent incisor that emerges at the age of 7 years will normally not fit harmoniously into the face until facial growth has been completed much later. The transition of the incisors is often followed more carefully by the child and parents than other processes of the development of the dentition because these changes occur in the anterior part of the mouth, can be easily followed, and above all have a marked effect on appearance. It is also noteworthy that incisor transition is marked by considerable variation. Parents frequently become concerned, fortunately unnecessarily so.

Various aspects of transition in the incisor region are considered below. Disturbances in transition and their causes are discussed. In particular the consequences of traumata to deciduous teeth are dealt with. Thought is given to supernumerary teeth, hypertrophic frena, large multiple diastemata, reverse overbite, thumb-sucking, and abnormal tongue and lip posture. Taking records and making observations are covered. Finally, differential diagnosis of a large maxillary central diastema is described.

Fewer problems come to light in incisor transition in the mandible than in the maxilla. In this chapter the accent lies therefore on the maxillary incisor transition. Problems in mandibular incisor transition will be dealt with as they arise.

8.2 Asymmetries in times and positions of emergence

In the mandible, little difference exists between left and right as far as it concerns the time when deciduous teeth are lost and the moment when their successors emerge in the mouth. Normally, there is also little difference in the position at which teeth emerge, as long as the teeth are properly formed and no crowding exists.

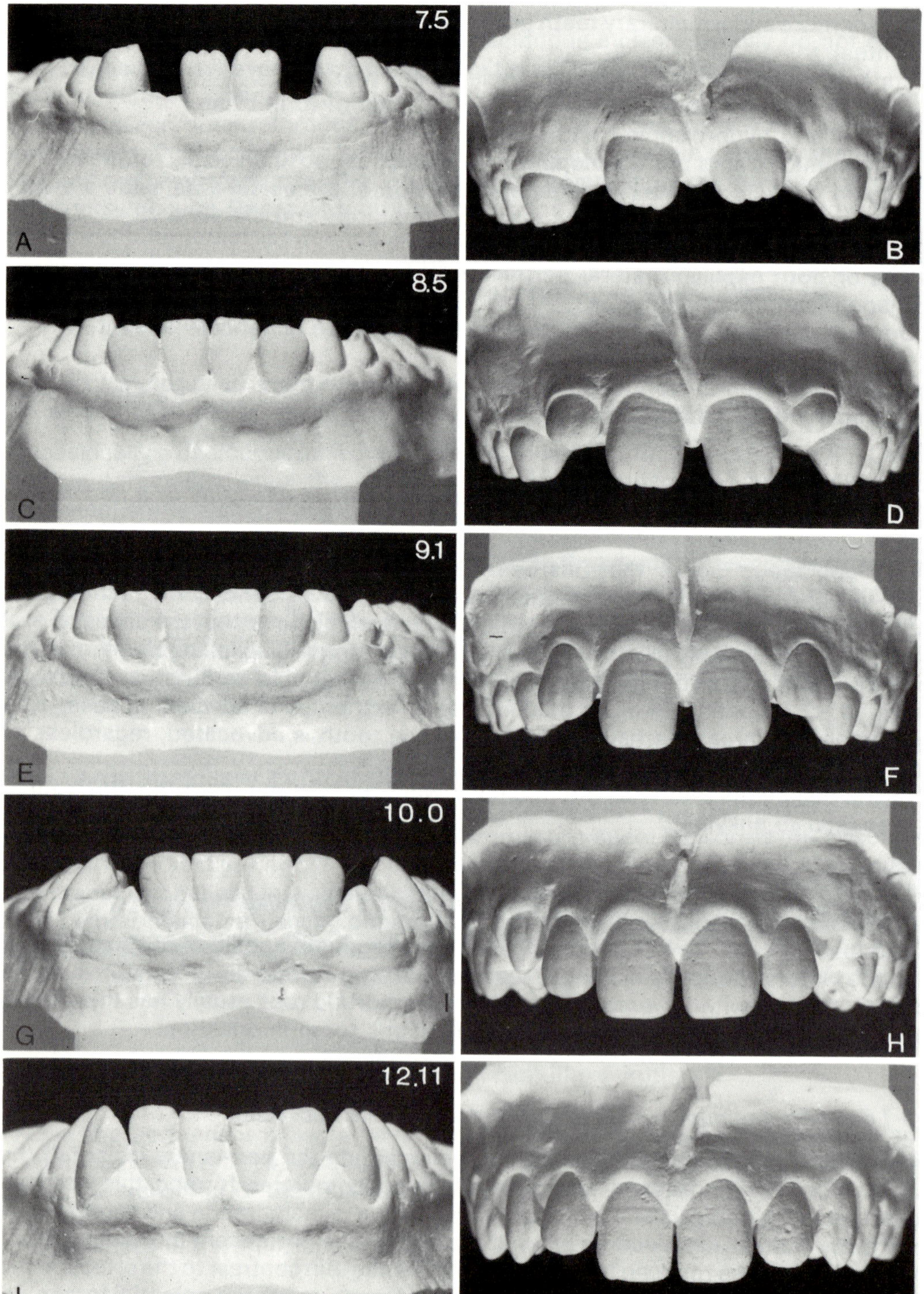

Figure 8-1

Fig. 8-1 Natural development of the dentition in a boy, showing changes in the mandibular and maxillary incisors during transition and some time after.

A, B *At the age of 7 years 8 months the two mandibular central permanent incisors have almost reached the level of the occlusal plane. They are in contact. The two maxillary central permanent incisors, which emerged later, are situated well apart and their crowns diverge.*

C, D *At the age of 8 years 5 months the mandibular lateral permanent incisors have emerged and almost reached the occlusal plane; there is mandibular incisor crowding.*
The maxillary lateral incisors have emerged without contact with the central incisors; their crowns diverge. The central diastema has become smaller.

E, F *At 9 years 1 month the distal surfaces of the mandibular lateral incisors are located labial to the mesial surfaces of the deciduous canines; the mandibular permanent incisors as a block are more labially placed than their predecessors were. The maxillary lateral permanent incisors have moved further occlusally. There is no contact anywhere between the four incisors. The central diastema has diminished further.*

G, H *At 10 years the mandibular permanent canines have emerged, more labially than where their predecessors had been. During the transition of the canines the lateral incisors' positions have improved. Also, in the maxilla the permanent canines have emerged recently; they likewise take up a position more labial than their predecessors. There is now contact between the central and lateral incisors. The central diastema is still narrower.*

I, J *At 12 years 11 months there is good contact between mandibular canines and lateral incisors. The mandibular incisors are in regular alignment.*
The maxillary canines have almost reached the occlusal plane. The central diastema is almost closed. The mesiodistal angulation of the incisors has improved ever since emergence until now, and this process continues.

This series of illustrations shows the spontaneous improvement in alignment over a period of more than 5 years and indicates that in the normal course of events there may be irregular situations that correct themselves and thus treatment of those conditions is definitely not acceptable. In general, the difference in times of emergence of corresponding mandibular and maxillary permanent teeth is greater than in this example. On average, maxillary teeth emerge about 1 year later than mandibular teeth. The numbers in the illustrations denote the age in years and months. (From Van der Linden.[226])

8.5.4 Loss of a deciduous incisor with displacement of its successor

As a result of trauma to the deciduous incisor, the permanent incisor may be displaced within the jaw. This leads not only to an abnormal position of the permanent tooth before emergence, it also changes its orientation with respect to the forming part of the tooth, which can result in a deviation in the long axis of the tooth (dilaceration). The displacement of the crown of the permanent incisor through trauma in the deciduous dentition is usually dorsal.[7] Subsequent formation of the tooth involves tissues that have not been displaced joined to those that have indeed been displaced. This produces a kink in the eventual form of the tooth. The size of the deviation is related to the extent of the displacement; the location of the deviation is related to the degree of formation reached at the time of the trauma. The deviation can occur in the crown, though usually it is in the root (Figs. 8-2 and 8-3).

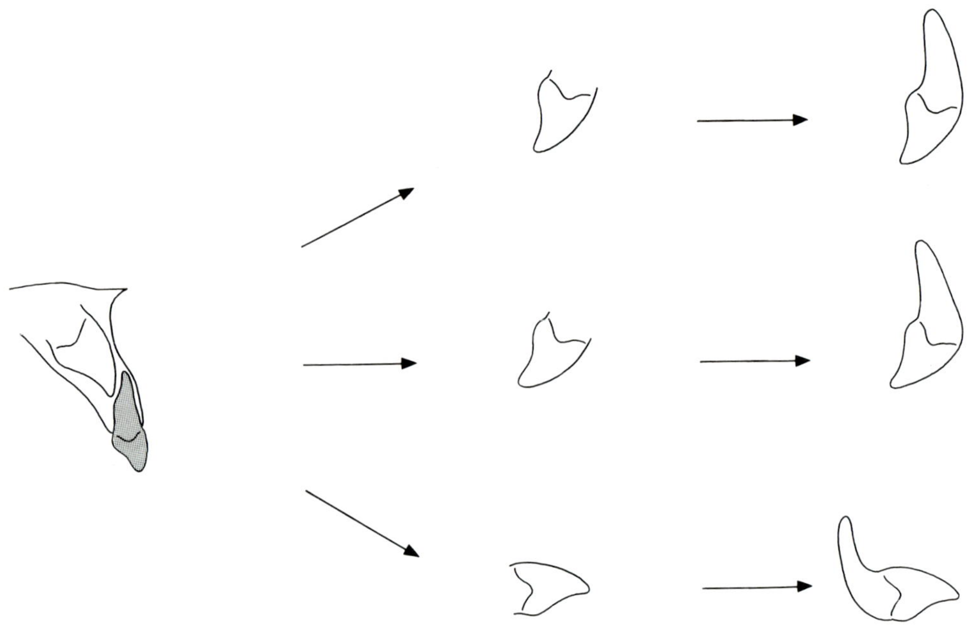

Fig. 8-2 Consequences of trauma to the predecessor, which displaces a central permanent incisor, related to the degree of displacement of the tooth.

A Situation at the moment of trauma.
B Depending on the extent and direction of the forces due to the trauma, the crown can be displaced more or less; the deciduous incisor may or may not be lost.
C Subsequent tooth formation leads to a kink in the tooth, because the forming part of the tooth has been slightly displaced, if at all. The extent of the deviation is related to the degree of displacement of the already formed part of the tooth.

The prognosis for preservation of the tooth will depend on the extent of the dilaceration. A central permanent incisor with an acute labial deviation of the crown will find its root apex penetrating the labial alveolar wall if the crown is brought into alignment with the rest of the arch. Moreover, there will often be excessive root resorption during the necessary tooth movement.

Maxillary central incisors can also be displaced cranially by trauma to their predecessors. This can result in the crown coming to lie more horizontally; the kink is then labial. Displacement of the permanent incisor crown is difficult to explain mechanically. Perhaps the displacement depends on the obstacle that is presented by scar tissue.[138] Clinically, maxillary central incisors with a labial kink cause more problems than those with a palatal kink, and they are also probably noticed earlier because of those problems.

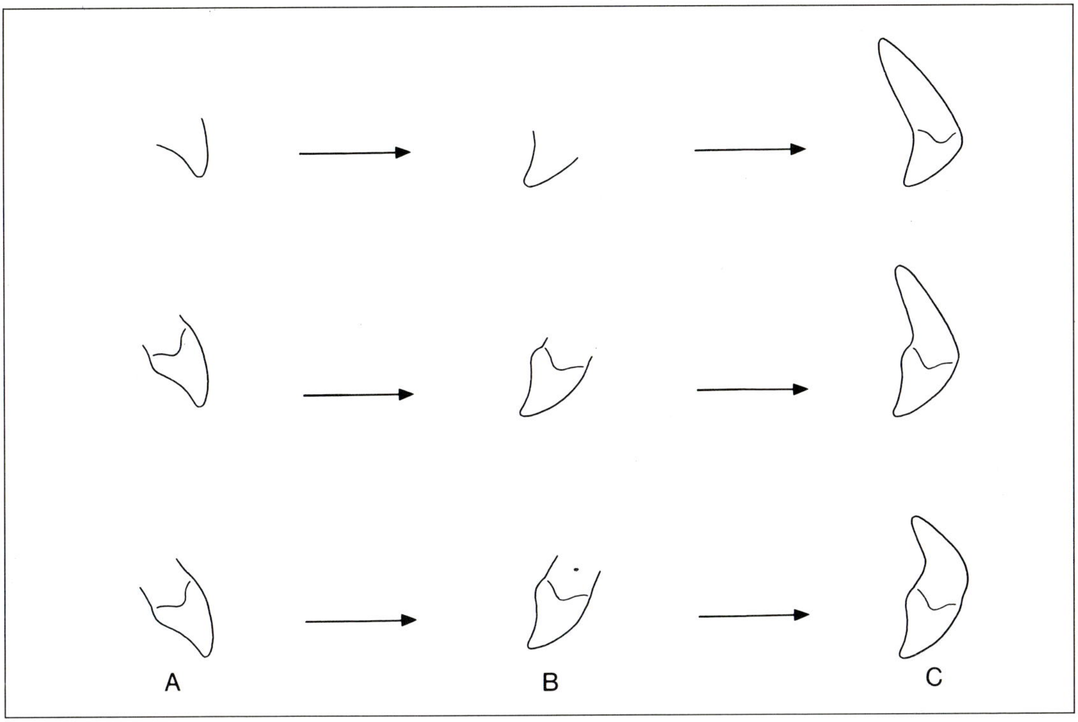

Fig. 8-3 Consequences of trauma to the predecessor, which displaces a central permanent incisor, related to the stage of tooth formation.

A Situation at the moment of trauma.
B Depending on the stage of tooth formation the locations of the deviation will differ.
C The remaining portion of the tooth is completed in its original location, or a location only differing a little from that. The dilaceration can be situated in the almost completed crown, or at different levels along the root.

Depending on the stage of tooth formation at the moment of trauma, the prognosis for retention of the tooth will differ. If the dilaceration is in the crown or the cervical third of the root, removal of the tooth is indicated.

When the displacement of a permanent incisor is minimal the incisor will emerge spontaneously, even if delayed. Of course it often penetrates the mucosa more labially and higher than normal. This leads eventually to a relatively longer clinical crown. If a tooth emerges outside the keratinised zone, no attached gingiva forms labially. High emergence of a central permanent incisor also occurs occasionally in cases when previous inflammation originating from the deciduous predecessor has been associated with a fistula.[30]

8.5.5 Intrusion of a deciduous incisor

A deciduous tooth forced into the alveolar process produces similar results to those mentioned previously (8.5.1, 8.5.2, and 8.5.3). The tooth will usually move occlusally back from its infraposition. After initially being lost from view it can reemerge; it often remains in infraposition subsequently.
It is usually pointless to try to determine what effect trauma in the deciduous dentition has had, before the time has arrived when the succedaneous teeth normally would have emerged. The critical matter is to decide whether the associated permanent tooth can later attain its normal position in the dental arch. A decision is required only if the appropriate time has arrived when, in the light of future therapy, the relevant permanent tooth needs to be surgically exposed or removed. Two considerations are essential in this respect. One relates to the manner by which further development of the dentition can be guided, in particular through inducing spontaneous changes by which part of the therapy can be achieved. The second consideration involves the consequences of intervention by oral surgery, particularly prevention of damage to teeth that are still developing. Furthermore, it is important to limit the extent of bone loss, especially where the labial and lingual walls of the alveolar process are concerned. The thin cortical plate does not fully return after removal.
On the basis of the aforementioned considerations, further investigation of the effect of an injury to the deciduous dentition on the morphology and emergence of a central permanent incisor is not indicated before the lateral permanent incisors are fully emerged. One should bear in mind that loss of a maxillary central deciduous incisor usually leads to a delayed emergence (about 1 year) of its successor.[101] Further, such a premature loss can, by the associated delay in eruption of its successor, unfavourably influence the spatial development of the maxillary arch, because eruption of the central permanent incisor plays a role in increased intercanine distance.[223]

8.5.6 Trauma followed by a periapical abscess on a deciduous incisor

Intrusion of a deciduous incisor, or trauma in general, can result in pulpal necrosis. The consequence is inflammation with bone loss periapically. If no treatment is instituted the process can spread extensively, because no connective tissue encapsulation of the apical inflammation occurs with deciduous teeth as it does with permanent teeth. Inflammation caused by the necrotic pulp tissue of a deciduous tooth can give rise to defective enamel formation in the as yet unerupted permanent tooth.[223] After trauma to a deciduous incisor one must watch for possible loss of vitality. The measures that need be taken have already been described in 8.5.1.

8.5.7 Midline supernumerary teeth

In the proximity of the median suture of the maxilla one or more supernumerary teeth occasionally can be found. They are usually conical or tear drop in form and can be oriented in any direction.[21] If they have a normal path of eruption and are not too abnormal in form (e.g., peg shaped) they can emerge near the midline. After emergence they can be extracted, in adherence to the rule that supernumerary teeth with no useful function should be removed directly after emergence. Further

development of the dentition can then proceed normally. Intervention to correct any effects of the earlier presence of a supernumerary tooth is generally unnecessary.
Midline supernumerary teeth that do not erupt spontaneously should be removed. The choice of the time to act depends on the same factors as those mentioned in 8.5.5. Despite the fact that in particular cases the early removal of the supernumerary tooth will assist spontaneous correction, it usually is best to delay it until there is no perceptible risk that the remaining teeth might be damaged.[233] That stage is reached when all four maxillary incisors are fully erupted and the roots of the central incisors are almost fully formed (age 10 to 14 years). If a supernumerary tooth interferes with the eruption of a central incisor, or if a follicular cyst develops around it, then early removal is indicated. After removal of a supernumerary tooth at an early age it is essential to pay attention to the possibility of delayed eruption of the teeth still to emerge in that area.
The effect that one or more supernumerary teeth in the midline may have on the alignment of the maxillary incisors is determined by their number, size, and location. One or two supernumerary teeth can be present without any sign being given by the permanent incisors.

8.5.8 Other supernumerary teeth

Occasionally a maxillary lateral permanent incisor is duplicated. In such cases the predecessor is often double as well. They are almost always adequately oriented and emerge normally.[75,93] If the crowns of the authentic and supernumerary teeth closely correspond in colour, form, and size, the decision as to which of the two should be extracted will be made essentially on the basis of root formation and position relative to the dental arch.

8.5.9 Abnormal shape or size of maxillary permanent incisors

Sometimes the crown of one maxillary central permanent incisor is significantly wider than that of the other side. More seldom the crown of one or both maxillary lateral incisors will be unusually large. Quite often one encounters the opposite, where the maxillary lateral incisors are very narrow. In such situations it is advisable, after all permanent incisors are in place, to make a tooth set-up for visualizing an optimal arrangement in three dimensions. Should other anomalies in the position of the teeth or jaws be present, the situation in the maxillary incisors must be seen in relation to the overall diagnosis and treatment planning. In those circumstances it might be appropriate to extract such incisors. Building up crowns by means of composite resins is a very practicable proposition. Abberations of enamel formation and size and form can readily be disguised.

8.5.10 Hypertrophic frenum

Some children exhibit a pronounced maxillary labial frenum that runs between the central incisors to the incisive papilla. If the upper lip is pulled outward, putting such a frenum under tension, the palatal tissues in the region of the incisive papilla may

blanch. If that tissue does not blanch then it can be assumed that a string of connective tissue does not run from the labial surface to the palate.
The great majority of frena, including those that originally ran from labial to palatal surface, gradually disappear naturally by the time of emergence and installation of the lateral permanent incisors and canines. The central diastema then closes. [16,43,160,228]
Extirpation of a frenum before the permanent canines have fully emerged is seldom indicated. Absence of gradual decrease of the diastema and of reduction of the labial frenum indicate the presence of other phenomena that can be responsible for the persistence of the central diastema. In this connection agenesis of lateral incisors or presence of a supernumerary tooth in the midline can be mentioned.
The aspects of differential diagnosis in this area are still to be dealt with.

8.6 Disturbances in the transition of mandibular incisors

Trauma to mandibular deciduous incisors is seldom seen. Supernumerary teeth also are less frequently observed in the mandible.[29] However, one does occasionally find an extra lateral incisor there. Such teeth are difficult or impossible to distinguish from the other teeth in shape, size, or colour. The problem can usually be solved simply by extracting an incisor. If it is not done, then as a rule, in otherwise normal circumstances, diastemata among the maxillary incisors remain.
The most common problem in the transition of the mandibular incisors is crowding of the permanent incisors. Primary crowding is nowhere so often evident nor so pronounced as in the anterior part of the mandible. Rotations and overlapping of the mandibular permanent incisors may be present even before emergence. After emergence the influence of tongue and lips can secure only a minimal improvement in their position.
Mandibular lateral permanent incisors always emerge a little more lingually in the dental arch than do central incisors. Subsequently, they take up their correct positions under the influence of the tongue if sufficient space is available. Sometimes the opportunity for this improvement does not happen until the posterior teeth begin to exfoliate.
The mandibular incisors distinguish themselves from the maxillary incisors in their ability to be moved across the median plane. The maxilla has a median suture, and the mandible does not. With a small anterior section of the apical area in the mandible, the crowding can be concentrated unilaterally. Mandibular incisors can for this reason emerge tilted mesiodistally. An erupting lateral permanent incisor can cause resorption of the root of its predecessor and of the adjacent deciduous canine (see Chapter 9).

8.7 Large multiple diastemata

When relatively ample room is present in the jaws (large anterior section of the apical area) the transition of the mandibular and maxillary incisors is usually untroubled. In such cases abnormal locations of the tooth germs of the incisors rarely occur. If they emerge too far labially or lingually they will subsequently assume a better position in the dental arch. After full eruption multiple diastemata may remain. In such circumstances it is irresponsible to indulge in active closure of the diastemata just because they exist. At the very least one should wait until all permanent teeth have erupted fully (with the exception of the third molars) and facial growth and maturation of the facial musculature are largely complete. Meanwhile, the diastemata may diminish spontaneously in the course of normal development. In addition, continuing growth of the face will lead to further enclosure of the dentition and the diastemata diminish in their obtrusiveness even if they do not change in size.

8.8 Reverse overbite

A previously normal situation in the deciduous dentition can be converted to a reverse overbite as the result of a slightly abnormal position or direction of eruption, giving rise to reversed incisal contact between the permanent teeth. With continuing eruption the affected teeth will diverge more from normal. Frequently a ventral forced bite develops with or without a lateral forced bite combined with it. Without question, it is preferable to prevent a reverse overbite. Usually the dentist is not confronted with it until the reverse overbite has been in existence for some time. In cases of sufficient space in the dental arch, a correction can often be achieved in a short time by using a tongue blade or an inclined plane fixed to the mandibular teeth. Because the first method operates reciprocally a simultaneous change in mandibular and maxillary teeth can be obtained that will enable a good sagittal overbite to develop. With an inclined plane the displacement is mainly limited to maxillary teeth.

Persisting deciduous incisors can lead to a reverse overbite. Such a development should be prevented and the deciduous teeth concerned extracted in time.

When a reverse overbite is encountered involving several teeth, attention should be given to a possible mandibular prognathism.

8.9 Thumb-sucking

The pressure exerted when intensive thumb-sucking and finger-sucking is indulged in leads to an open bite in the deciduous dentition, a frequently asymmetric eversion of the maxillary incisors, a protrusion of the alveolar process, and sometimes a linguoversion of the mandibular incisors. The frequency and vigour of the abnormal habit determine to a large extent the degree of deviation. When the deciduous incisors exfoliate but the habit continues, a comparable abnormality in the conformation of the permanent incisors will develop.

In general, it is worthwhile breaking a sucking habit about 6 months before loss of the deciduous incisors is due. Then the associated deviations can begin to correct before transition. On the other hand, it has yet to be proven that continuing with an abnormal sucking habit up to the second transitional phase leads to permanent detrimental consequences. If a child is in a position of being able, without creating other problems, to cease a sucking habit before transition of the incisors, then every effort should be devoted to that objective. But when there is clear evidence that such is not the case, it is better not to make a fuss about it, because later cessation can still produce spontaneous correction of any disturbances in the arches.

8.10 Abnormal tongue posture

Some children hold their tongues between their mandibular and maxillary incisors, which can lead to premature cessation of vertical eruption. Tongue interposition can also be associated with eversion of the incisors. Transition of the incisors in such instances will be adapted to the position of the tongue.
Such a tongue position makes itself evident when speaking. Tongue interposition can be considered the principal etiological factor in an anterior open bite when cessation of a sucking habit is not followed by further eruption of the affected incisors.

8.11 Interposing lower lip

In extreme Class II/1 anomalies in young children the lower lip rests behind the maxillary deciduous incisors. In such instances facial orthopedic therapy in the deciduous dentition using a functional appliance (activator) should be considered. Most situations where the lower lip interposes are only apparent after two to four maxillary permanent incisors have emerged. These teeth take up a more labial position than their predecessors and have a more labial inclination. The same applies to mandibular incisors, but to a lesser extent. Interposition of the lower lip after transition will give rise to further increase in the labial position and inclination of the maxillary incisors and reduction of those of the mandibular incisors. The incomplete establishment of the root length amplifies the tipping effect. Moreover, the maxillary permanent incisors can now overerupt because adequate vertical support from the lower lip is lacking.
Treatment of Class II/1 anomalies in which the lower lip lies behind the maxillary incisors should be started earlier than when this is not so. This conclusion does not only depend on the above changes in labiolingual position and inclination and overeruption of the maxillary permanent incisors. The danger of trauma to the prominent incisors is also important. Further, the severity of the sagittal discrepancy between the dental arches, which in these instances is usually a full premolar crown width, demands a relatively early start in orthodontic therapy also. An activator is often an appropriate appliance to alter the vulnerable and unfavourable situation. Further discussion of different factors that are important in the prevention and cure of lip interposition will be covered in Chapter 12.

8.12 Anamnesis and examination

When disturbances occur in the transition of the incisors one must first enquire whether or not any members of the family have suffered from agenesis, supernumerary teeth in the midline or elsewhere, or teeth of anomalous form. Furthermore, it needs to be discovered if an injury has been suffered in the past that involved the front of the mouth. One should look for evidence of abnormal habits in sucking or other things. It should be remembered that question-asking may not elicit the necessary information. For example, frequently poking a pencil between the maxillary incisors may be the reason for a central diastema inexplicably remaining open, but if the question is asked "do you suck your thumb?" it is unlikely that the child will say, "no, but I poke a pencil between my teeth."

After the position and inclination of the teeth, the occlusion, and the soft tissue influences have been inspected, the examination should be broadened using a mouth mirror. The alveolar process should be felt with the fingers to test the presence and location of as yet unerupted permanent teeth and to detect possible abnormalities. By holding the alveolar process with the fingers of one hand and trying with the other hand to move the deciduous and permanent teeth that are present, a clearer picture of the position, form, and length of the matching roots can be obtained. Careful palpation can yield much useful information.

Radiographs should only be taken when the desired information cannot be obtained by other means and are necessary at that moment to make a responsible decision as to whether to take action.

When only an abnormality of incisor transition is apparent, it is seldom indicated to take radiographs until all the maxillary incisors have emerged or should have done so. At this point it makes sense to consider whether panoramic radiographs would be more useful. One should weigh the inherent lack of detail in the orthopantomogram against the advantage of greater coverage of the jaws and the more limited skin dose. For example, one can immediately ascertain if all premolars are developing when an orthopantomogram is available. Bite-wing radiographs can also often provide that information but would not be first choice if knowledge of the apical regions is required. A small midline supernumerary tooth can easily be seen on a periapical film, whereas an orthopantomogram often shows that region indistinctly.

8.13 Differential diagnosis of a large maxillary central diastema

On the basis of the records and examination of the patient one can try to reach a differential diagnosis regarding the presence of a large diastema between the maxillary central permanent incisors. The following possibilities should be taken into account:

1. Injury in the deciduous dentition. The effect of injury is usually asymmetric and seldom results in failure of a central diastema to diminish in size.
2. Abnormal location of tooth germs. Certainly where the anterior section of the apical area is large, the maxillary central permanent incisors might be laid down a

9.2 Morphological differences between mandible and maxilla

In the mandible permanent teeth can cross the midline even before emergence. There is no longer a partition between right and left halves of the jaw once the symphysis is calcified before the emergence of the deciduous incisors. The crowding in the mandible can concentrate itself, as it were, on one side. In the maxilla the median palatal suture remains in existence and cannot be crossed by teeth. The crowns of the maxillary central incisors can, after emergence, migrate mesially and tip. But the roots do not cross the suture. Hence, unilateral spontaneous early loss is seen more often in the mandible than the maxilla.
In the mandible the crowns of the central permanent incisors are narrower than those of the lateral incisors, hence a lateral deciduous incisor seldom is lost prematurely from the mandible. On the other hand, premature resorption and loss of the mandibular deciduous canine occurs relatively often. In the maxilla with its wide central permanent incisors, premature loss of the lateral deciduous incisor is quite likely. The root of the deciduous canine in the maxilla resorbs prematurely less often than in the mandible. This difference stems primarily from the greater space available for the emerging maxillary lateral incisor to migrate as compared to the limited space in the mandible. Further consideration will not be given here to the underlying difference between the jaws respecting the positions of the permanent teeth before emergence, their crown dimensions, and the size of the anterior section of the apical area. These aspects have been treated extensively in preceding chapters.

9.3 Consequences of premature loss through resorption

The early creation of extra space in the dental arch assists improvement of the positions of the permanent incisors already present or as yet unerupted. Rotations can self-correct, overlaps can reduce. Against this is the fact that the increase in the intercanine width that normally ensues in association with the transition of the incisors does not occur after premature loss of deciduous teeth that are essential for this increase. The available arch length is usually negatively influenced by the premature loss of deciduous incisors and canines. Unilateral premature loss, or bilateral loss with a significant time difference between times of loss, leads to a deviation of the midpoint of the dental arch (Figs. 9-1 and 9-2).
Displacement of a tooth before formation is complete can give rise to deformation of the root. This can be seen in a mandibular lateral permanent incisor after unilateral premature loss of a deciduous canine.[227]

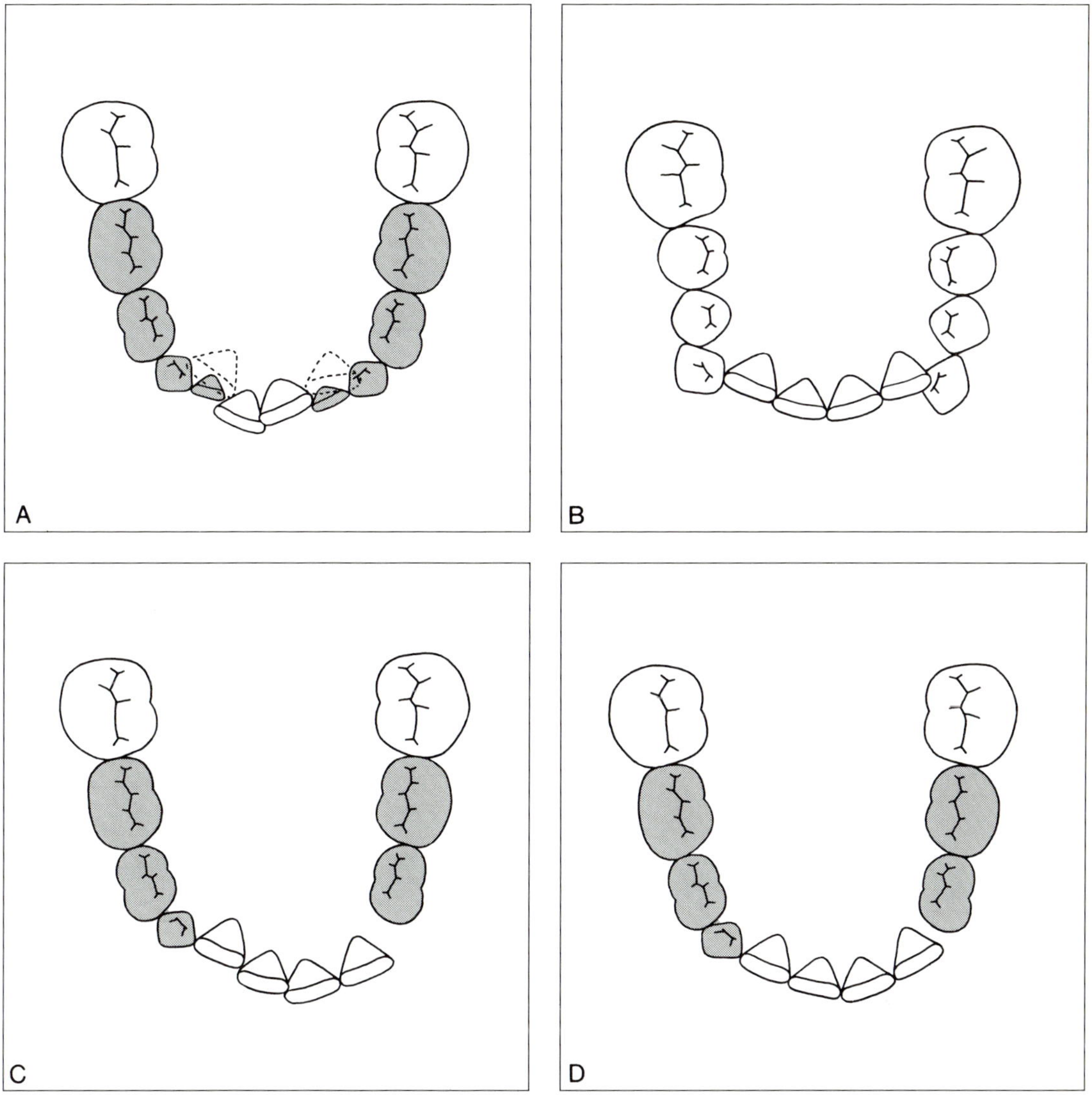

Fig. 9-1 Changes in the mandibular arch associated with premature loss of deciduous canines resulting from resorption.

A Lateral permanent incisors in a crowded dentition can emerge in a better position if, before their emergence, the deciduous canine and lateral deciduous incisor have exfoliated.
B Later there is insufficient room in the dental arch for the permanent canine. Moreover, the mandibular incisors have tipped lingually.
C Unilateral premature loss through resorption of a deciduous canine is associated with an asymmetric arrangement of the mandibular permanent incisors.
D Subsequently the mandibular incisors move further to the side of the premature loss; the midpoint of the dental arch deviates still more.

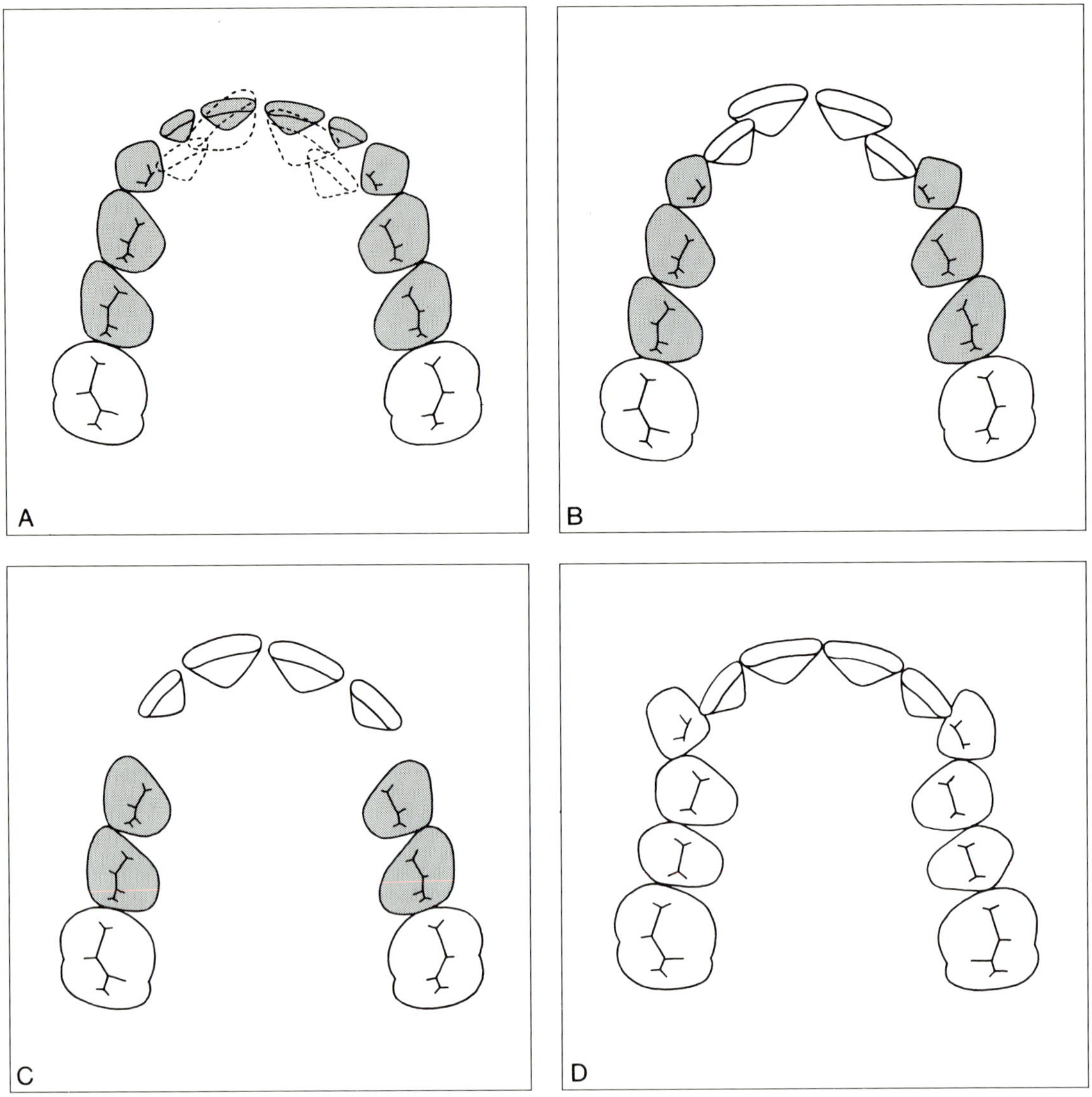

Fig. 9-2 Changes in the maxillary arch associated with premature loss of deciduous teeth resulting from resorption.

- *A* *Central permanent incisors in a crowded dentition can emerge in a better position if, before their emergence, the lateral and central deciduous incisors have exfoliated.*
- *B* *The lateral permanent incisors will generally emerge palatally; there is insufficient room for them in the dental arch.*
- *C* *If not only the lateral deciduous incisors but also the deciduous canines are exfoliated early because of resorption, the lateral permanent incisors can emerge into the arch.*
- *D* *Subsequently there is insufficient space in the dental arch for the permanent canines, which usually will emerge on the labial aspect of the alveolar process.*

9.4 Symptoms of impending premature loss through resorption

Lack of diastemata in the deciduous dentition indicates a small anterior section of the apical area, and abnormal crowding can develop with the emergence of the permanent incisors.[225] Premature exfoliation can be expected.
Emergence of a central permanent incisor across the midline of the mandible can point up a displacement of the midpoint of the arch that has already been present before the teeth emerged. Account then needs to be taken of the likelihood of early resorption of the root of the deciduous canine and its premature loss on the side where there is most crowding.
Resorption of the deciduous teeth is associated with increased mobility. Early increase in mobility indicates that premature loss is imminent. A difference between left and right sides would suggest that unilateral exfoliation is likely. This also applies to a midpoint deviation of the dental arch combined with crowding.

9.5 What to do in cases of (impending) unilateral early loss

In cases of imminent or actual premature loss it is desirable to prevent increased asymmetry and to reduce the existing one if feasible. Most patients with premature loss will later require orthodontic treatment. Asymmetries between arches are awkward to correct. Preventing or reducing their extent by guiding the development of the dentition is desirable. Sometimes extracting the corresponding deciduous tooth on the other side will provide a good influence. Above all, rotations and overlaps will improve.
When cases of unilateral early loss can be anticipated, one should consider removing the contralateral deciduous tooth before the other one exfoliates. In this way one provides the possibility of early spontaneous correction of the position of the permanent incisors. As well, it must be decided if one should wait on the actual loss of the other deciduous tooth, letting it determine its own time for exfoliation, or determine the moment of removal. Complicating factors that should be considered in this regard will be dealt with shortly.

9.6 Indications and contraindications for extracting deciduous canines

The disadvantages connected with premature extraction of deciduous canines are more numerous and serious than the advantages. Only in special cases is it wise to remove one or more deciduous canine(s) prematurely.

9.6.1 Indications for extracting deciduous canines

The most important indication for early removal of deciduous canines is serious crowding of permanent incisors. Symptoms are rotations, overlapping, and deviations of the midlines of the arches. Timely elimination of deciduous canines has the

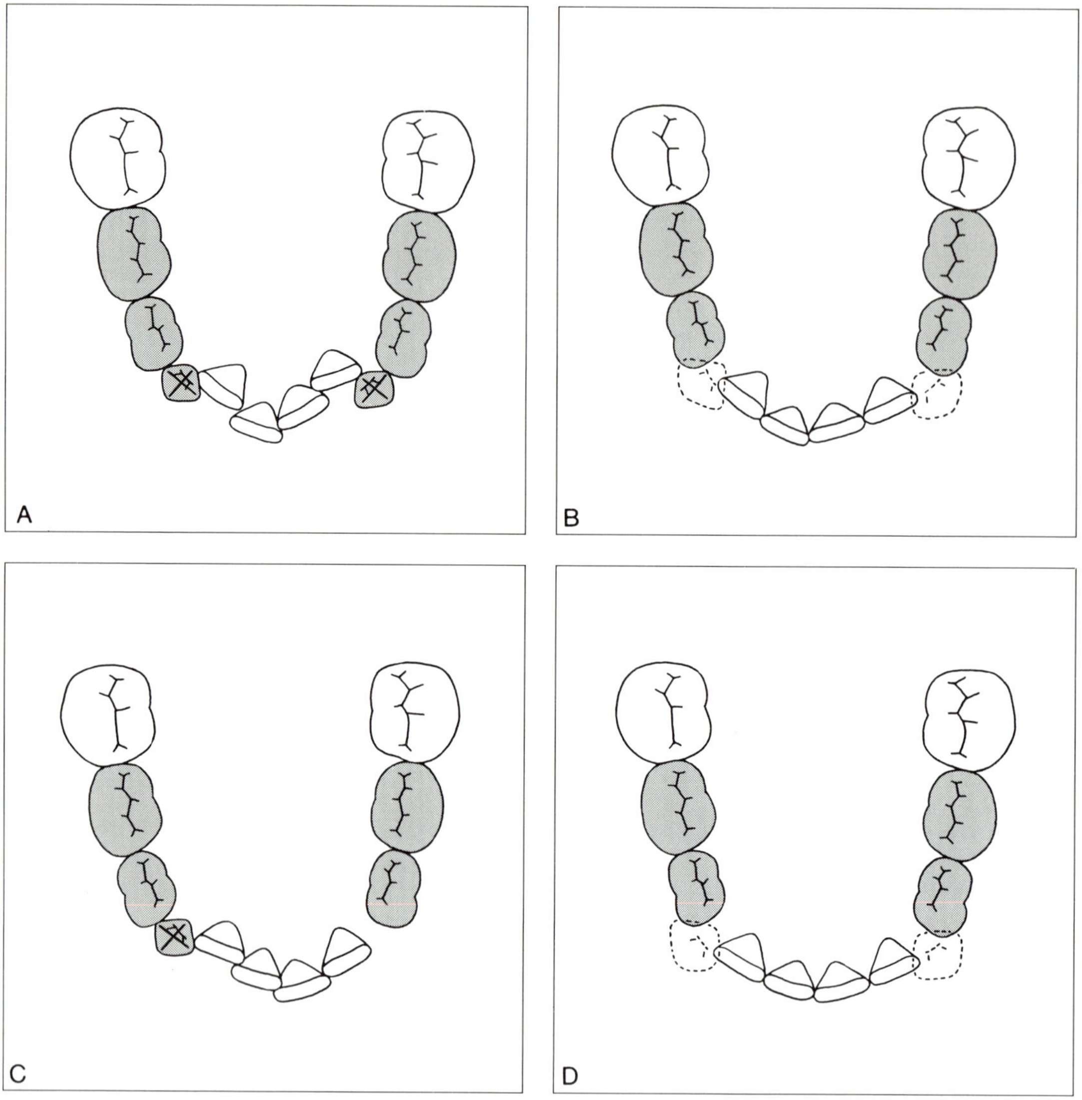

Fig. 9-3 Spontaneous improvement in the alignment of permanent incisors after extraction of mandibular deciduous canines.

A *Timely extraction of deciduous canines in a case of crowding leads to a better position of the lateral permanent incisors. In an asymmetric arrangement of the mandibular incisors it is worth considering removing the canine on the side where there is least crowding before removing the one on the other side.*

B *Subsequently there is too little room for the permanent canines; moreover the mandibular incisors have tipped lingually.*

C *When a deciduous canine is exfoliated on one side because of premature resorption, extracting the canine on the other side will lead to an improved position of the mandibular incisors.*

D The deviation in the midpoint of the dental arch will be reduced; the spaces remaining for the permanent canines are too small. Extracting deciduous canines merely shifts the problem elsewhere. Subsequently the crowding in the canine region must be relieved and the mandibular incisors moved forward to their original positions.

advantage that the above symptoms will improve spontaneously. This facilitates subsequent orthodontic treatment (Figs. 9-3 and 9-4). Moreover, periodontal conditions can improve. This applies particularly when a mandibular central permanent incisor standing in labioposition exhibits gingival stripping.[9]

If the premature removal of deciduous canines is followed by serial extraction, the permanent canines can emerge within the dental arch. This is more favourable periodontally than emerging labially. The buccal bone will be thicker; the attached gingiva will be wider. The same favourable effect can occur also when, in instances where no permanent teeth were removed, adequate space for the unerupted canines is provided in time. From the periodontal point of view in the long term, teeth emerging within the dental arch have the most favourable prognosis, better than those emerging lingually but even more so than those emerging labially or buccally.

If there are indications for extracting mandibular deciduous canines, it is better to wait until the lateral permanent incisors have emerged before proceeding. In the maxilla it is sometimes desirable to start sooner, particularly when marked rotations exist. The difference between maxilla and mandible in the mechanism of increased intercanine width is yet another reason to let the lateral permanent incisors in the mandible emerge in contact with the deciduous canines. In the maxilla this is not important.[223] A deviation of the midline of a dental arch is an indication for removing a deciduous canine at an earlier stage (Fig. 9-3).

Although asymmetric loss of a deciduous canine is a sign of crowding, it is an indication for extracting the deciduous canine on the other side; the argument for this has been given previously.

Sometimes a lateral or ventral forced bite involving deciduous canines can be an indication for extraction of those teeth. Generally, occlusal grinding should be given preference in dealing with forced bites, unless extraction is required for other reasons. In Class II/1 anomalies with crowding of the maxillary incisors, a ventral forced bite can be produced if one or both maxillary lateral permanent incisors emerge palatally. To correct such a forced bite these teeth must be moved forward. The room needed to achieve this can mostly best be obtained by extracting both maxillary deciduous canines.

Occasionally permanent canines emerge labially, lingually, or mesially when persistent deciduous canines provide an obstruction to reaching a better position. It will be obvious that the retained teeth should be removed. That particularly applies when a maxillary permanent canine emerges high labially, because it otherwise will exhibit an abnormally long clinical crown.[139] If it emerges above the keratinised zone, attached gingiva is less likely to form labially. This also applies to mandibular canines.

effectiveness of that procedure depends on the original convexity of those surfaces, and this usually is limited.
The alternative of occlusal grinding in forced bites has been dealt with above.

9.8 Preventing or later correcting detrimental effects of extracting deciduous canines

Detrimental effects should be prevented or corrected when attempting to preserve an intact permanent dentition. Whether one should try to prevent unfavourable sequelae or decide to correct them at a later stage will depend primarily on the local conditions in the dental arches, sagittal relation between the arches, overjet and overbite, lip position, facial musculature, and profile.

9.8.1 Preventing detrimental effects

The lack of broadening of the deciduous intercanine width as a consequence of premature loss or extraction of maxillary lateral deciduous incisors or mandibular deciduous canines is unavoidable. The same applies to a certain degree to the retroclining and lingual displacement of the incisors when permanent mandibular teeth are removed later.
Unfavourable consequences can only be avoided by employing orthodontic appliances directly after the teeth are exfoliated. Such therapy is seldom advisable. One can instead accept the development of an undesirable situation with the objective of correcting it later when it is appropriate to initiate the orthodontic therapy that the overall treatment plan requires.
The effect of retroclination of the mandibular incisors in Class II/1 anomalies is most undesirable. One can attempt to counteract it by employing an activator or other appliance that operates in the same way, directly after the extraction of the deciduous canines. That applies particularly to cases of an (impending) lower lip behind the maxillary incisors as the associated large sagittal deviation calls for early treatment of the Class II/1 anomaly.

9.8.2 Correcting detrimental effects

In Class II/1 anomalies with a disto-occlusion of a half premolar crown width, the undesirable consequences of extracting maxillary deciduous canines can be resolved later in an elegant fashion by employing headgear therapy. The effect of a headgear applied to the maxillary first permanent molars in increasing the total arch length can not only restore the missed broadening of the intercanine width but also gain the space required.
In the mandible one can attempt to regain the arch length in a similar way, using a Denholz appliance or a 0.045-in. buccal arch. An attendant advantage of this approach is that the vestibular musculature is held away from the mandibular teeth and as a result spontaneous improvement can better follow under the influence of tongue pressure.

One can also try to regain lost space, even compensating for the missed broadening of the intercanine width, by using a lingual arch in the mandible.
With the use of full fixed appliances it is usually possible to regain what space has been lost as the result of premature loss of deciduous canines. This also applies to regaining the increase in arch width that did not take place earlier.

9.9 Supplementary remarks

Rotated permanent incisors have a marked tendency to relapse after orthodontic treatment. Spontaneous correction of rotations that occur after premature extraction of deciduous canines shows less relapse. If, unexpectedly, these spontaneous corrections do not occur, it is advisable to use orthodontic appliances to overcorrect the rotations and, along with normal means of retention, to cut through the supraalveolar fibres of the periodontal membrane.[227] By attending to rotation correction early in treatment, the remainder of the treatment time is an extra retention period.[24]
Many factors are involved in deciding whether to treat without extraction of permanent teeth. A number of these, but not all, have been dealt with in the discussion on premature loss or extraction of deciduous canines. Further, it sometimes occurs that cases where extraction of the deciduous canines was intended to be the first step in the the serial extraction procedure show a morc favourable development than was expected and removal of first premolars is not carried through later on.
Extraction of deciduous canines is a simple procedure. The improvement in incisor alignment that follows usually greatly satisfies the child and parents. Shortsightedness in this brings ill consequences. If one has not taken account of the further development of the dentition from the beginning, one appears to have been performing a trick. Eventually there will be no room for the permanent canines. Above all the overjet and overbite have increased abnormally. Ultimately, any treatment must now involve loss of four premolars. This has, among other things, the consequence that usually a good dental correction can only be obtained by using comprehensive fixed appliances. Moreover, account has to be taken of a dished-in face. This appearance of premature aging can be very disturbing. The patient for whom this treatment is being planned will of necessity be quite young, and it is difficult to predict how the treatment will affect the profile at a later age.
In trying to prevent undesirable consequences one must realise that orthodontic treatment that begins early normally lasts a long time, because it is necessary to supervise the dentition until it is complete. This demands a considerable endurance of the patient and his or her family, which is not always possible. Extracting deciduous canines may involve a considerable lengthening of treatment time. It is only desirable in a few specific situations.
In doubtful cases one should either wait and/or consult a colleague whose experience is as extensive as possible. Only after a full analysis and formulation of a complete treatment plan should deciduous canines be extracted.
To conclude, a general dentist should never decide to extract deciduous canines without involving the orthodontist. Timely consultation is encouraged.

Chapter 10

Agenesis of One or Both Maxillary Lateral Permanent Incisors

10.1 Introduction

The failure of one or both maxillary lateral permanent incisors to form usually comes to light after an examination instituted because there are problems in the transition of the maxillary incisors (see Chapter 8). The child and the parents are usually not prepared for it.

In this chapter the symptoms are given that can point to agenesis of maxillary lateral permanent incisors. The space conditions in the dental arch that are important in treatment are dealt with. Advantages and disadvantages of orthodontic and prosthodontic space closure are explained. Special consideration is given to the esthetic aspects of placing the permanent canine alongside the central incisor. The different possibilities for prosthodontic closure are discussed. The role played by the dental arch relations in deciding on the treatment mode is clarified. Possibilities for influencing the development of the dentition in good time are indicated. Unilateral agenesis is treated separately. Retention and postretention problems are brought up.

10.2 Diagnosing agenesis of maxillary lateral permanent incisors

Agenesis may not come as a surprise in families with members whose maxillary lateral permanent incisors never formed or formed in miniature. In history taking, one should remember to enquire about the occurrence of agenesis in the family. Further, one should be alert to agenesis of maxillary lateral permanent incisors when:

1. Lateral deciduous incisors are missing
2. Lateral deciduous incisors are still present and exhibit only little mobility 1 year after emergence of the central permanent incisors
3. Eighteen months after the emergence of the central incisors (and exfoliation of the lateral deciduous incisors) the mucous membrane has not yet been penetrated by the lateral permanent incisors
4. An unusually large central diastema exists
5. The size of the central diastema does not reduce or reduces only a little
6. Palpation of the alveolar process does not reveal the presence of lateral permanent incisors

Certainty about the presence or otherwise of unerupted teeth is only obtained radiographically. This means should only be used when there is no other clear sign of formation.
The long-term planning of the case determines when it is essential to know if teeth are present or not. This is enlarged upon in section 10.8. In general one must have positive information 1 year before the second transitional period is due.

10.3 Space conditions in the dental arch

In cases of missing lateral incisors where a marked crowding in the maxillary dental arch would exist if all permanent teeth were present, the most obvious treatment objective is to achieve contact between the central incisors and the canines.
Maxillary permanent canines are formed with a mesial angulation, certainly in instances of a small anterior section of the apical area. Their path of eruption conforms with this. In the absence of the maxillary lateral permanent incisors, the canines can emerge particularly far mesially and contact the central incisors. In such instances the lateral deciduous incisors exfoliate as their roots resorb at the approach of the permanent canines. When the anterior section of the apical area is large, a more mesial emergence of the permanent canine can be encouraged by early removal of the lateral deciduous incisors and persistence of the deciduous canines. The latter can be extracted later, unless long-term retaining is aimed for. Indeed, in situations of crowding, retaining the deciduous canines is not indicated.
In imminent cases one can artificially reduce the available arch length in the involved quadrants by removing the maxillary second deciduous molars early. Their extraction should preferably be executed a good 6 months before the adjacent first deciduous molar is due to exfoliate. Subsequently, the first permanent molar migrates and rotates mesially.
It is better to extract the first deciduous molar at an earlier moment, when rotation of the maxillary first permanent molar should be prevented and only a limited reduction of arch length is needed.[189]
If no crowding exists, and particularly if excess space prevails, achieving contact between canines and central incisors (with or without retention of the deciduous canines) is not the only solution. Closing the space through prosthodontics should also be considered. In arriving at the best solution the relation between the dental arches is an essential variable (see 10.7).

10.4 Orthodontic versus prosthodontic closure

On the basis of purely dental arguments it is preferable to avoid prosthodontic appliances as much as possible.[150,214] One should realise that the dentition of the patient involved must function for many years yet. Hence, the long-term planning should strive to keep a substantial part of the natural dentition intact during the patient's entire lifetime. In that light, it makes a considerable difference if an initial prosthesis is provided at the age of 18 years as compared with 48 years.

As a standard solution it is best to aim for closing the anterior spaces with contact between permanent central incisors and canines. Contraindications for such a decision are:

1. An extreme surplus of space in the maxillary arch
2. A Class I anomaly with no crowding in the mandible
3. A dished-in profile
4. Esthetic problems (see 10.5)
5. A Class III anomaly

When there is much room in the maxillary dental arch and a contraindication to arrive at a continuous arch of permanent teeth without diastemata, it is reasonable to attempt to retain the deciduous canines as long as possible. As has already been pointed out, the permanent canines can emerge in the place where the lateral permanent incisors should have emerged, especially when there is a great deal of space. Often in such circumstances the deciduous canines do not resorb and exfoliate. Certainly, when the resorption of the deciduous canine roots is limited, these teeth can last many years. If they are lost at a later stage, at least the period during which a prosthodontic appliance has to be provided is correspondingly reduced. Moreover, a better prosthodontic restoration is possible in this situation than where the space to be filled is between the central incisor and canine.
The possibilities for prosthodontic restoration are broadened by the use of bonded composite resins. Bridges made using this method, particularly if employing a cast palatal splint fixed to the abuttments, can remain in place over a long period.

10.5 Esthetic aspects of positioning the permanent canine alongside the central incisor

Whether or not the appearance of a canine placed alongside a central incisor is acceptable in the permanent dentition depends on several factors. How much of the incisor area is displayed when speaking or smiling is important.[133] A relatively large canine crown next to a central incisor of below average mesiodistal width certainly is not a harmonious arrangement. This applies also to a marked labial convexity of the canine crown. A canine with its mesioincisal angle far away from the cusp tip also is not attractive in appearance when positioned alongside the central incisor. Discontinuity in the incisal edges of the four front teeth is unsatisfactory.
Some of the above reservations can be overcome by grinding. The point of the canine always needs flattening, and if possible should be changed into an incisal edge. Some palatal grinding is frequently desirable to reduce the labiolingual thickness. Aligning the canine with a mesial tilt can produce a better effect.
Another objection can be the colour. Maxillary permanent canines are usually darker than central incisors.
The shortcomings of using maxillary canines as lateral incisors apply more to boys than girls, because there is a sex distinction in size, colour, and form of canines. Girls have canines that are relatively narrower, whiter, and more of the form of lateral incisors than do boys.

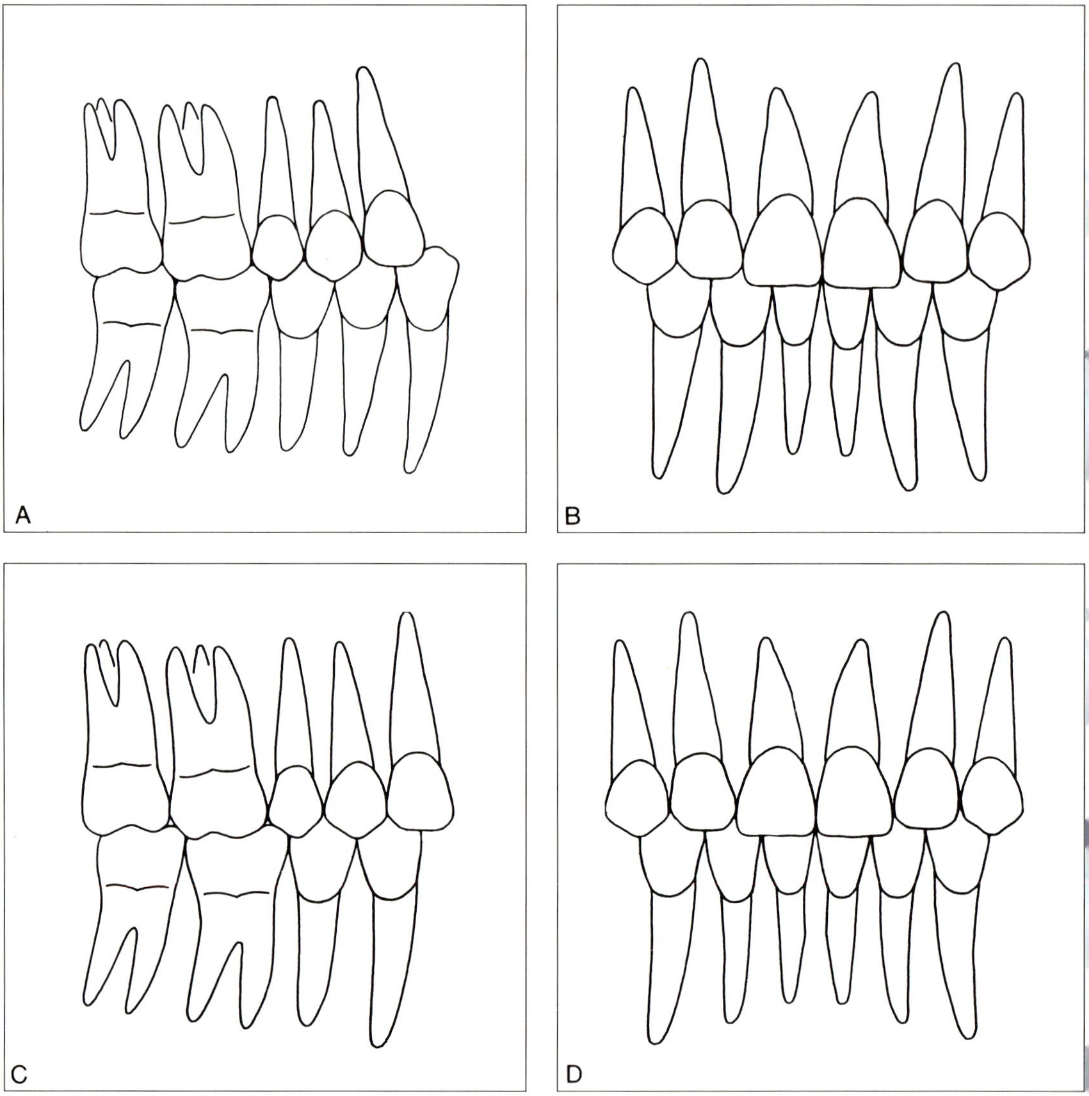

Fig. 10-2 Class I anomaly with bilateral agenesis of maxillary lateral incisors, in which compensating extractions are used in the mandible.

A, B In cases with extreme crowding in the mandibular anterior region, extraction of two mandibular incisors can be considered. Which teeth are chosen depends on their original positions and the tooth size discrepancy (TSD). Here the mandibular lateral incisors have been removed.

C, D If the crowding is concentrated more in the posterior regions of the mandibular arch, the first or second premolars are more appropriate for removal. Here the mandibular first premolars have been sacrificed.

In such situations it is suggested that possible alternatives be looked at using a diagnostic set-up. By this means one can also see if crowns need to have mesiodistal diameters adjusted in order to secure a good occlusion and an acceptable esthetic result.

If mandibular premolars should be sacrificed, systematic extractions according to the principles of serial extraction therapy are preferred. The benefits of this procedure are maximised when the first step (extraction of the deciduous canines) is undertaken approximately a year before the beginning of the second transitional period.
At that time it is in general still possible to move the maxillary dental arch sufficiently mesially in relation to the mandibular arch. After emergence the premolars can subsequently arrive at the desired interdigitation.

10.9 Unilateral agenesis of a maxillary lateral permanent incisor

The combination of two maxillary central permanent incisors with just one lateral incisor is usually unsatisfactory, particularly when spaces remain and when the incisal edges are at different levels. The effect is even worse when the existing lateral incisor has an anomalous form. However, a mere deviation of the midline of the dental arch is often not noticed.

Several solutions can be distinguished when aiming for a more or less symmetrical arrangement of the maxillary anterior teeth with coincidence of the contact point between the central incisors and the median plane of the maxilla:

1. Extraction of the existing maxillary lateral permanent incisor occasionally can be considered, namely when this tooth is abnormally formed (e.g., peg-shaped lateral incisor) and/or has a defective root. Above all, if one is dealing with a situation of crowding, or a Class II/1 anomaly, this solution is even more appropriate (Fig. 10-1B).
2. In a case of unilateral agenesis of a maxillary lateral permanent incisor one must also consider removing a maxillary premolar on the other side, naturally followed by orthodontic treatment in most cases (Fig. 10-3A).
3. Retention of the deciduous canine can be appropriate on the basis of the factors set out previously and can be a suitable remedy in situations of unilateral agenesis of a maxillary lateral incisor (Fig. 10-3B).
4. Mesial displacement of the maxillary teeth on the side of the agenesis leads in a Class I anomaly to a disto-occlusion at that side. The neutro-occlusion on the other side remains as it was. The procedures given previously for bilateral agenesis must now be applied unilaterally (Fig. 10-3C). In practice that is by no means simple. A less optimal sagittal interdigitation of premolars and molars sometimes has to be accepted. That applies particularly when the one maxillary lateral incisor has a narrow crown. The associated tooth size discrepancy (TSD) will not provide a good occlusion without further adjustment.
5. A prosthodontic solution to the problem is more likely to be the answer in a case of unilateral than bilateral agenesis. The substitution concerns only one tooth; the associated negative aspects are correspondingly less significant (Fig. 10-3D).

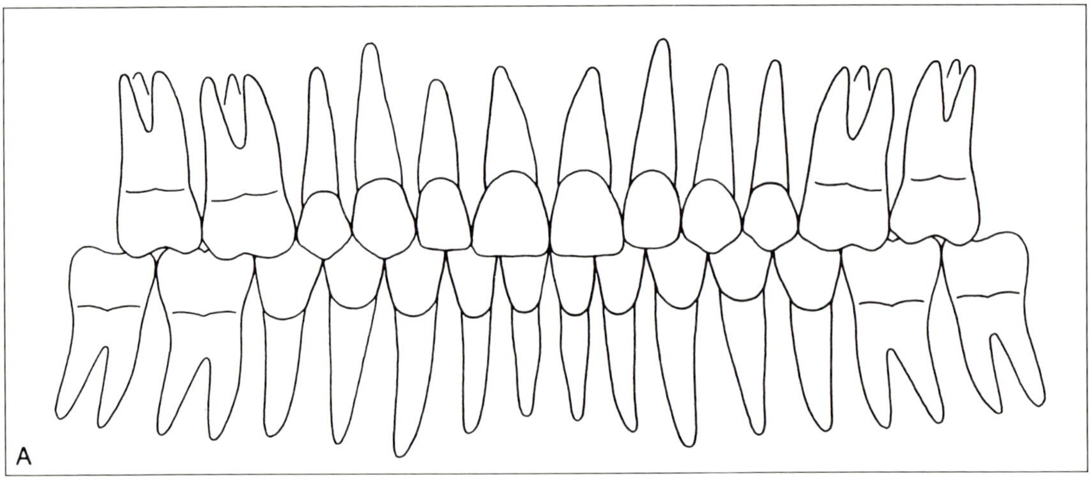

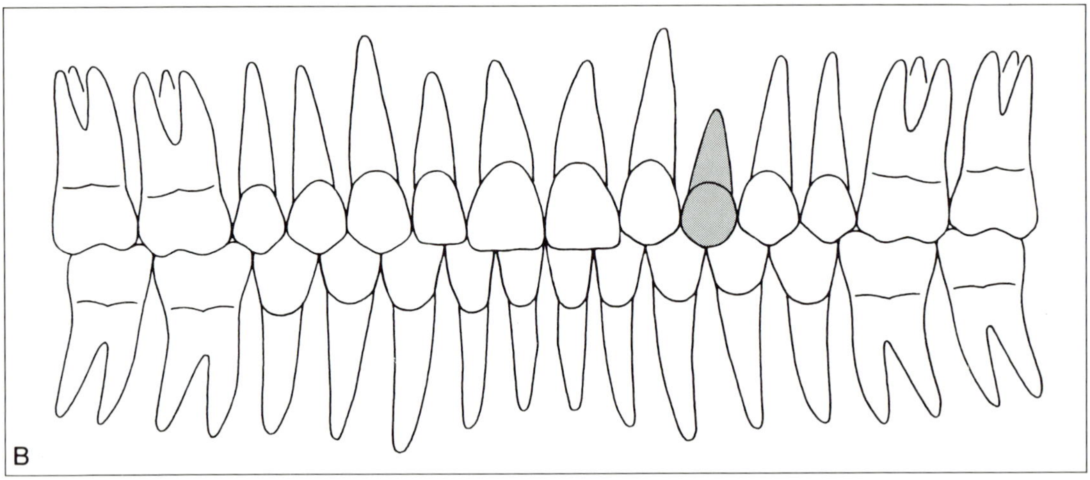

Fig. 10-3 Some possible modes of treatment for unilateral agenesis of a maxillary lateral permanent incisor.

- *A Extraction of a maxillary premolar on the other side with production or maintenance of a disto-occlusion of the molars on each side.*
- *B Retention of the deciduous canine on the side of the agenesis, which then occupies the place between the permanent canine and the first premolar.*
- *C Establishment of a disto-occlusion of the molars on the side of the agenesis with neutro-occlusion on the other side.*
- *D The space resulting from the agenesis is not dealt with orthodontically but prosthodontically.*

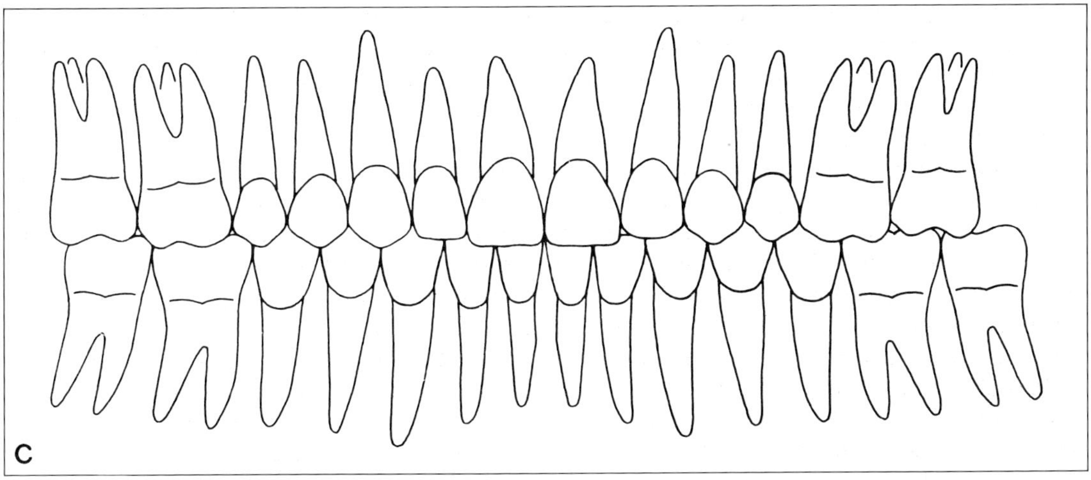
C

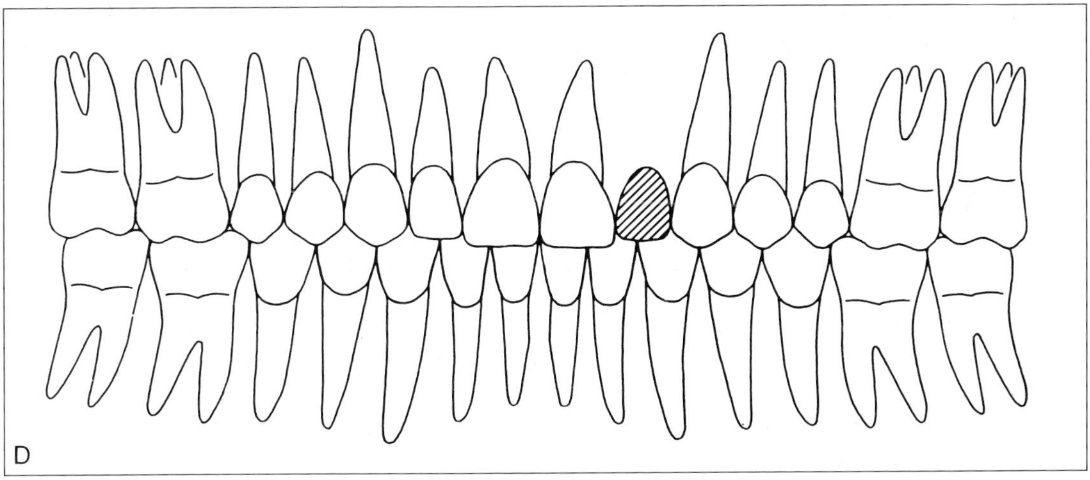
D

10.10 Retention and postretention problems

Diastemata reappear in most cases of agenesis of one or both maxillary lateral incisors that have been treated without prosthodontic replacement. Despite long periods of retention, frenectomy, and section of the supraalveolar fibres, the central incisors usually will not remain in contact. There are few changes following completion of orthodontic treatment that patients object to as much as a central diastema. Perhaps

this is because when looking in a mirror it is in the centre of the field of vision. In normal personal contact one seldom looks directly at another's face in that fashion. All in all, a patient usually has a different point of view of a central diastema than the people around him or her. They seldom find the diastema to be obvious or bothersome in the way some patients do.
With the help of composite resins it is possible to join the two central incisors together in a simple noninvasive procedure. This can be done either by flowing composite resin around the contact point or by bonding a metal strip or wire to the palatal surface of the teeth. In both cases it is advisable for the patients to keep their removable retainers. Should the fixed retention break, resuming use of the removable appliance immediately will prevent reappearance of the diastema. Subsequently the fixed retention can be repaired. It cannot be emphasised too much that when fixed retention is used every effort should be used by both patient and dentist to avoid plaque retention. Strict oral hygiene is essential, and the retentive device should be constructed so as to avoid as much as possible any situations that favour the collection of plaque. The metal strip or wire should be placed free of the gingiva but also clear of the occlusion. In addition, the bonded areas should be small, with no excess composite resin. The surfaces should be kept as smooth as possible, and in particular the junction of the composite resin and enamel surfaces should flow smoothly.

10.11 Supplementary remarks

The maxillary anterior teeth are the most important teeth from an esthetic point of view. The patient's standards of expectation will vary with the degree of defect visibility. The level of the lips in smiling and speaking is pertinent in this regard.
In choosing the best remedy for these problems, the long-term result must be considered. The clinical crown length generally increases with advancing age because of movement apically of the supporting tissues of the teeth. On the other hand, the lip positions in older people are different from those of younger people, exposing less of their maxillary incisors when speaking or smiling. It is wise, knowing the tendency of diastemata to return, to emphasise this when discussing objectives with the patient before commencing treatment. It helps also to spend time developing the patient's sense of perspective so that realistic treatment aims can be adopted. Explanations after treatment relapses are more or less useless, but as part of the treatment plan they are evidence of experience.

Chapter 11

Trauma and Loss of One or More Maxillary Permanent Incisors

11.1 Introduction

Loss of one or more maxillary permanent incisors directly or indirectly as the result of trauma is a shocking experience for the patient and patient's family. It often requires dental first aid and subsequent dental intervention. Questions as to what future treatment will be required soon arise.

The long-term planning and related treatment usually are better placed in the hands of an orthodontist than a general dental practitioner. The latter does, of course, need the knowledge to collaborate intelligently in the long-term planning and to contribute his or her wider knowledge of the patient and patient's family circumstances.

In this chapter consideration will be given successively to replantation, loss of a tooth either directly after trauma or at a later time, variations in loss, the time when trauma occurred, setting up of a treatment plan, particularly in regard to the dental arch relationships, principles of treatment, guidelines for the positioning of substituting teeth, and ultimately the problems of retention and the postretention period.

11.2 Replantation of an avulsed tooth

When a permanent tooth is dislodged in an acccident and the alveolar process is reasonably intact the tooth should be replaced as soon as possible. This is recommended not only for psychological reasons but primarily because it is often the most effective treatment from a dental point of view. However, every minute counts. After 30 minutes outside the alveolar process the prognosis for lasting success is already unfavourable, especially when the tissues around the tooth dry out.[6] Finding the lost tooth very quickly is essential. This needs to be followed by the patient cleaning the root by sucking it in his or her mouth (or as second choice with milk or by rinsing it under a tap). Directly afterwards the tooth should be pushed back into place and held fast as well as possible. If that cannot be done, the patient (or parent) should keep the tooth in the mouth under the tongue until a dentist or oral surgeon can be reached who can replant it. If the above routine cannot be followed for unavoidable reasons, the next best thing is to place the tooth after cleaning it, but without interfering with the root surface (which should by no means be rubbed), in a cup with milk or in a water-soaked sterile gauze pad or other soft material, and seek professional help.

Professional dental attention is required for provision of a splint. This can be accomplished using composite resin reinforced with steel wire. This is better than ligating a preformed stainless steel wire splint in place with metal ligatures, which until

recently was the preferred approach. Because the traumatized tissues may bleed, it may not be easy to maintain the perfectly clean field necessary for reliable bonding, but it is much easier on the patient, who has already suffered enough, than any other approach.
An antitetanus injection is essential if the patient is not currently protected. It will soon be necessary to perform a root canal treatment. Trauma involving damage of gingival tissues makes plaque removal more difficult and painful. By rinsing with a chlorhexidine solution, plaque accumulation can be reduced and healing enhanced.
Only after ample time has passed can an assessment of the future life of the replanted tooth be relied on. They seldom last more than 10 years. In devising a long-term treatment plan therefore, one must take account of the likely unfavourable prognosis, certainly when the tooth has been out of the alveolus for a long period and has become dry. Extraction of such teeth should be envisaged and planned for.

11.3 Loss without replantation

When avulsed teeth have not been replanted or subsequently have been lost, the loss is difficult for the patient and parents to cope with. They are anxious to know what must be done and what the end result will be. They will rightly ask their family dentist for information and advice. His or her task is to give them guidance about the possibilities and limitations of the treatment available both in general dentistry and orthodontics. Moreover, another aspect of the dentist's task may be, if required, to provide a temporary prosthodontic appliance to camouflage the defect. Such an appliance should not interfere with spontaneous changes that may benefit orthodontic therapy.

11.4 Teeth unable to be saved after trauma

If a tooth has suffered trauma but has not been knocked out, it may still be impossible or undesirable to retain it. This applies particularly to teeth of which the pulp vitality has been lost with a root which is only partly formed, especially where the root canal diverges at the apex. However, in certain cases apexification can still be obtained by filling the root canal with calcium hydroxide. When this treatment fails and a wide divergent apex remains, extraction is indicated. This also applies to teeth with one or more fractures. Extraction must also be considered when a major part of the crown has been fractured, because repair will have long-term limitations.[4-6]
Fortunately in many cases of trauma to maxillary incisors it is feasible to preserve the involved teeth. Teeth that have been well treated endodontically can be moved orthodontically without concern. If there is any reason to anticipate apical root resorption, the root canal filling might be placed a little short of the apex.[201]
Where a major fracture of the crown has occurred apical to the gingival margin, the provision of a crown restoration is improved and facilitated by first extruding the tooth in question. Such a procedure may also be useful with minor fractures, not just in the provision of a crown but also in building up the defect with composite resin.
After trauma (particularly intrusion), teeth may develop ankylosis. In such cases alveolotomy with "en bloc" surgical relocation of the involved teeth can be considered, particularly for adults.

11.5 Variations in the loss of maxillary permanent incisors

In most cases trauma will involve one or two central incisors in the maxilla. In proportion, this will occur much more often in cases of large overjets than in normal incisor relationships. In addition, injuries to maxillary anterior teeth occur most in the age range of 7 to 10 years, and more often to boys than girls. It seems clear that the lack of lip coverage for the maxillary incisors will also contribute to their vulnerability. Injuries involving only a lost lateral incisor are rare.[4,39,118,149]

11.6 Age at injury

It makes a difference if the trauma occurs in the first transitional period or (much) later. When loss of an incisor has occurred at an early age it is still possible to guide the development of the dentition (see 10.8), but such is not the case when an incisor is lost from a complete permanent dentition. In that situation a prosthodontic solution is more likely to be sought, although it is still possible to close the space using orthodontic appliances.

11.7 Setting up a treatment plan after trauma

The moment when trauma occurred determines the time when it will be possible to make a diagnosis and formulate a treatment plan. Shortly after the accident a long-term treatment plan should be made. From this come measures that may be instituted prior to the use of appliances. Those measures will not be described further here but are found in Chapter 10. The train of thought that forms the basis of the treatment plan required after loss of maxillary incisors is largely the same as that involved in cases of agenesis of one or two maxillary lateral incisors. For example, extraction of a second (or first) deciduous molar should be considered on the side on which one central incisor has been lost.
With the traumatic loss of a maxillary incisor the possibility of transplanting an unerupted premolar should also be considered. This applies particularly when two incisors on one side have been lost. It is not possible to move a tooth across the median suture in the maxilla. The possibility of transplanting a tooth later does not detract from the importance of quickly replanting an avulsed tooth. Even if transplantation will be performed later, it will be better if a socket already exists from the replanted tooth than if it has to be constructed in a partly resorbed alveolar process. The indications and procedures involved in transplanting teeth can be found in the specialist fields of orthodontic and surgical treatment.[103,104,112,152,200,231]
Moving a lateral incisor into the place of a lost central incisor usually involves building up the crown of the lateral incisor to a size more in keeping with its location. Thanks to the availability of composite resins and veneers of other tooth-coloured restorative materials, this alteration can be realised nowadays without grinding the tooth and without fear of pulp damage.[72a,182,183,183a] Surgical adjustment of the cervical gingiva

can be performed if the clinical crown height is too small and the gingival contour does not match that of the adjacent teeth.[243] Finally the possibility of placing a metallic implant to substitute for a lost incisor is mentioned. This approach should be considered particularly when two incisors on one side have been lost. However, facial growth should be completed before the implant is inserted.

11.8 Dental arch relations and loss of maxillary incisors

Generally speaking, the remarks made concerning dental arch relations and agenesis (see 10.7) also apply to this situation. Because most cases involving trauma to incisors exhibit molar disto-occlusion, a solution involving preservation or emphasis of this condition will usually be the most convenient.
Table 11-1 and Fig. 11-1 present a survey, if incomplete, of the standard orthodontic solutions to the problems related to loss of one or more maxillary incisors. Reference to the information given in Chapter 10 makes further description unnecessary. However, perhaps with excess zeal, a number of basic principles are recalled in the next paragraph.

11.9 Basic principles concerning traumatic loss of maxillary incisors

A prosthodontic replacement should be avoided if at all possible. The disadvantages involved in orthodontic treatment and the subsequent general dental treatment procedures are usually less than those related to a prosthodontic solution. Of course, the latter may require some orthodontic therapy as a part of it. The pros and cons are naturally more apparent if the situation that may be expected many years ahead is taken into account.
However, if in achieving a completely closed dental arch a clear deterioration of the profile and change in facial animation would ensue, a solution providing for prosthodontic replacement should be given more weight.
Should there be a Class II/1 anomaly it will generally be advantageous to keep the existing molar disto-occlusion or, if needed, to exaggerate it. If the profile is such that it is particularly necessary to reach a neutro-occlusion, then two mandibular teeth will need to be sacrificed. Class I anomalies that do not require mandibular extractions can be changed into a molar disto-occlusion in the course of eliminating the maxillary spacing. Certain interventions into the development of the dentition can simplify subsequent appliance therapy (e.g., extraction of maxillary second deciduous molars, serial extraction).
After orthodontic treatment it is necessary to determine whether or not the maxillary teeth, which have ended up in a position they would not ordinarily have assumed, will require adjustment. Sometimes in these situations compensating reduction of approximal enamel thickness in the mandibular incisors is called for (stripping).
Making a diagnostic set-up by which different possibilities can be studied in a realistic format is usually an indispensable aid in reaching a correct conclusion. This applies in particular to instances when mandibular teeth have to be sacrificed.

TABLE 11-1
Standard solutions in treatment after loss of one or more maxillary permanent incisors (see Fig. 11-1).

Tooth lost	Anomaly	Standard solution
11, 21	Class II/1	Teeth 12 and 22 in place of 11 and 21. *(1)* Keep molars in disto-occlusion (Fig. 11-1A); *(2)* extract two mandibular teeth and correct disto-occlusion to neutro-occlusion (Fig. 11-1B).
11, 21	Class I	Teeth 12 and 22 in place of 11 and 21. *(1)* Extract two mandibular teeth and keep molars in neutro-occlusion (Fig. 11-1B); *(2)* place molars in disto-occlusion (Fig. 11-1A).
11	Class II/1	Tooth 12 in place of 11. *(1)* Extract tooth 24 and keep molars in disto-occlusion (Fig. 11-1C); *(2)* or 22 (Fig. 11-1D).
11	Class I	Tooth 12 in place of 11. *(1)* Extract tooth 24 and extract two mandibular teeth, keeping molars in neutro-occlusion (Fig. 11-1E); *(2)* or extract 22 (Fig. 11-1F); *(3)* secure molar in disto-occlusion right (Fig. 11-1G); *(4)* extract tooth 24 and secure molars in disto-occlusion (Fig. 11-1H); *(5)* or 22 (Fig. 11-1I).
11, 12, 21, and 22	Class II	Teeth 13 and 23 in place of 12 and 22 and keep molars in disto-occlusion (Fig. 11-1J).

Fig. 11-1 (see page 222) Standard solutions after loss of one or more maxillary permanent incisors (see Table 11-1).

A The maxillary lateral incisors have been moved to the place of the missing central incisors; the molars are in disto-occlusion.
B The lateral incisors have been moved to the place of the missing central incisors; both first premolars (or two other mandibular teeth) have been removed; the molars are in neutro-occlusion.
C The right lateral incisor has been moved to the place of the lost central incisor; the left maxillary first premolar has been removed; the molars are in disto-occlusion.
D As in C, but now with extraction of the maxillary left lateral incisor instead of the first premolar.
E As in C, but now with extraction of both mandibular first premolars; the molars are in neutro-occlusion.
F As in D, but now with extraction of both mandibular lateral incisors; the molars are in neutro-occlusion.
(Legend continues on page 225)

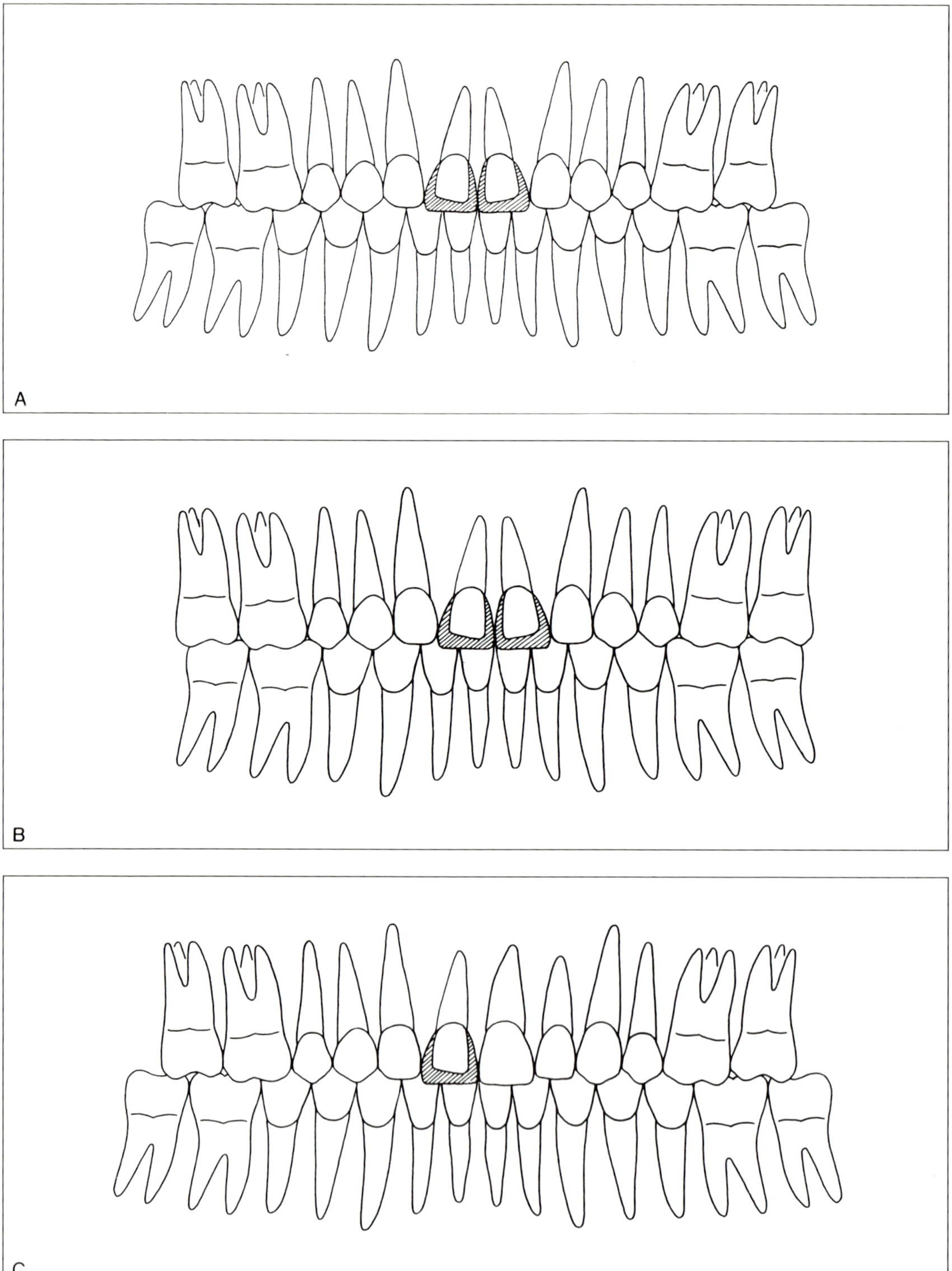

Figure 11-1

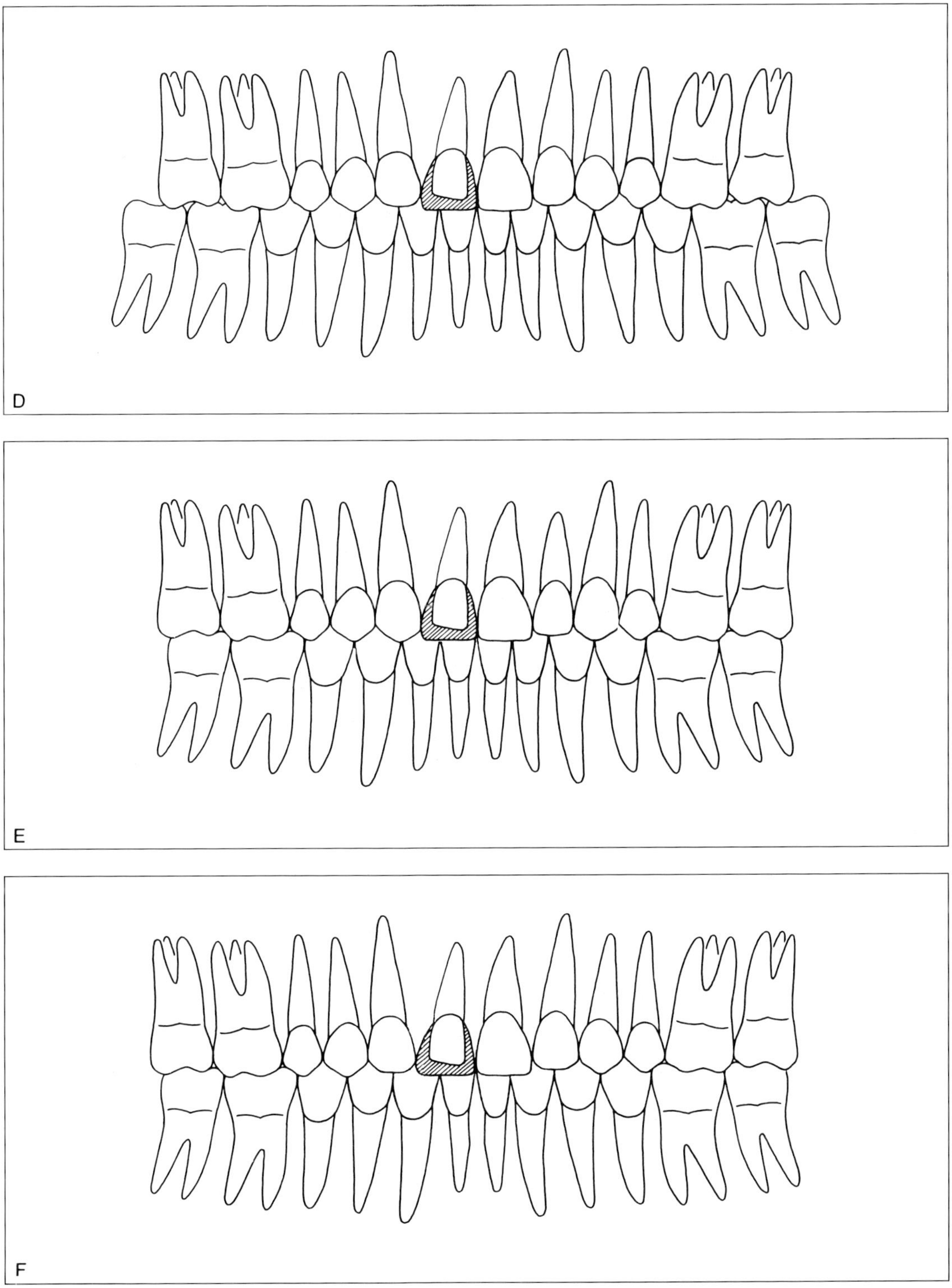

Figure 11-1

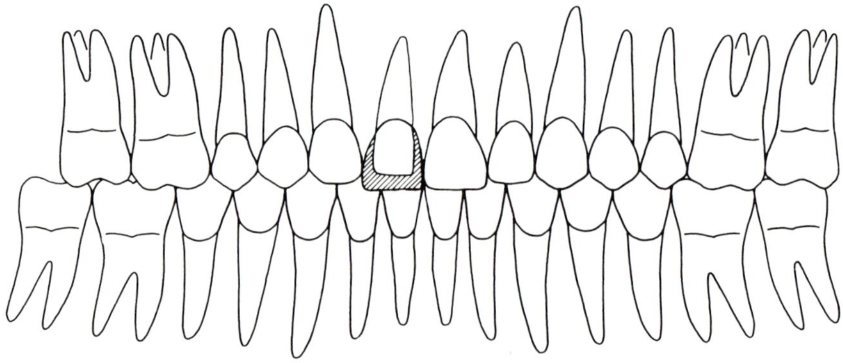

G

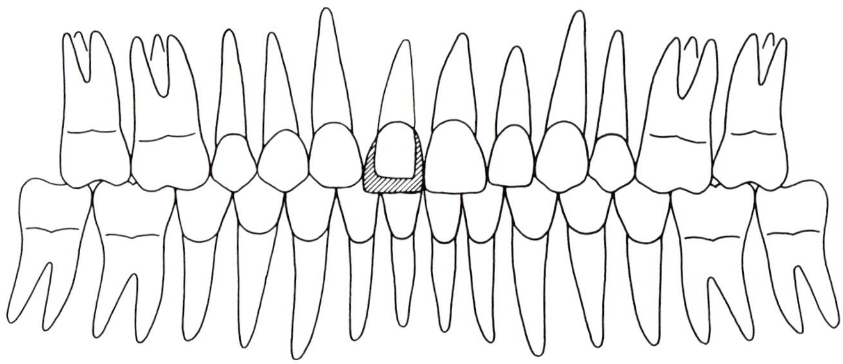

H

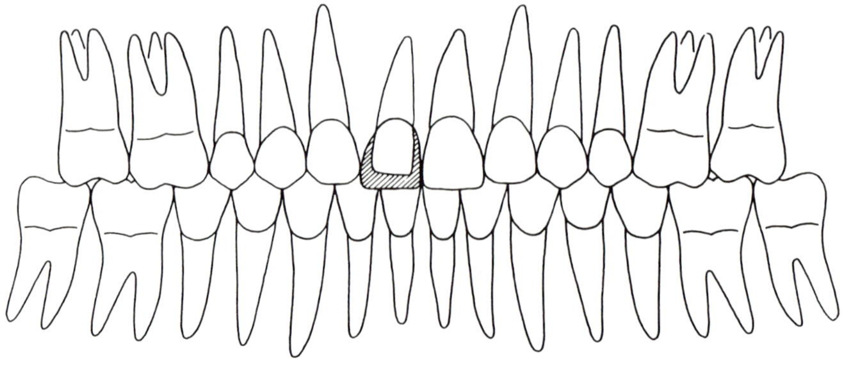

I

Figure 11-1

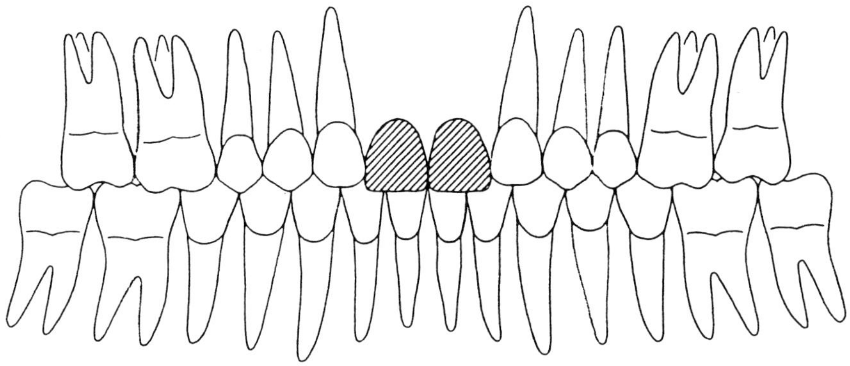

J

Figure 11-1

(Legend 11-1 continued)

G *The maxillary right lateral incisor has been moved to the place of the lost central incisor; on the right, the molars are in disto-occlusion and on the left, in neutro-occlusion.*

H *As in G, but with extraction of the maxillary left first premolar; on both sides the molars are in disto-occlusion.*

I *As in H, but now with extraction of the maxillary left lateral incisor instead of the first premolar.*

J *The maxillary canines have been moved into the place of the missing lateral incisors; the central incisors have been replaced prosthodontically; the molars are in distro-occlusion.*

11.10 Guidelines for positioning substituting teeth

When space due to loss of maxillary permanent incisors is closed by displacing teeth, the results depend mainly on the location and orientation of the substituting teeth and the adjustments made in crown form by grinding and building up by composite resins. Further, the result obtained can deteriorate considerably as relapse occurs. Particularly, opening of spaces and change in angulation can lead to an unacceptable appearance.[183a]

The esthetic features of the arrangement of maxillary anterior teeth can be divided in vertical, transverse, and labiopalatal aspects.

The most essential vertical feature is how much of the teeth becomes exposed in speaking and smiling. The incisal borders practically always show. Asymmetrically arranged teeth should not be accentuated by unevenness of the incisal borders, that in those cases should form one straight line. Not all individuals expose the cervical borders of the teeth. Individuals with a high gingival line are critical in that respect in contrast to those who do not show the cervical one third of the crowns of the maxillary anterior teeth.

Often dentists and orthodontists place too much emphasis on the impressions given by dental casts and intraoral colour photographs or slides. The conclusions derived from these observations frequently do not coincide with the patient's ideas. For example, a deviation of the midlines of the two dental arches is often not noticed by patients. Also, an irregularity in the course of the cervical borders is not a problem for most patients if they do not expose it.

Deviations in the transverse direction depend largely on the degree in which they show up, particularly in the patient's view. Midline deviations and asymmetrical tooth arrangement are often camouflaged when the incisal line is straight, crown width ratios are within the acceptable range of variation, and the incisal thirds of the crowns conform in shape and colour with what is expected to be seen.

In labiopalatal direction, the thickness of the crowns at different levels and the location of the cervical borders play a major role. In cases of vertical and sagittal contact between the mandibular and maxillary anterior teeth, consideration of the shape and position of the palatal surfaces of the maxillary teeth is essential, as are articulation movements. However, these points do not apply to open bite cases.

Also, the contour of the labial surface must be taken into account. A maxillary canine can be too bulky when placed at the location of a missing lateral incisor, especially when the central incisor crowns have a small labiopalatal dimension. In addition, the anteroposterior orientation of the cervical border should be considered and mostly requires a palatal tipping of the apex of a canine that substitutes for a lateral incisor to achieve better esthetics.

To secure optimal results, special guidelines must be applied for the location of substituting teeth and the prevention of relapse, including loss of atypical angulations. It is of utmost importance to prevent the occurrence of an ugly central papilla and its retraction that leads to an empty space between the central incisors at the cervical region. Further, substitute teeth should be positioned so that they can be built up to match the crowns of the lost teeth. In addition, the course of the cervical borders, when visible, must be esthetically pleasant.

Loss of teeth is associated with reduction of alveolar bone. Treatment approaches and techniques that increase the chance for irritation of the soft tissues and the reduction of alveolar bone should be avoided. Especially when a tooth with a large mesiodistal dimension is lost, the bone reduction may create a problem, particularly adjacent to the midpalatal suture, which cannot be crossed. Moving a root over the midsagittal plane to the other side of the jaw will not encounter limitations in the mandible, unlike in the maxilla where the suture will become displaced when a root is moved to the other side. Subsequently, the suture tends to return to its original orientation, resulting in tipping back of the root unless prevented by an adequate permanent retention device.

Some of the problems that can be encountered in the treatment of patients with loss of one or more maxillary incisors are emphasized in Figs. 11-2 through 11-9, and suggestions are given on how to avoid these problems and how to arrive at optimal results.

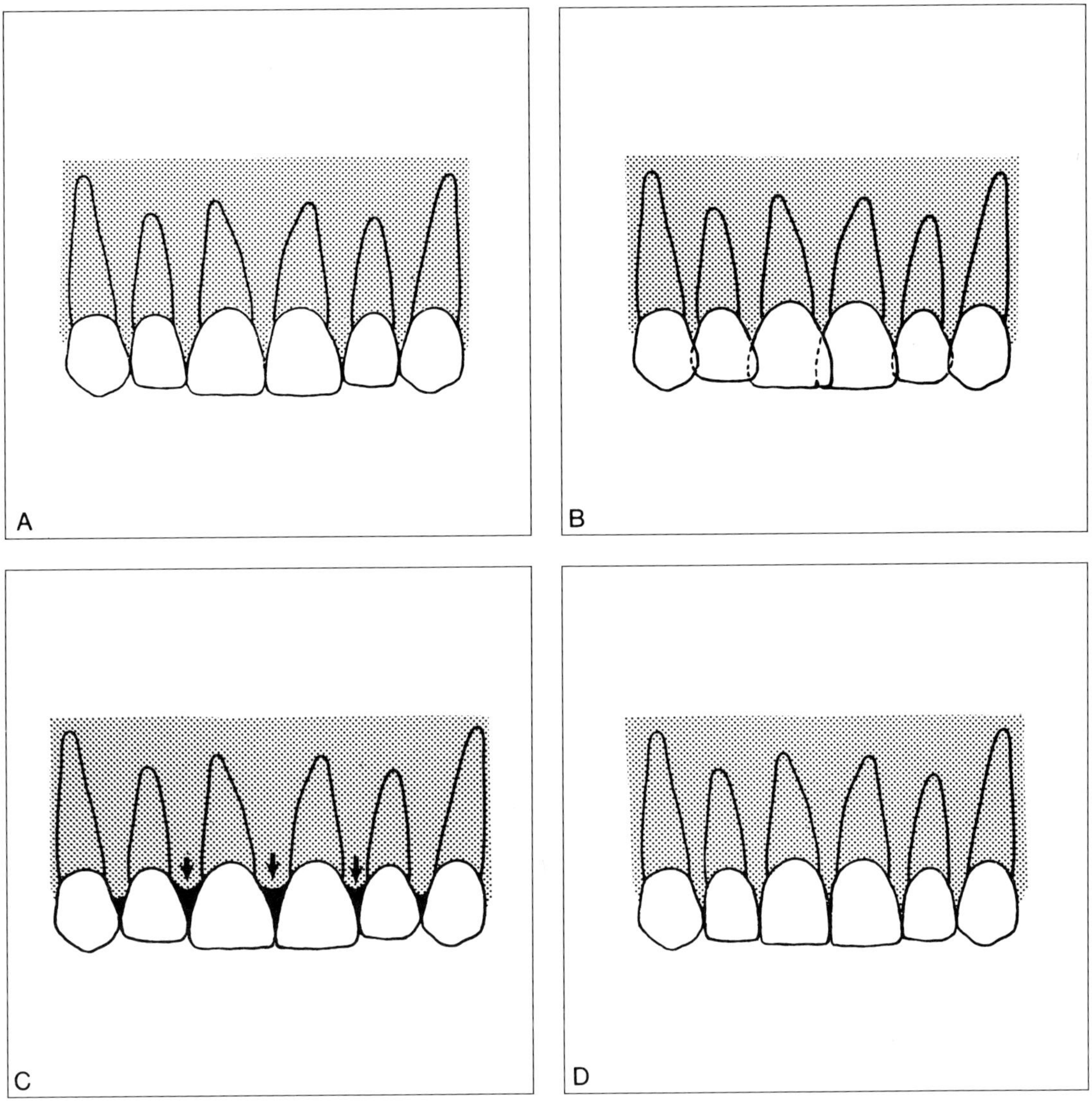

Fig. 11-2 The effect of mesiodistal crown dimensions and tooth form on the shape and presence of interdental papillae.

A Average normal tooth forms and arrangement favour normal interdental papillae.

B In cases of extra-wide incisors, combined with crowding and overlapping, the distances between adjacent cervical borders are small and adequate papillae are usually present.

C Alignment of the teeth illustrated in B will lead to considerably increased distances between adjacent cervical borders. Frequently the papillae will not enlarge and adapt sufficiently. The papillae will retract with, as a consequence, empty triangular spaces between the teeth in the cervical region. This development is more likely to occur in adults than children.

D Reshaping tooth forms by reducing the interproximal enamel thickness will eliminate the increased distances between adjacent cervical borders and diminish the chance of ending up with empty interdental spaces.

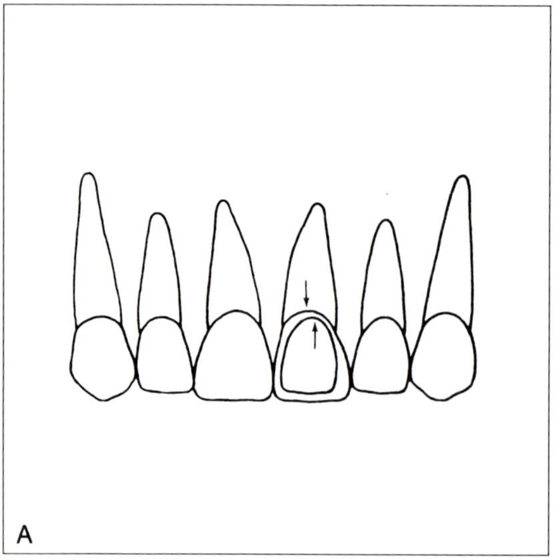

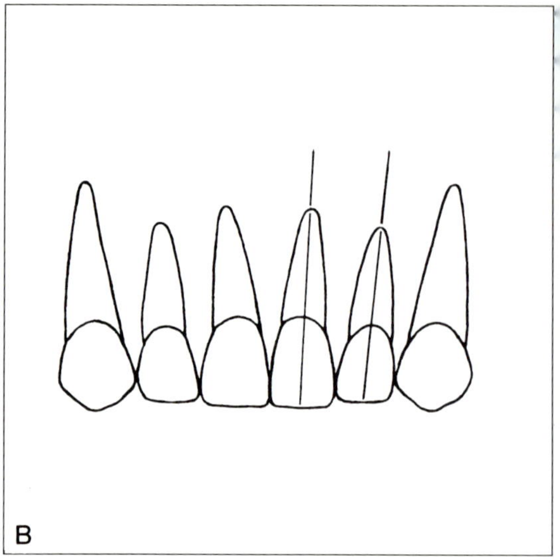

Fig. 11-3 Differences between maxillary central and lateral incisors in crown form and angulation.

A The highest point of the clinical crown of a central incisor is located mesial to its centre line, that of the lateral incisor distal to it. This difference is associated with the convex distal surface of the central incisor. Both aspects are illustrated by the drawing of the crown of the lateral incisor within that of the central incisor.

B The lateral incisor is more angulated than the central incisor, which enhances the differences in crown shape leading to a more distal location of the highest point of the crown of the lateral incisor.

Fig. 11-4 The effect of the angulation of a lateral incisor substituting for a central incisor and of the width of the other lateral incisor on the esthetics of the maxillary anterior region.

A Normal arrangement and angulation of anterior teeth.

B When a substituting lateral incisor is placed in its standard angulation, the buildup of the crown will have its highest point too far distally and deviate in shape from the adjacent true central incisor. The right canine has been reshaped to substitute for the right lateral incisor and to match the left lateral incisor.

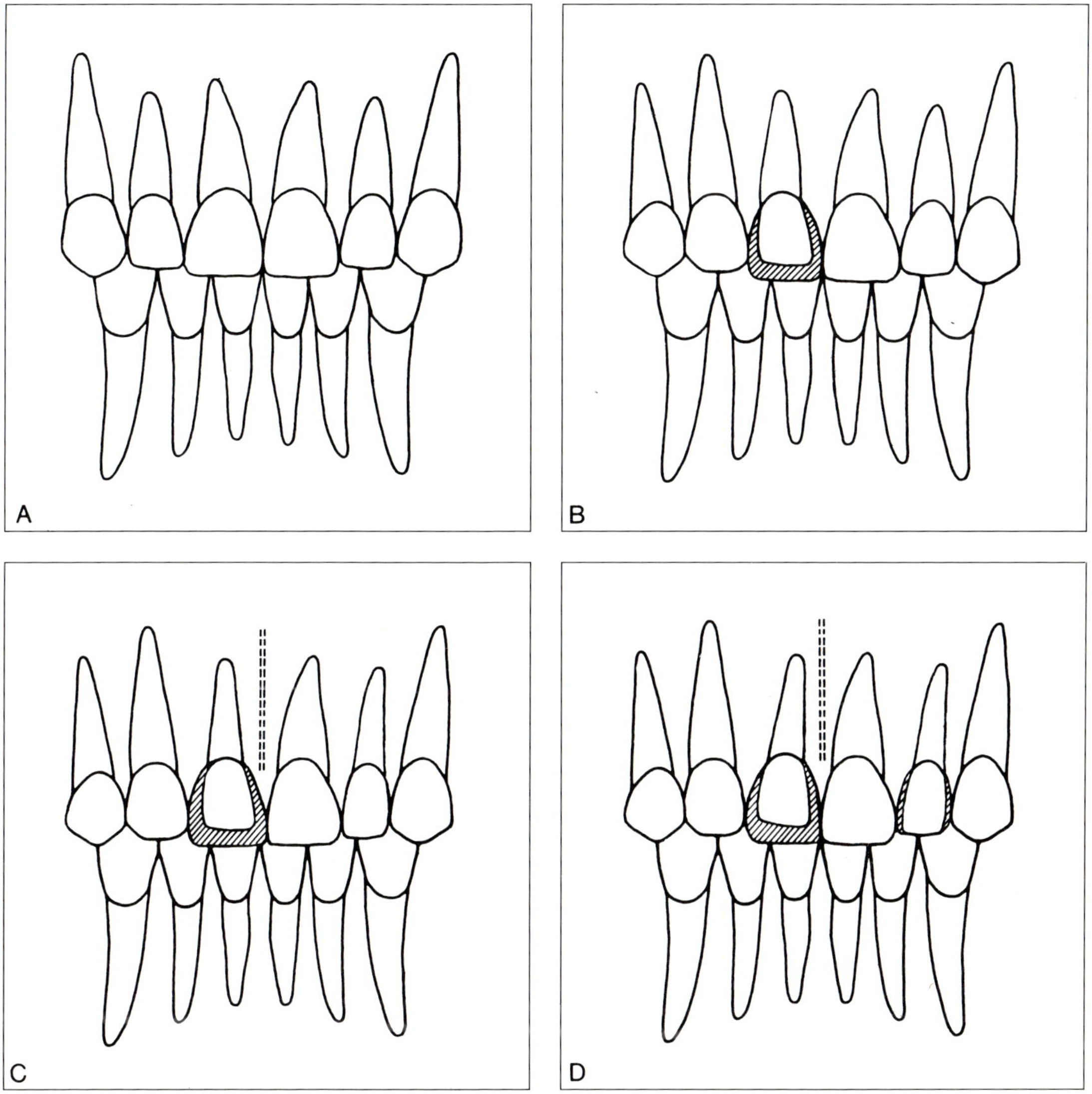

Figure 11-4

C A small left lateral incisor cannot be matched by the right canine. In addition, the buildup on the substituting right lateral incisor must be extra wide to compensate for the small left lateral incisor. Consequently, the midlines of the dental arches will not coincide.

D The situation in C will result in a better appearance when the left lateral incisor crown is extended. Midlines can then coincide and the buildup on the right lateral incisor can match the adjacent crown in width. Note that the mesial surface of the right lateral incisor root is parallel to the suture, allowing for a buildup with the highest point of the clinical crown mesial of the center line.

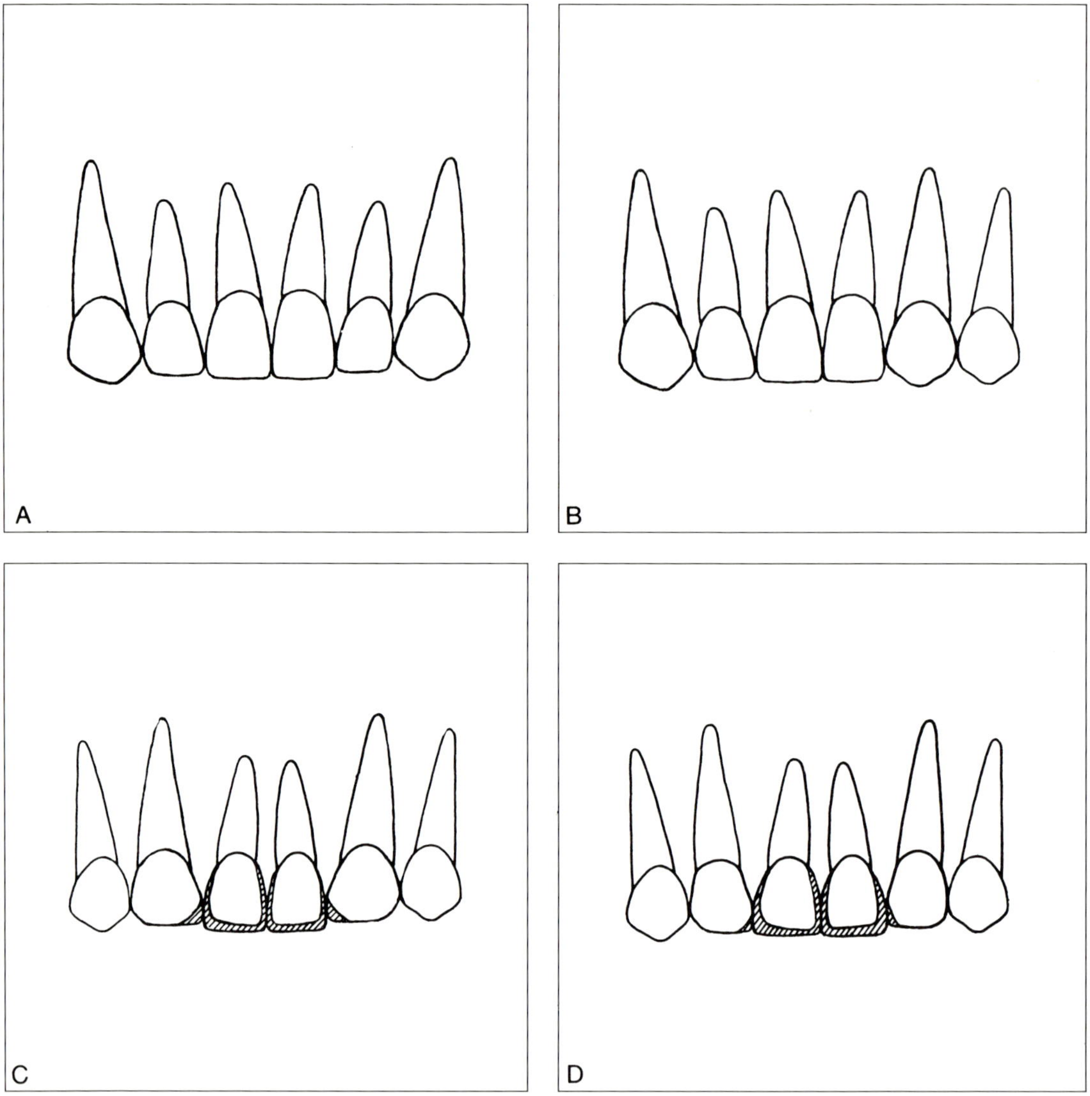

Fig. 11-5 The effect of excessively wide canines on the esthetics of the maxillary anterior region in cases of missing incisors.

A Normal arrangement and angulation of anterior teeth.
B An extra-wide canine can look oversized when it substitutes for a missing lateral incisor.
C Buildups on lateral incisors that substitute for central incisors will look strange and ugly when they are adjacent to large (and darker) canines, even if their mesial corners have been built up.
D Mesiodistal reductions of the canines and larger buildups on the substituting lateral incisors will lead to a more acceptable appearance. Note the parallel orientation of the mesial surfaces of the roots of the substituting lateral incisors.

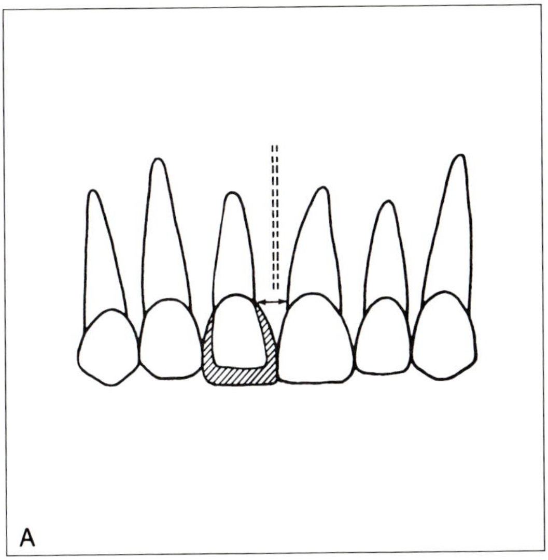

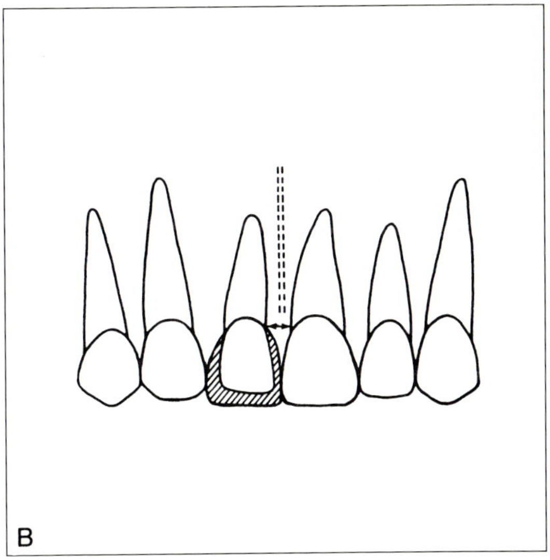

Fig. 11-6 The effect of the angulation of a substituting lateral incisor on the crown form and on the central papillae.

A Standard angulation will result in a large distance between the adjacent cervical borders in the median plane (double arrow) and in a tooth buildup that does not match the central incisor crown.

B A parallel orientation of the mesial surface of the substituting lateral incisor with the median suture will lead to a short distance between the adjacent cervical borders and allows a buildup that can resemble the missing crown.
Note that better crown forms are also achieved when the remaining space is mainly located at the distal side of the substituting lateral incisor and little at the mesial side.

Fig. 11-7 (see page 232) The effect of the angulation of two lateral incisors that serve as substitutes for missing central incisors on the central papilla and on crown forms.

A The effect of the angulation of substituting lateral incisors on the central papilla is even more important when both central incisors need to be replaced. The distance between the adjacent cervical borders (double arrow) will be extra large when the normal angulation for lateral incisors is accepted.

B By putting both mesial surfaces parallel and close to the median suture, a normally shaped, healthy, and long-lasting central papilla can be achieved.

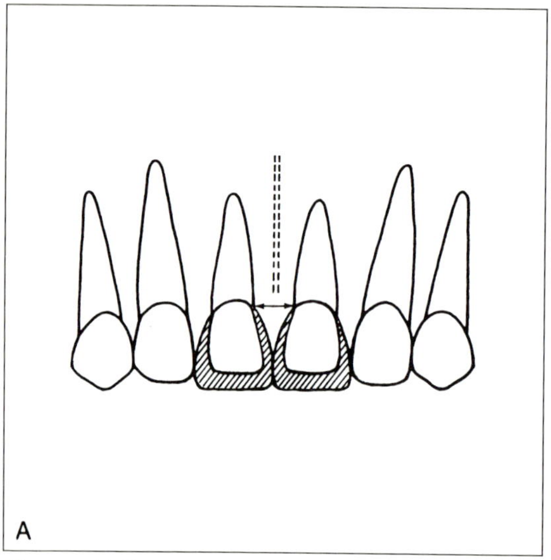

Figure 11-7
(Legend on page 231)

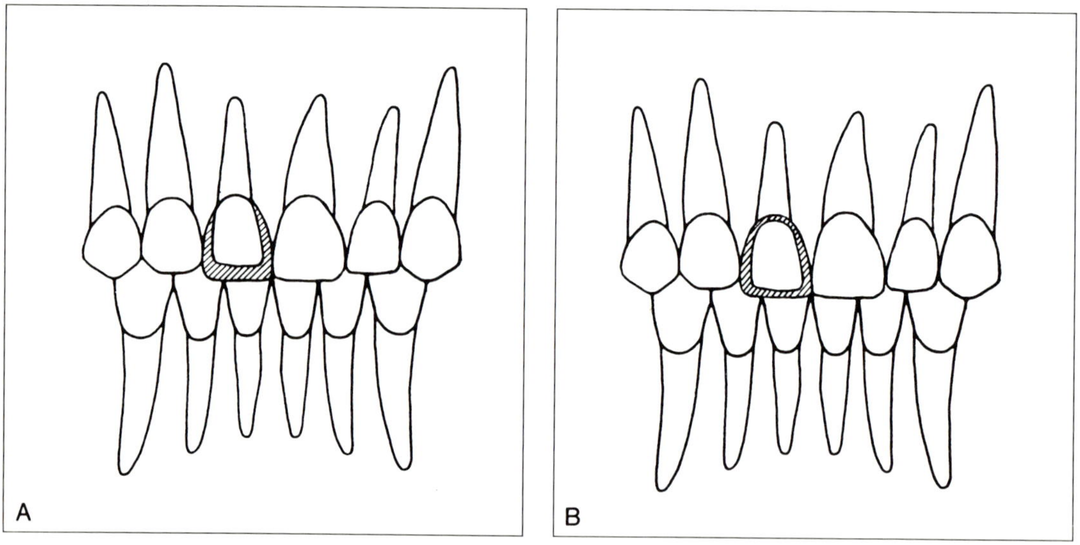

Fig. 11-8 Methods to increase the clinical crown height of a lateral incisor that must serve as a central incisor.

A By lining up the cervical borders of the anterior teeth the artificial crown does not have to be extended in an apical direction.

B Extrusion of the lateral incisor usually should be followed by palatal grinding and by gingivectomy to arrive at comparable clinical crown height. The buildup of the crown must extend more apically. Further, the chances to arrive at a good central papilla are reduced. In addition, relapse of the extruded tooth will result in unevenness of cervical borders and of the incisal line.

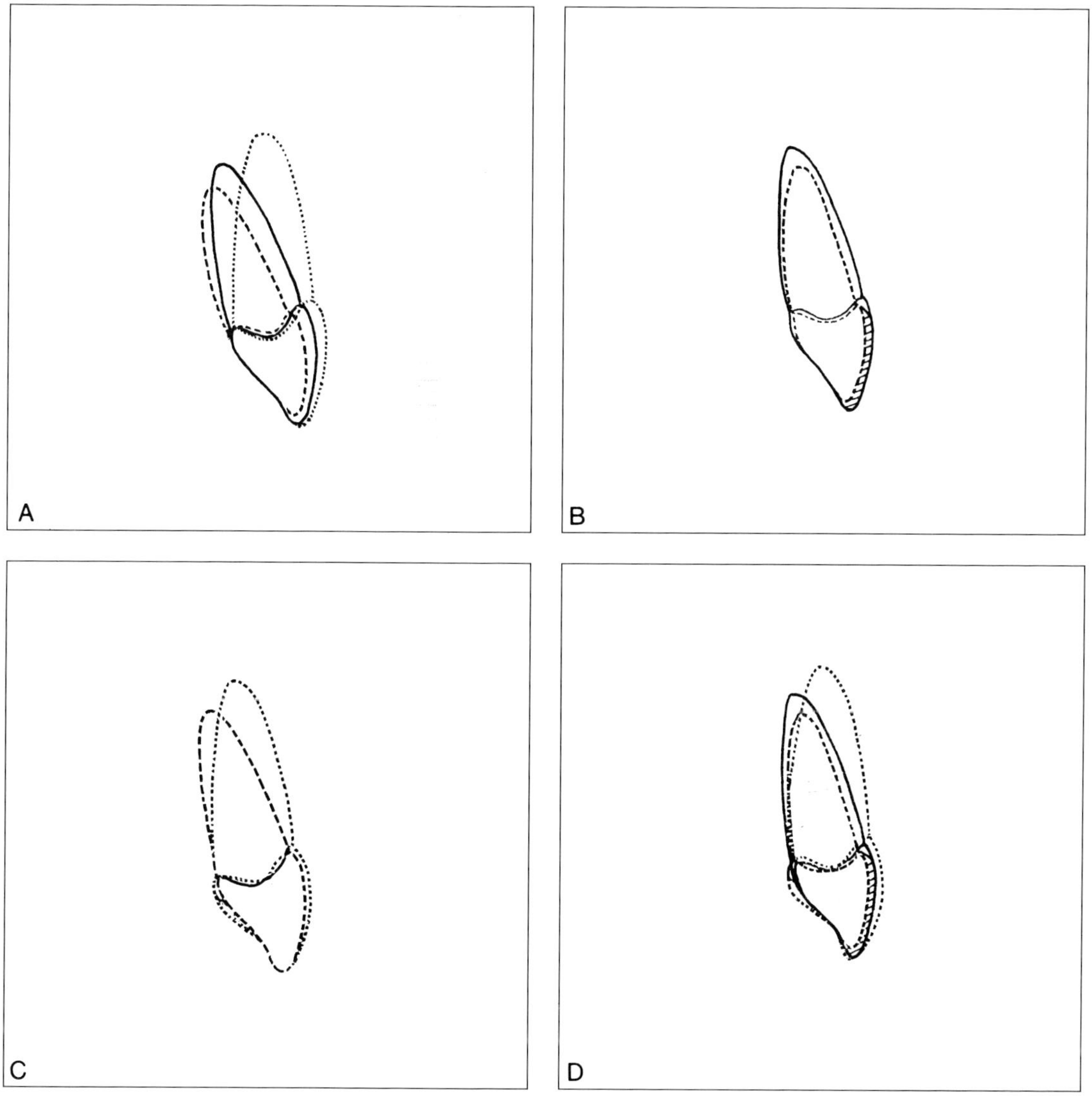

Fig. 11-9 The effect of palatolabial crown dimensions and inclinations on the anteroposterior position of cervical borders.

A Superimposed palatal surfaces of a normally situated central incisor, lateral incisor, and canine reveal the differences in thickness and inclination.
B When a lateral incisor takes the place of a central incisor its inclination must be more upright.
C A canine that substitutes for a lateral incisor must be reduced palatally and its apex tipped lingually.
D A lateral incisor that substitutes for a central incisor and a canine that replaces a lateral incisor must be adapted in form and inclination to match those on the other side.

11.11 Retention and postretention problems

Remarks on this subject made in Chapter 10 concerning agenesis of maxillary lateral incisors apply here also. Maxillary incisor arrangements lacking one or more teeth are seldom stable after orthodontic treatment. Lateral incisors that are moved near to the midline have a great tendency to return distally, which also applies to changes in angulation. In these cases long periods of retention and section of the supraalveolar fibres are of little help.
When one considers any relapse to be unacceptable, then it is necessary to convert to permanent retention with a multistranded wire attached with composite resin that encompasses sufficient adjacent teeth (Fig. 11-10). This wire has to be placed prior to the removal of the fixed appliances or on the same day. The use of a Hawley retainer for an intermediate phase prior to applying a multistranded wire should be avoided. Changes in angulation of substituting teeth cannot be preserved with a removable retainer even if precautions for that purpose are incorporated in the design.

11.12 Supplementary remarks

Children who lose one or more maxillary permanent incisors through trauma experience a serious injury; that also applies, and usually even more, to the parents. The way in which the dentist deals with this, since he or she often is the first expert consulted, is most important. Apart from first aid, in which replantation is a desirable element, giving information on future treatment possibilities is of great value in providing sympathy and support.
At a later stage, when the consequences of the trauma and the possible treatment aims are discussed in more detail, using examples from the records of comparable patients who have already been treated can be most useful in clarifying points and producing reassuring evidence for the future. A diagnostic set-up is outstanding in its value in demonstrating to the patient and parents the result the treatment seeks to achieve.

Fig. 11-10 Retention procedures for corrections of anterior teeth with substitutes.

A The created atypical angulation of the right lateral incisor has a strong tendency to relapse. To prevent this relapse permanent retention by bonding a multistranded wire to the palatal surfaces is a necessity. At least both adjacent teeth must be incorporated, and frequently also an extra one, because the risk for opening of spaces or other unacceptable changes has to be countered.

B Depending on the original situation, the types of corrections performed, and the alterations in tooth crowns realised, the extension of the retention wire must be determined. It is often advisable to incorporate four anterior teeth.

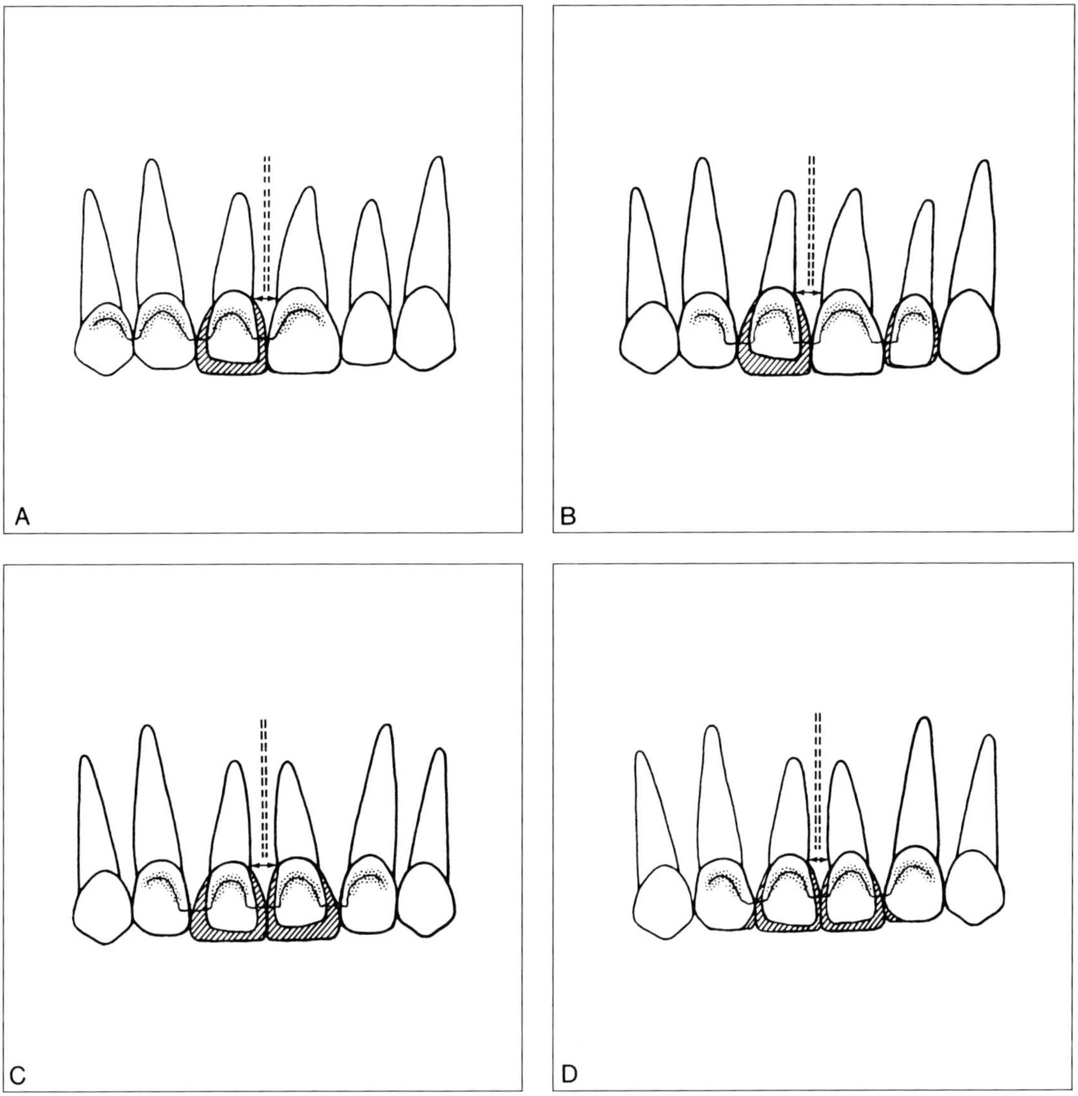

Figure 11-10

C Special care should be given to adequate retention of the angulation and position of two substituting lateral incisors because each has only one normally aligned neighbouring tooth.

D Substitutes that need only limited buildups also must be retained permanently. Note that the situation in D is more favourable than in C because the distances between the adjacent cervical borders are shorter. Also compare these distances in A and B in relation to the angulation and crown sizes.

Chapter 12

Abnormal Lip Positions After Transition of the Incisors

12.1 Introduction

A closed mouth with normal lip contact is associated with nasal breathing, provision of labial support for the maxillary and mandibular incisors, and vertical support for the maxillary incisors. The orofacial region can function and mature normally.
However, there is great variability in lip positions, embracing the way in which upper and lower lips touch each other and the relation between lips and teeth. In this connection important factors are the size, shape, and mutual relations of the bony structures directly behind the lips, the alignment and occlusion of the incisors, and the size and activity of the lips.
After first briefly describing normal lip position, this chapter will cover different lip situations as they relate to various orthodontic deviations; in this regard the emphasis is on Class II/1 anomalies. Subsequently the discussion leads to changes that occur in lips and lip posture during growth and maturity. The diagnosis and detection of deviant lip positions and preventive and therapeutic measures that can be used are covered.

12.2 Normal lip position

Postnatally, a baby's mouth at rest is closed. The jaws are relatively little developed, the alveolar processes are not yet built up, the tongue lies partly between the arches of the jaws, and there is ample lip tissue to maintain mouth closure.
In the period from birth to the first transitional period, normal mouth closure is maintained. The rapid growth of the jaws and development of the teeth seldom give rise to a situation wherein the available tissue is inadequate to provide good lip seal. This problem arises usually only after the maxillary permanent incisors have been in the mouth some time, and the development of the lips is relatively behind that of the dentition. The normal pattern of development is for the permanent incisors to emerge more labially than their predecessors so that, if the development of the lips is slower, the deficiency is emphasised. The mouth then is not closed when at rest; the lips can only meet if active muscle force is used.
Incomplete lip seal is only seen in a small proportion of children. This situation will improve gradually unless other anomalous circumstances prevail. A few years later the lips have caught up to the underlying tissues in their growth, and a proper seal can be achieved once more.

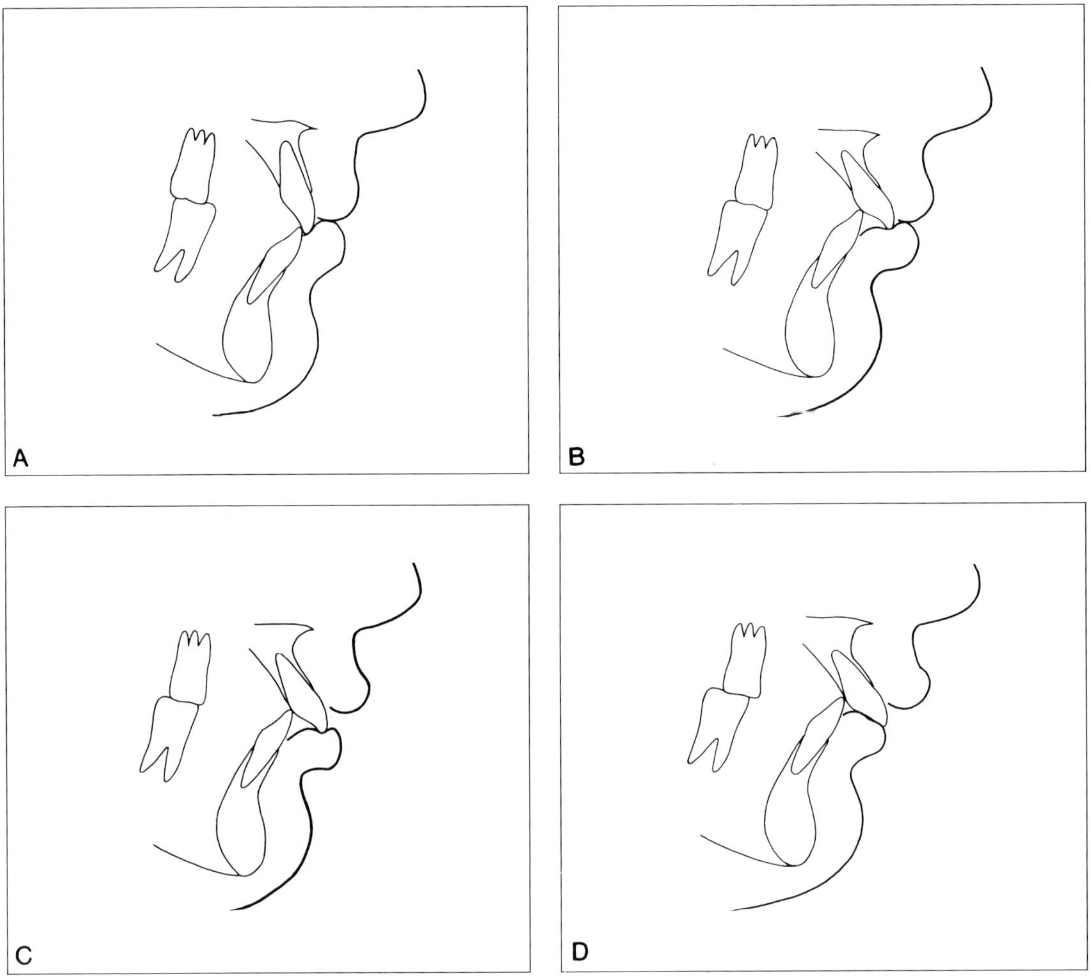

Fig. 12-1 Variations in lip position.

A Normally the upper lip lies against the maxillary incisors and the lower lip lies against the mandibular incisors and the incisal edges and part of the labial surface (1 to 3 mm) of the maxillary incisors. The anterior surface of the lower lip is slightly dorsal to that of the upper lip.

B In mild Class II/1 anomalies with disto-occlusion of half a premolar crown width (1/2 P.W.-disto) and moderate overjet and overbite, normal lip positions can exist with the lower lip no further dorsal than usual; the plica mentalis is deeper however.

C Class II/1 anomalies of moderately large extent (3/4 P.W.-disto) and correspondingly increased overjet and overbite can still permit the lower lip to contact the maxillary incisors incisally.

D In serious Class II/1 anomalies (1 P.W.-disto) with their associated incisor relationships, the lower lip often will be found dorsal to the maxillary incisors. The maxillary incisors can come into supraposition as the result of overeruption.

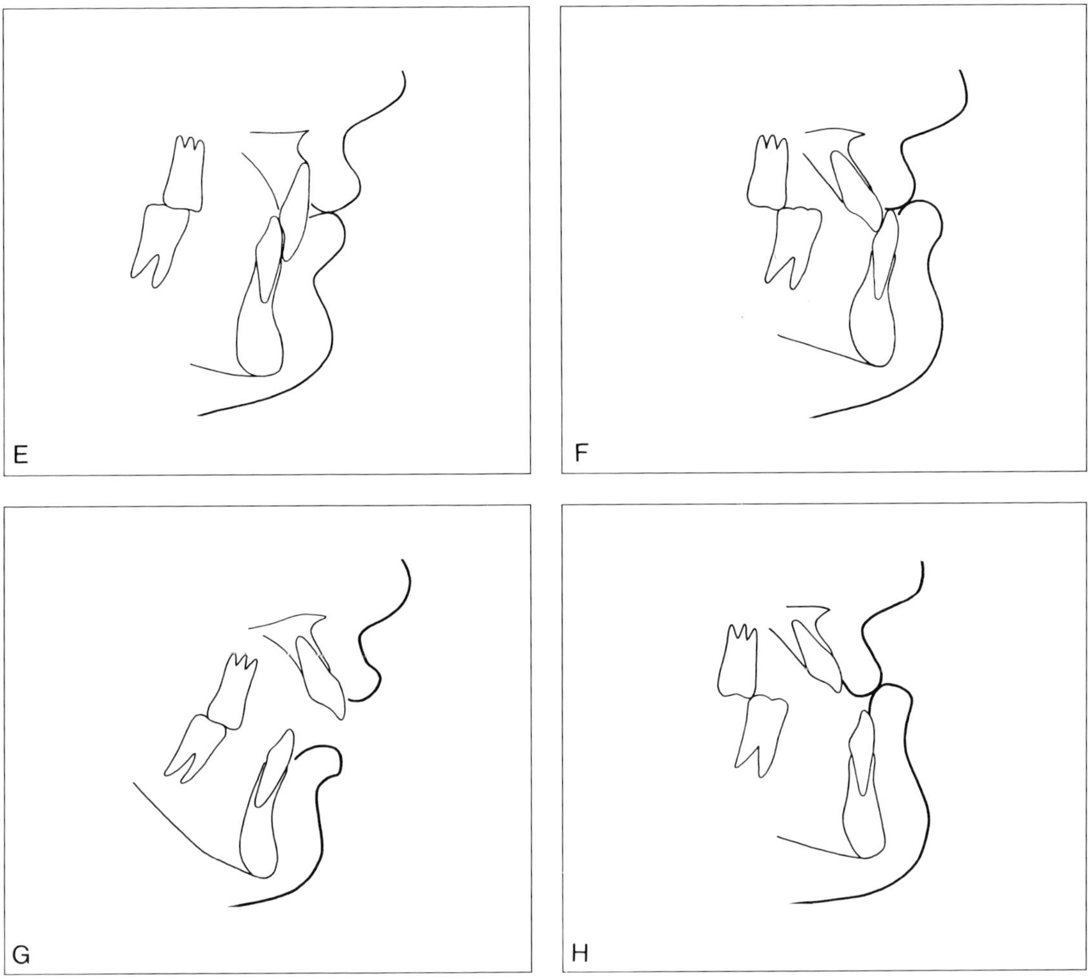

E *Class II/2 anomalies always show a high lip line. The maxillary central incisors are excessively covered by the lower lip. The lips maintain a positive lip seal at rest. The anterior surface of the upper lip is slightly ventral to that of the lower lip.*

F *In Class III anomalies the anterior surface of the lower lip is ventral to that of the upper lip. The larger the reversed overjet, the more pronounced is that effect. Even in pronounced Class III anomalies, the lips achieve satisfactory closure in most cases, because the maxillary incisors are everted and the mandibular incisors are retroclined. If the mandible is held in rest position the lower lip is usually less prominent than when the teeth are in occlusion.*

G *Open bite anomalies with disto-occlusion and excessive lower face height often are associated with an open mouth. The lips are slightly active and short, particularly the upper lip.*

H *Open bites combined with Class III anomalies usually display a closed lip relation. However that is not the case when there is restricted nasal breathing; an open mouth is then a vital need (for adequate respiration).*

When there is an adequate overjet and overbite with normal lip posture, the maxillary central incisors are to a large extent covered by the upper lip. The lower lip lies against the mandibular incisors and partly against the incisal edges and labial surfaces of the maxillary incisors. The lip line (stomion) is at a level 1 to 3 mm cervically from the incisal edges of the maxillary central incisors. The lower lip supports the maxillary incisors labially and vertically; the upper lip works only labially (Fig. 12-1A).

12.3 Lip positions in Class II/1 anomalies

The mouth is closed until the first transitional period, in Class II/1 cases as well as normal ones. In rare instances with a pronounced overjet (e.g., excessive thumb-sucking) the lower lip can be found to lie palatal to the maxillary deciduous incisors.
After emergence of the maxillary permanent incisors an abnormal lip position can arise from a large overjet (Fig. 12-1B to D). Moreover, the lower lip can take up a position between the maxillary and mandibular incisors, which influences further development in a deleterious way (Fig. 12-1D).
The lip position found after transition of the incisors will depend on a complex interplay of facial growth, development of the dentition, and functional influences. The picture is more simply and clearly interpreted by dividing the whole into a number of factors. These are set out in drawings (Figs. 12-2 to 12-13). In succession there are: the morphology of the craniofacial skeleton (Fig. 12-2); direction of growth in the face (Fig. 12-3); quantity of lip tissue (Fig. 12-4); height of the lip line (Fig. 12-5); path of eruption of the incisors (Fig. 12-6); diastemata in the deciduous dentition (Fig. 12-7); size ratio between crowns of deciduous and permanent incisors (Fig. 12-8); rotations of permanent incisors (Fig. 12-9); early resorption and exfoliation of deciduous teeth (Fig. 12-10); increase of the intercanine width (Fig. 12-11); deviant habits (Fig. 12-12); and premature loss of deciduous molars (Fig. 12-13).
It seldom occurs that just one of the 12 factors will lead to positioning of the lower lip palatal to the maxillary incisors. Rather, such a situation mostly occurs because of a combination of several factors that are interdependent or causally related. For example, there is a connection between the available room in the maxillary dental arch and the increase in intercanine width. In addition, the path of emergence of the maxillary central incisors depends on the height of the lip line.[60] Further, the bulk of lip tissue is related to the form of the craniofacial skeleton and the direction of growth. Some factors can exercise favourable influence whereas others are deleterious. Mutual effects can either enhance or neutralise each other. When many unfavourable factors are involved, the lower lip will most likely come to rest against the palatal surfaces of the maxillary incisors. What may appear to be trivial details can tip the scales one way or the other.
If the lips are closed, the location of the anterior aspect of the lower lip is determined not by the mandibular incisors but by the maxillary incisors. The size of the overjet appears to have no demonstrable influence on the anteroposterior relation of the anterior surfaces of the upper and lower lips when there is a normal lip seal. However, the depth of the plica mentalis does increase proportionately as the overjet becomes larger.[35]

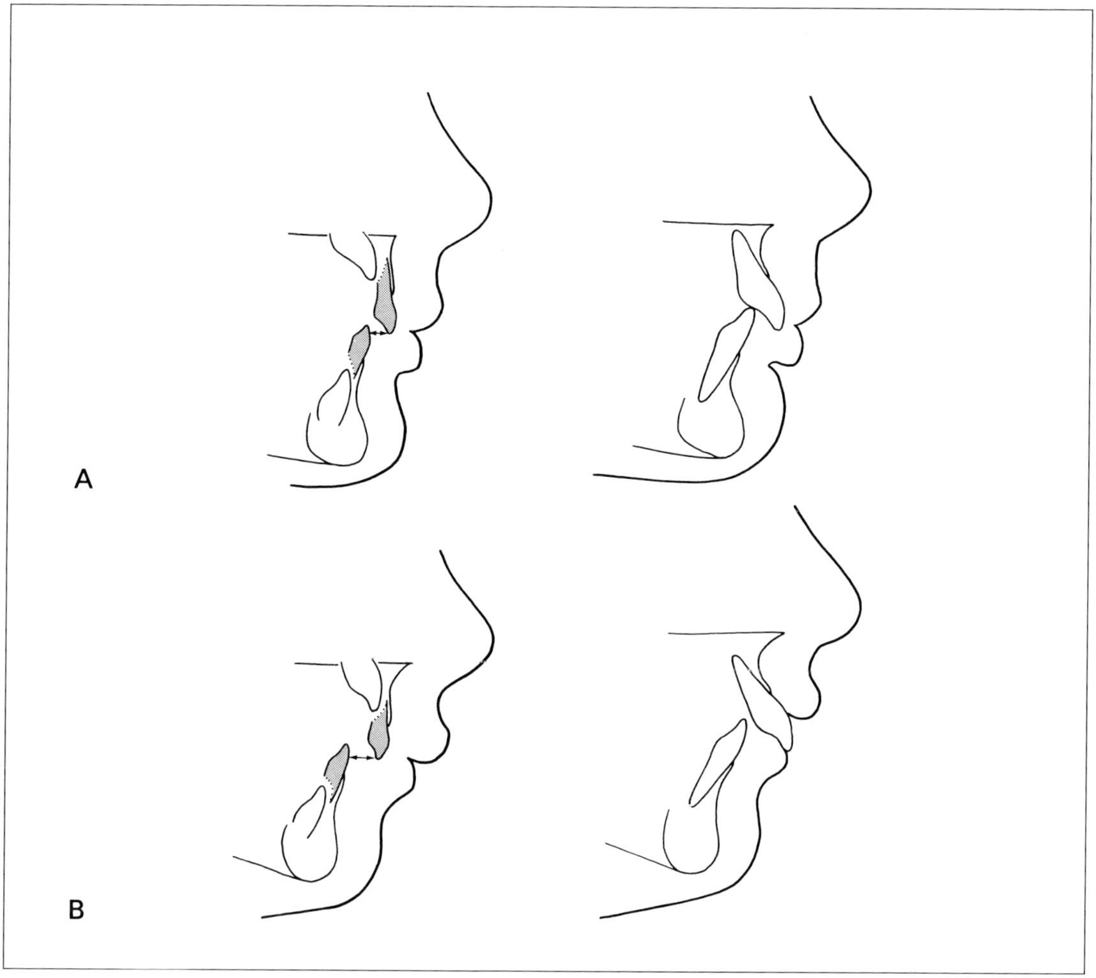

Fig. 12-2 Influence of craniofacial morphology on lip position in Class II/1 anomalies. (From Van der Linden.[219])

A With a mild distorelation of the jaws, a shallow lower face height, and a low mandibular plane angle, a closed lip relation will usually remain after incisor transition.

B With a pronounced distorelation of the jaws, an increased lower face height, and a steep mandibular plane angle there is a great likelihood that the lower lip will lie dorsal to the maxillary incisors after incisor transition.

A

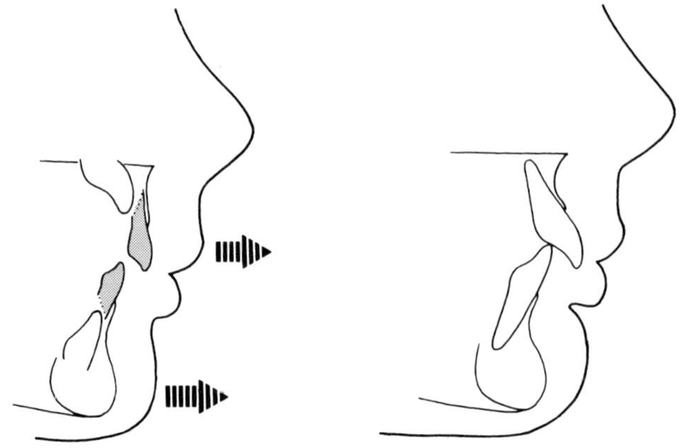

B

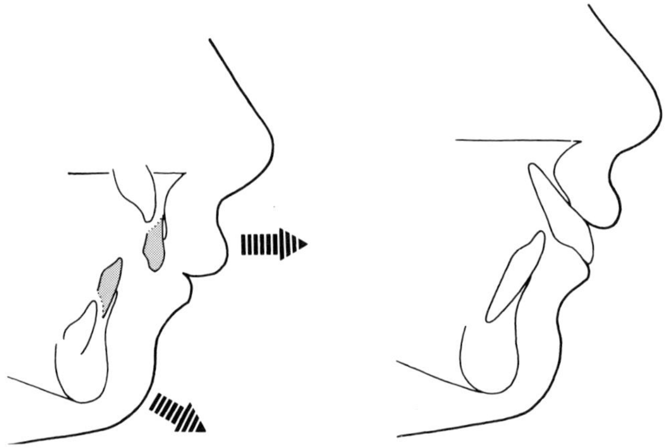

Fig. 12-3 Influence of facial growth direction on lip position in Class II/1 anomalies. (From Van der Linden.[219])

A Where growth of the lower face is principally horizontal, and where the mandible grows more ventrally than the maxilla, a closed lip posture will remain after incisor transition.

B Where the growth of the face is more vertical, the lower lip can come to rest dorsal to the maxillary incisors, particularly when the mandible grows less ventrally than does the maxilla.

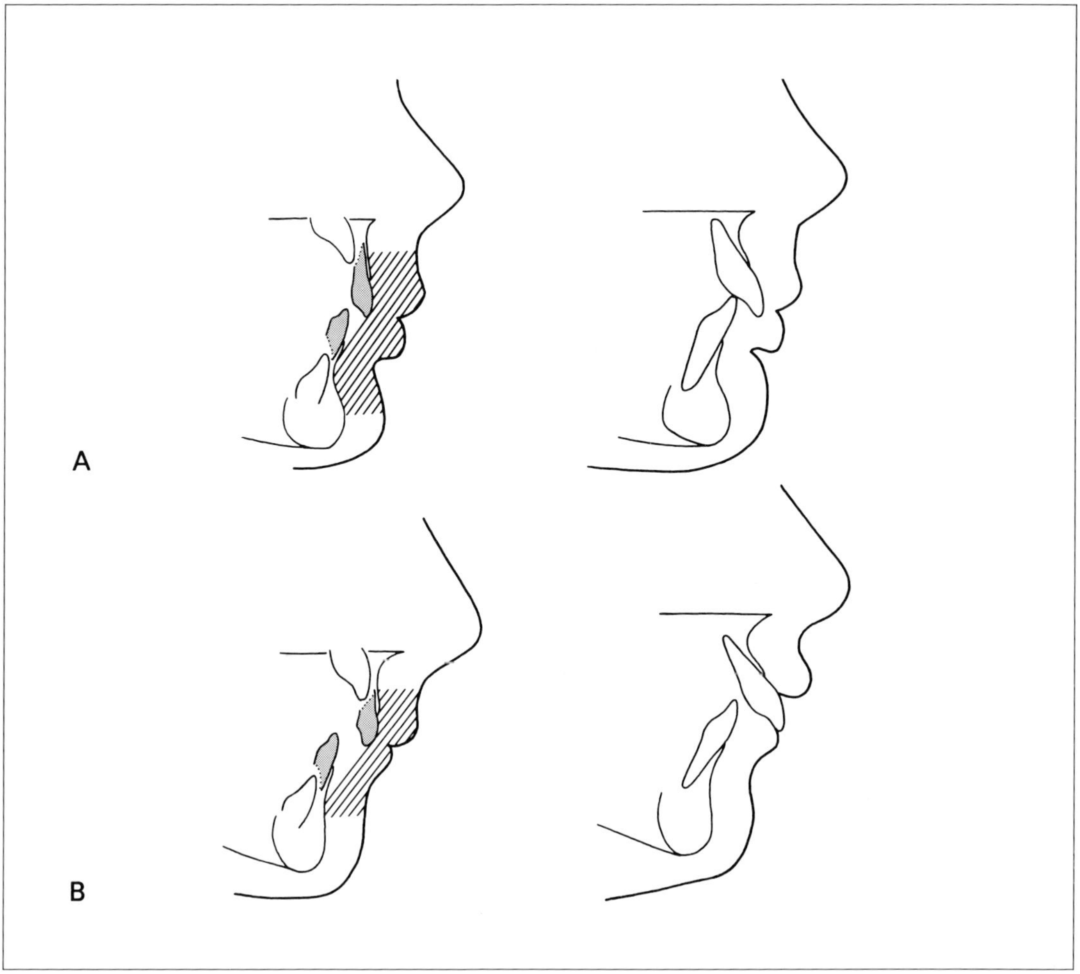

Fig. 12-4 Influence of the bulk of lip tissue on lip positions in Class II/1 anomalies. (From Van der Linden.[219])

A Children with voluminous lips will continue to cover their permanent maxillary incisors with their lips even though they have assumed a more labial position than their predecessors.

B If the lips are proportionately short and thin, the tendency for the lower lip to fall behind the maxillary incisors will be increased after incisor transition. The upper lip will only partly cover the maxillary incisors.

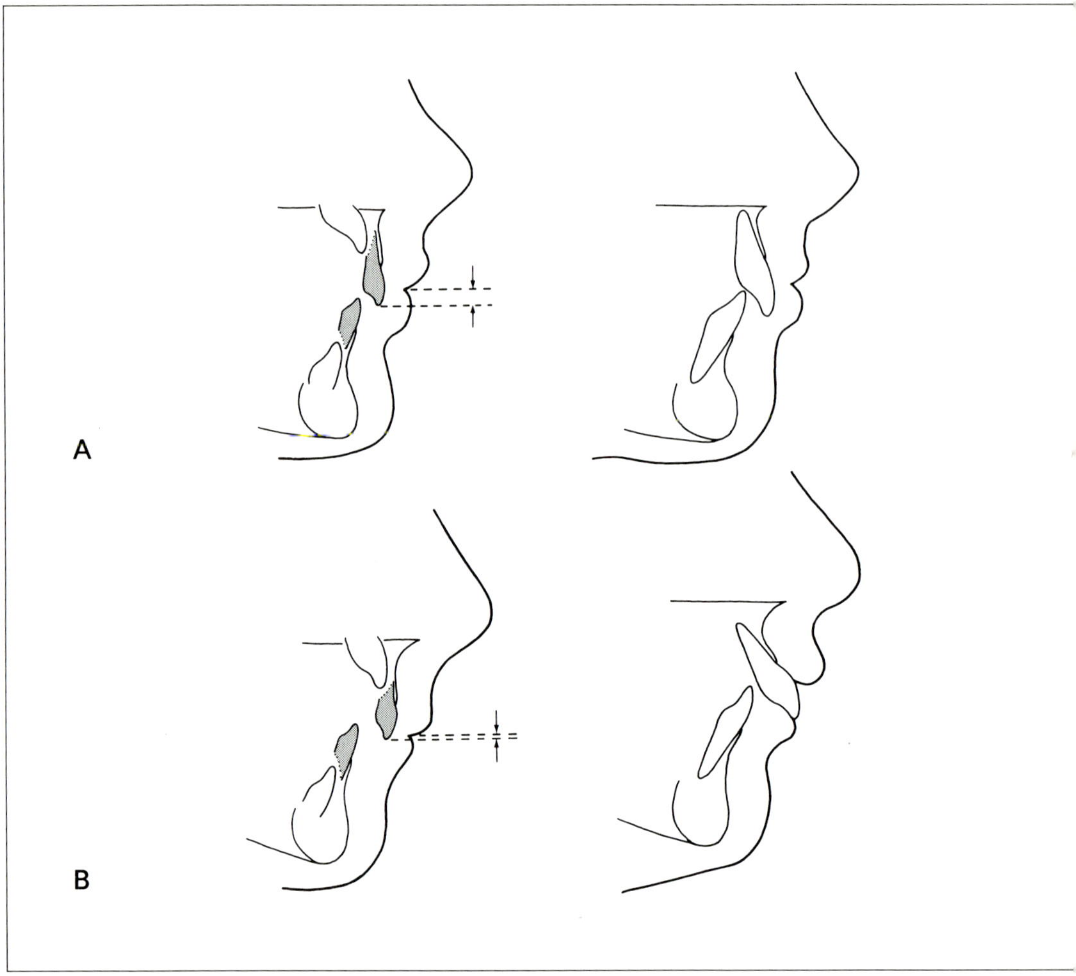

Fig. 12-5 Effect of height of lip line on lip position in Class II/1 anomalies. (From Van der Linden.[219])

A Where there is a high lip line the erupting maxillary incisors will come into contact with the lower lip earlier and as a result move less labially than they would otherwise. The closed lip relation remains.

B Where there is a low lip line the influence of the lower lip on the inclination of the erupting maxillary incisors is relatively minor. Moreover, a short lower lip will more easily contact the maxillary incisors palatally after transition than would a long lower lip.

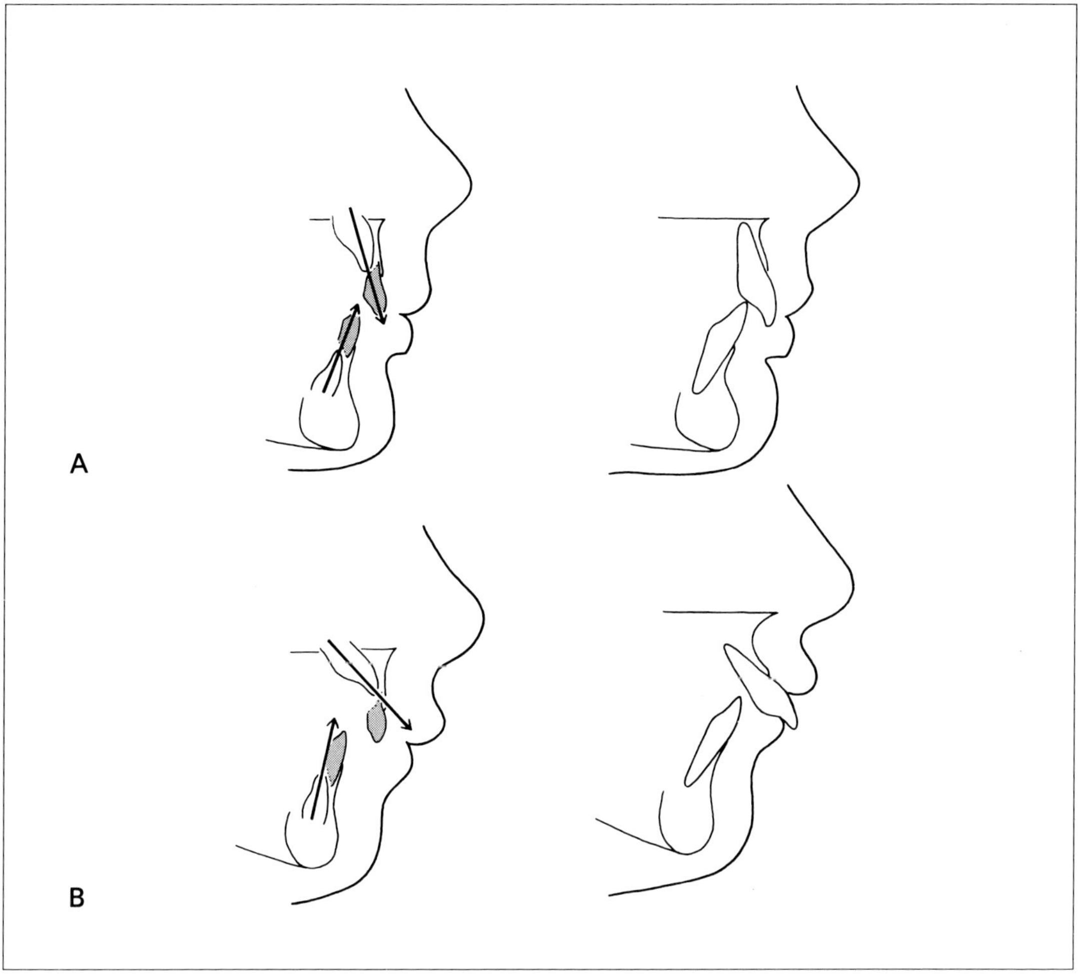

Fig. 12-6 Effect of path of eruption of incisors on lip position in Class II/1 anomalies. (From Van der Linden.[219])

A Eruption of maxillary incisors less labially and mandibular incisors more labially than usual gives rise to a relatively limited overjet and overbite. The closed lip relation remains.

B If the maxillary incisors erupt more labially and the mandibular incisors more lingually than usual, a large overjet and overbite will develop. The lower lip can then come into contact with the palatal aspect of the maxillary incisors.

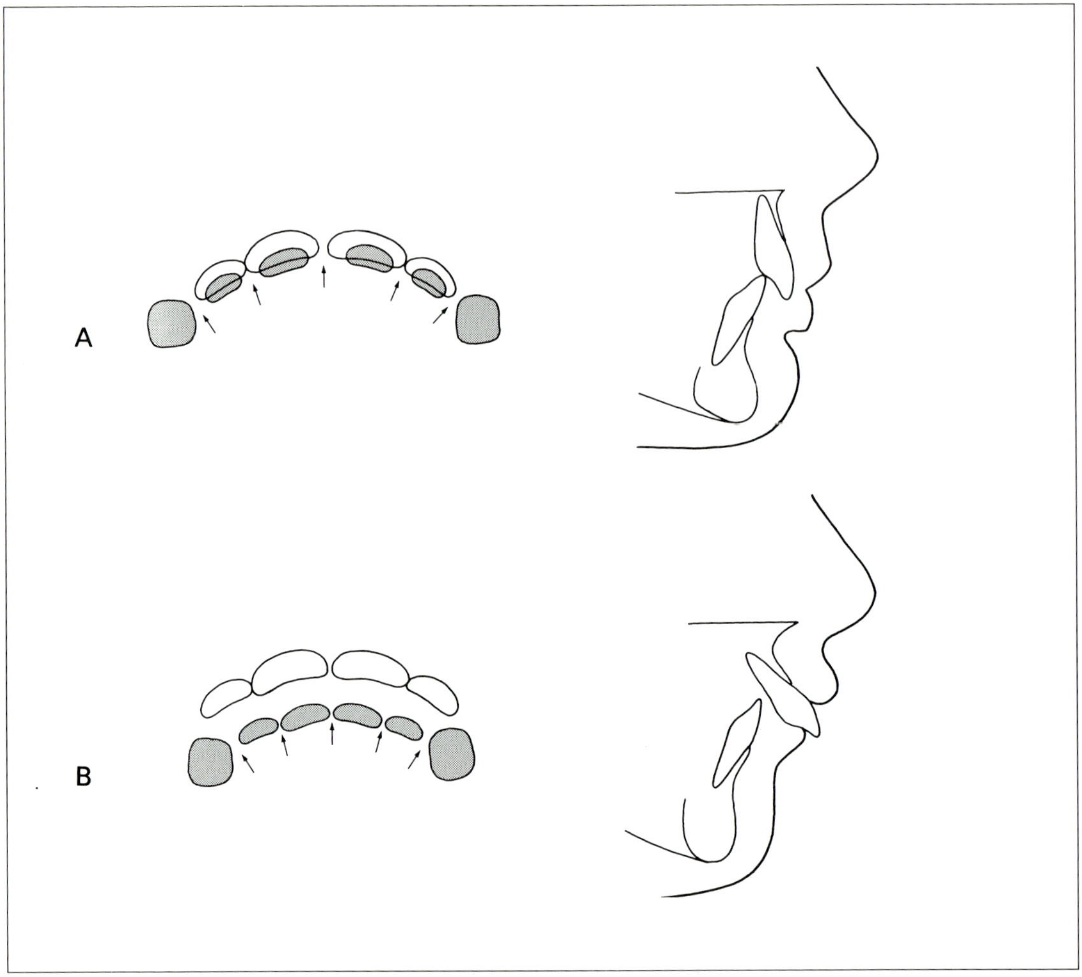

Fig. 12-7 Influence of diastemata in the deciduous dentition on lip position in Class II/1 anomalies. (From Van der Linden.[219])

A When large diastemata exist between deciduous incisors in the maxilla, the permanent incisors will take up positions little further labially in the dental arch than where their predecessors were. The closed lip relation remains.

B When there are few and small diastemata in the maxilla, or a total lack of them, the permanent maxillary incisors will emerge relatively far labially and move substantially further ventrally than the position of their predecessors in the dental arch. The lower lip can then come to lie behind the maxillary incisors.

A

B

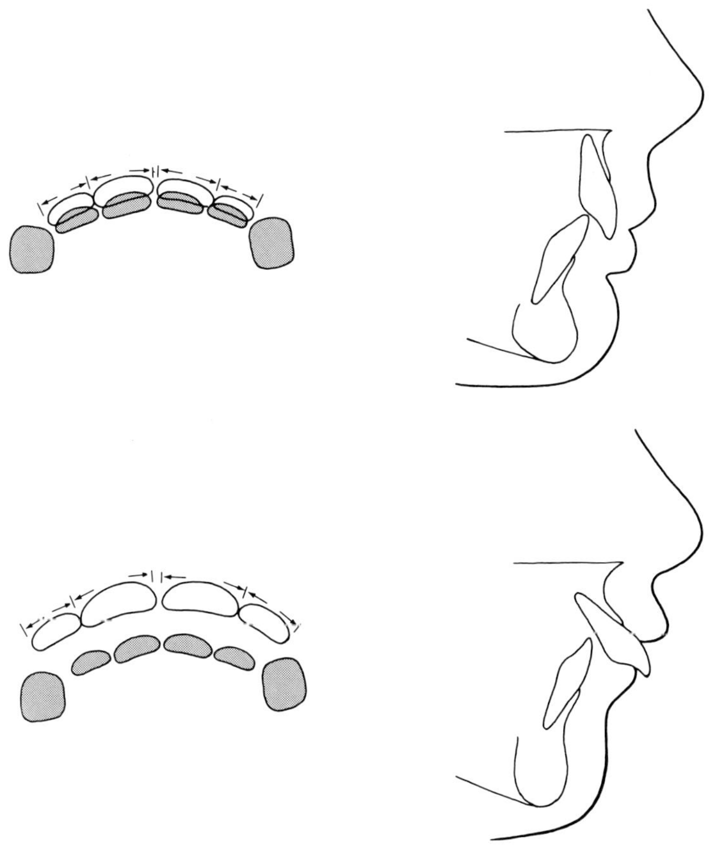

Fig. 12-8 Influence of the size relationship between the crowns of deciduous and permanent incisors on lip positions in Class II/1 anomalies. (From Van der Linden.[219])

A When the mesiodistal crown diameters of the maxillary permanent incisors are little greater than those of their predecessors, the former will take up positions only slightly more labial in the dental arch than where the deciduous incisors were.

B If the maxillary permanent incisors are considerably broader than the deciduous incisors, then they will take up positions further labially in the arch. The lower lip can then lie behind the maxillary incisors, especially when the size difference is less in the mandible.

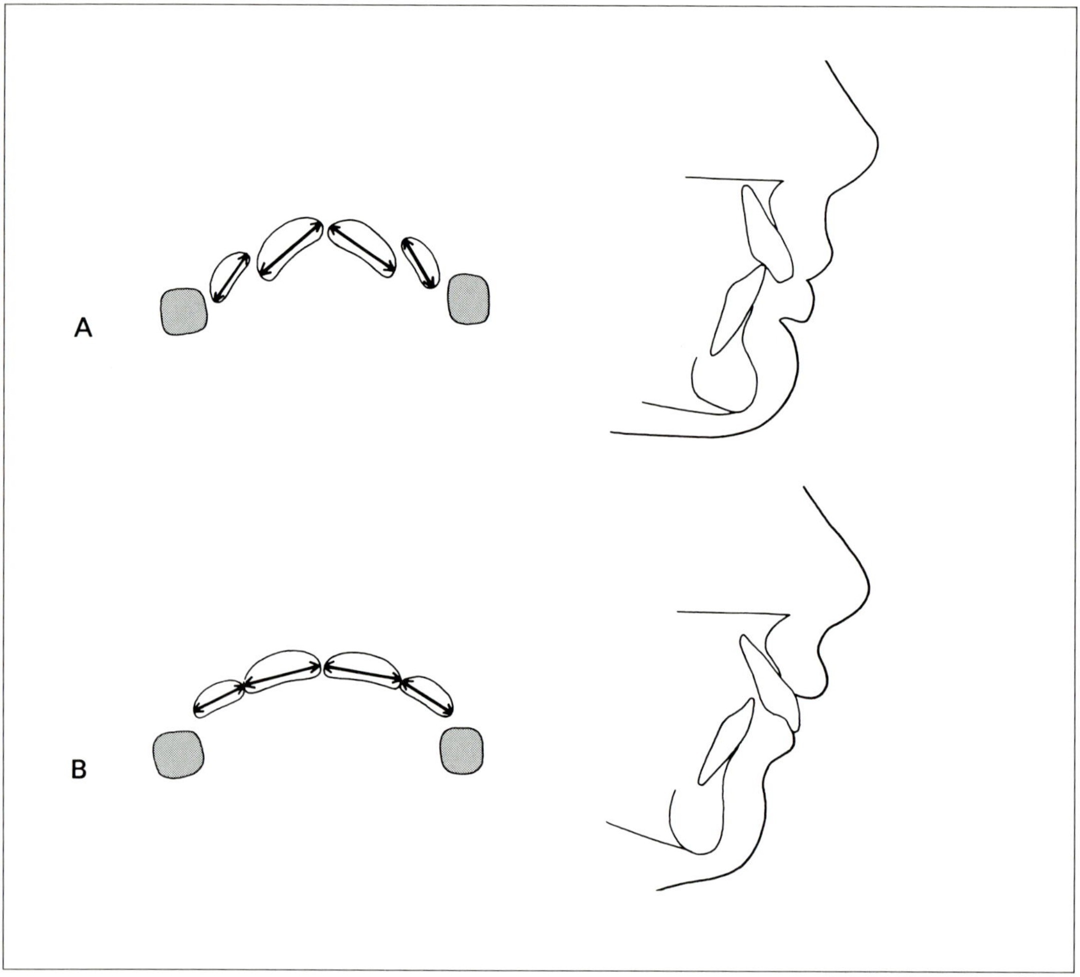

Fig. 12-9 Effect of rotation of permanent incisors on lip position in Class II/1 anomalies. (From Van der Linden.[219])

A Permanent maxillary incisors that emerge rotated require less space in the arch and usually erupt less far labially. The situation with the lips will not change.

B In corresponding circumstances but without rotations, the lower lip will rest behind the maxillary incisors sooner.

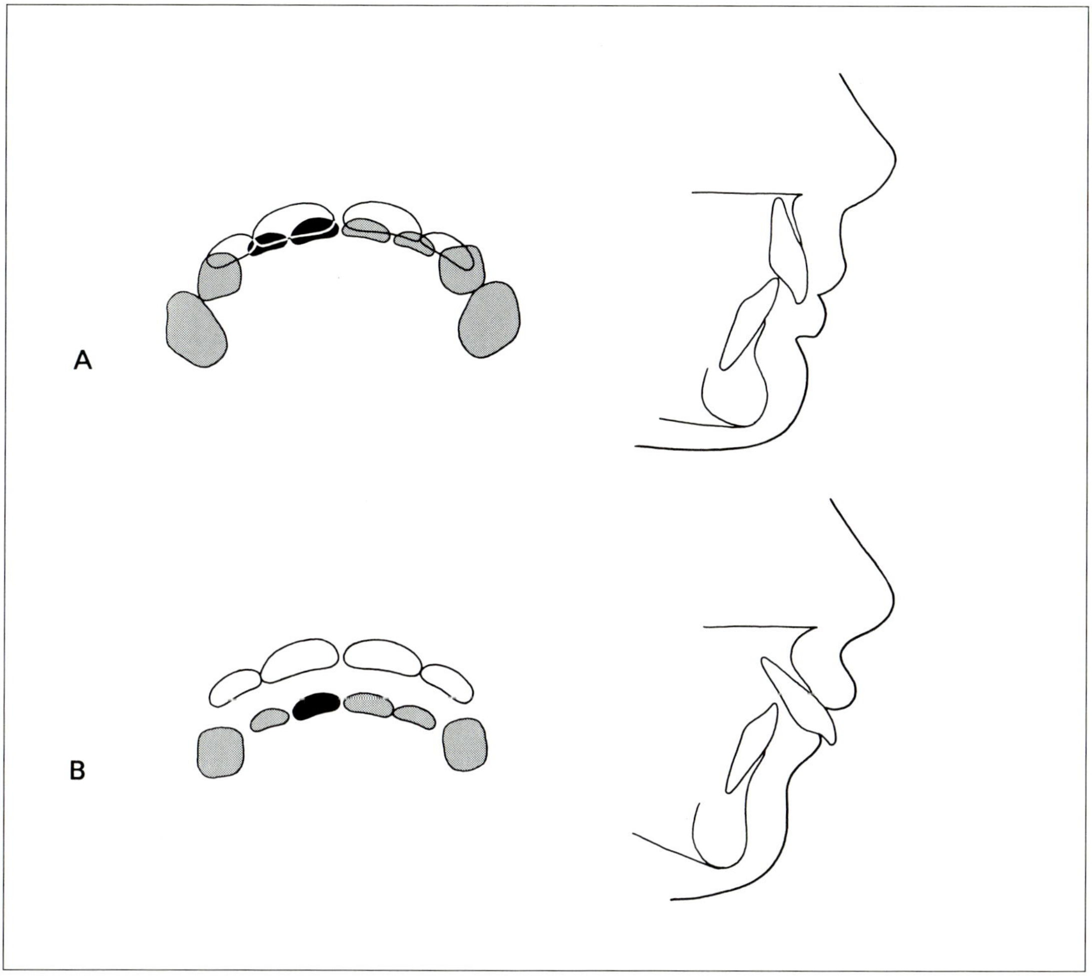

Fig. 12-10 Influence of premature resorption and exfoliation of deciduous teeth on the lip position in Class II/1 anomalies. (From Van der Linden.[219])

A *A central permanent incisor will erupt less far labially when prior to emergence the predecessor and also the adjacent lateral deciduous incisor are lost. The lip relations will not change.*

B *If premature resorption does not occur in cases of crowding, the incisors will emerge relatively far labially. The lower lip can then rest behind the maxillary incisors.*

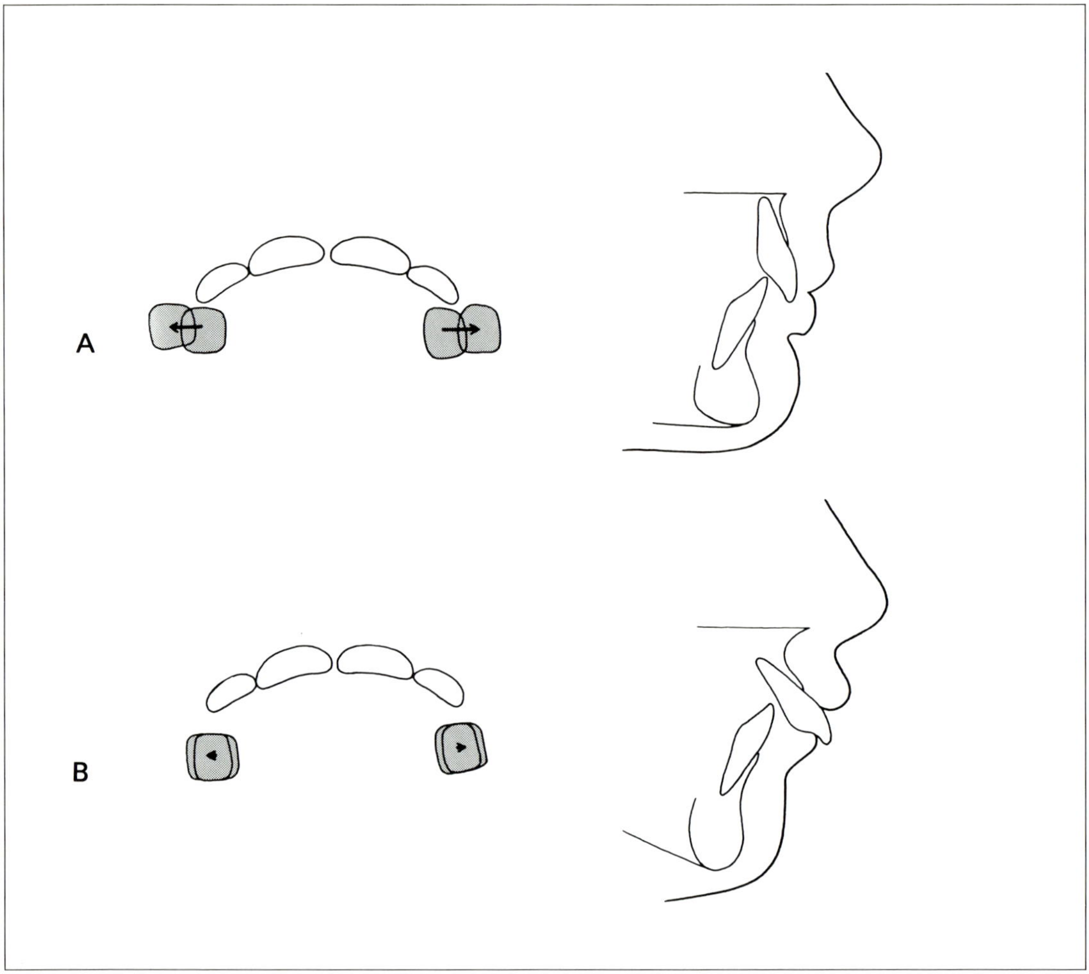

Fig. 12-11 Influence of increased intercanine width on lip position in Class II/1 anomalies. (From Van der Linden.[219])

A A considerable increase in intercanine width provides ample increase in space for the maxillary permanent incisors, which in consequence will emerge less far labially. The existing lip positions will be maintained.

B Where the increase in intercanine width is minimal the maxillary incisors are positioned more labially in the arch. The lower lip will then be more likely to rest behind the maxillary incisors.

A

B

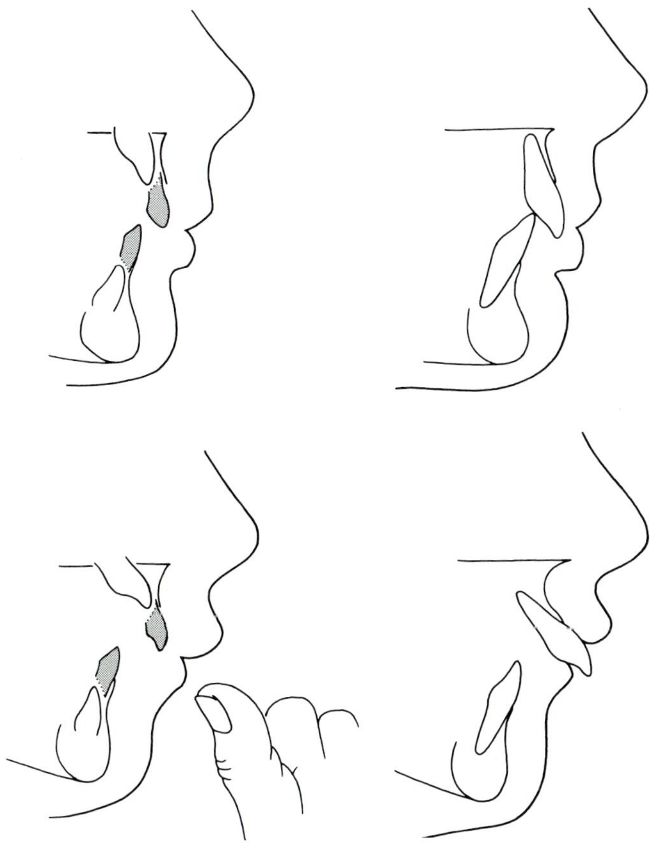

Fig. 12-12 Influence of abnormal habits on lip position in Class II/1 anomalies. (From Van der Linden.[219])

A The absence of abnormal habits supports the preservation of lip closure.

B Thumb-sucking or finger-sucking, lip-biting, and other abnormal habits can displace erupting maxillary permanent incisors labially and the mandibular incisors lingually. The lower lip will then be able to lie against the palatal aspect of the maxillary incisors after transition.

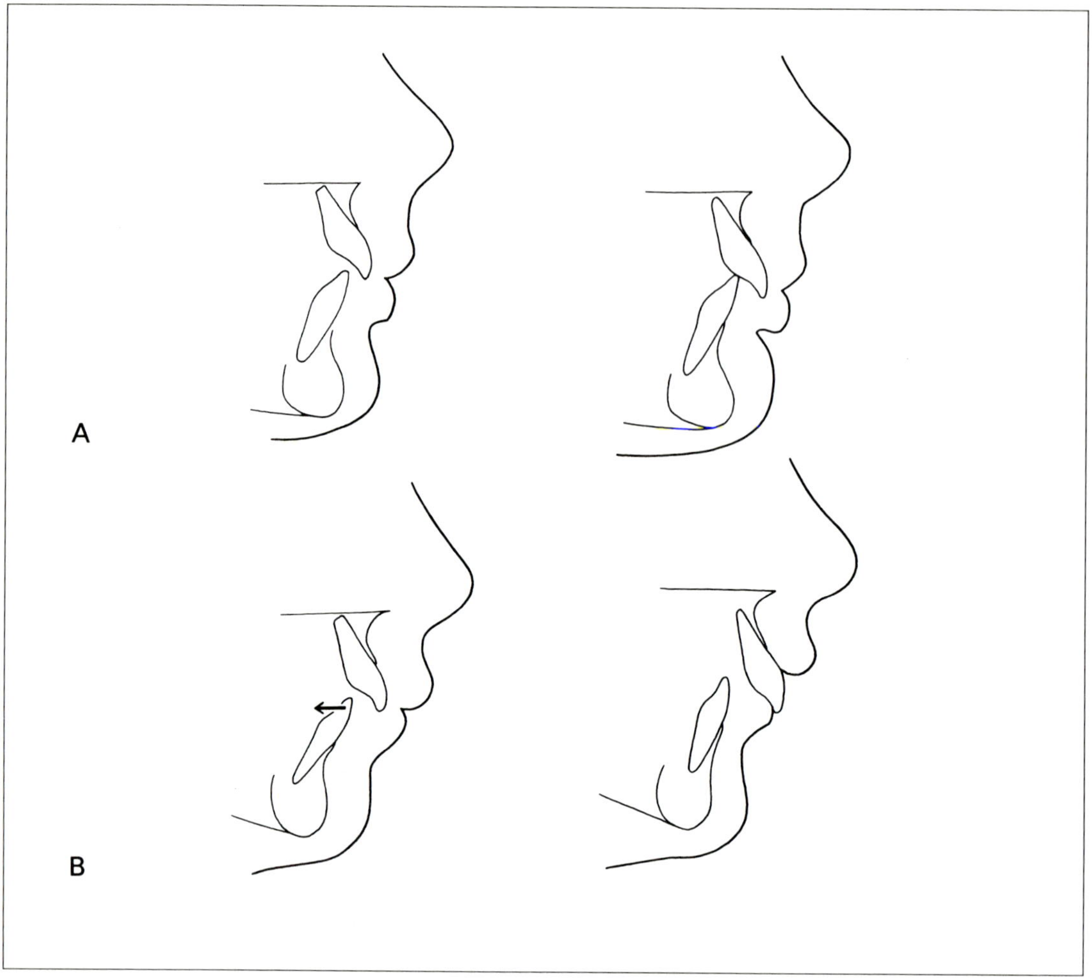

Fig. 12-13 Influence of premature loss of deciduous molars on lip position in Class II/1 anomalies. (From Van der Linden.[219])

A *When the mandibular deciduous molars retain their original mesiodistal dimensions with only minor reductions until the time of their replacement by the premolars, the mandibular incisors will not tip lingually. The lip positions will be maintained.*

B *When premature loss of mandibular deciduous molars or a significant part of their crown material occurs, the mandibular incisors can tip lingually with the danger of the lower lip coming to lie behind the maxillary incisors. Premature loss of maxillary deciduous molars has relatively little effect on maxillary incisor positions.*

12.4 Lip positions in Class II/2 anomalies

Characteristic of Class II/2 anomalies is a high lip line, which lies not at the incisal third of the crowns of the maxillary central permanent incisors but at the cervical third or even higher (Fig. 12-1E). The high lip line is the primary cause of Class II/2 anomalies and of Class I anomalies with Class II/2 symptoms (deckbites or coverbites). Orthodontic treatment without correction of the high lip line is unstable. The lower lip will tip the maxillary incisors back again after such treatment.[226] The high lip line in Class II/2 anomalies is associated with a short upper lip and often with a shallow lower face height, a prominent chin, and excess of soft tissue (Fig. 12-14).

12.5 Lip positions in Class III anomalies

The degree of mesiorelation of the jaws and the size of the reversed overjet largely determine the position of the lips in a Class III anomaly (Fig. 12-1F). The lower lip projects ventrally to the upper lip, something that also occurs when the incisor occlusion is merely edge-to-edge, because the lower lip is thicker than the upper. Because in serious Class III anomalies the mandibular incisors are tipped lingually and the maxillary incisors are tipped labially, a normal lip seal usually is possible. Generally, the situation regarding the lips will be affected by the rest position of the mandible. The larger the freeway space, the more the ventral aspect of the mandible becomes displaced caudally as it rotates back from habitual occlusion into the rest position. Consequently the lower lip falls back in relation to the upper lip and may even provide a normal profile when the patient is relaxed.

12.6 Lip positions in anterior open bites

In open bites that have been caused primarily by thumb-sucking, a normal lip relation can exist at rest. However, if there are other factors involved, the lip position can indeed be abnormal. Where an open bite is caused by interposition of the tongue, frequently the lips are held apart. Naturally, in mouth breathers the lips are always open.

Open bites often are associated with disto-occlusion; the mouth then is generally held open (Fig. 12-1G). Open bites with mesio-occlusion often do show complete lip closure, but not always (Fig. 12-1H).

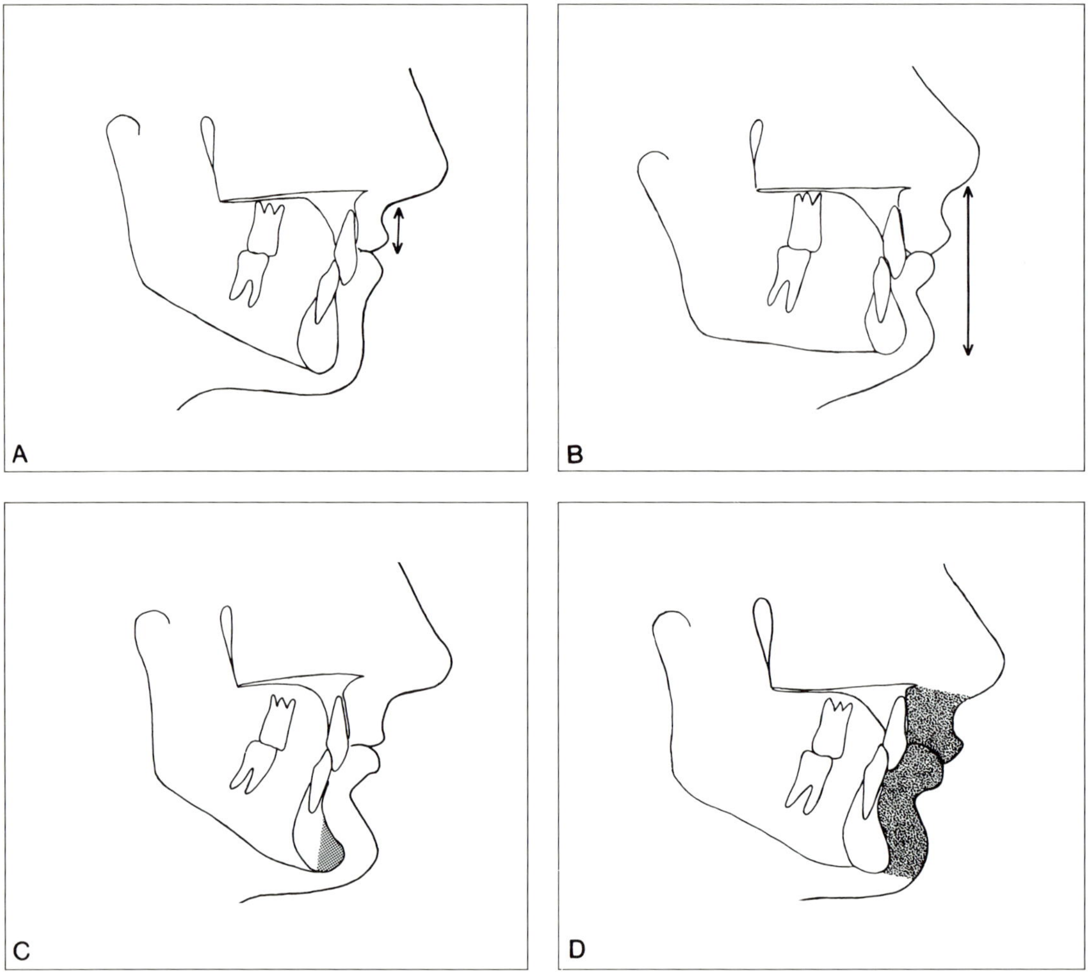

Fig. 12-14 In a Class II/2 anomaly four aspects, singly or combined, can present themselves. (From Van der Linden and Boersma.[226])

A A relatively short upper lip.
B A shallow lower face height with a more or less horizontal lower border of the mandible and a small angle of the mandible.
C A prominent bony chin.
D Excess of soft tissue.

12.7 Age changes in lip position

The increase in lip length that overcomes the backlog in vertical growth of the lower third of the craniofacial skeleton occurs principally between ages 9 and 13 years. Lack of lip seal after transition of the incisors can revert to complete closure during this process. In this period, and also for some years afterwards, the lips grow together more than the lower part of the face grows vertically, so that the lower lip becomes longer than the upper,[234] while both lips increase approximately equally in sagittal cross section.[128]

After adulthood is reached, changes continue in the morphology of the craniofacial skeleton, position of the teeth, and soft tissues (Fig. 12-15). The profile becomes straighter, the upper lip becomes longer and thinner, and the prominence of the lower lip increases. The lip line descends relative to the maxillary incisors.[14] Further, the mobility of the upper lip decreases with age; in smiling and speaking the maxillary incisors show less, the mandibular incisors show more.

Because lip growth only begins to catch up with vertical growth of the lower part of the face after completion of transition, it is the permanent incisors that dominate the face before and during adolescence. Only in following years does the dentition retreat into the face, due on the one hand to the continued forward growth of the jaws and the associated uprighting of the incisors, and on the other hand to the relatively greater increase in lip length. This development operates to change the open lip posture to a complete lip seal, and draws attention away from the dentition and any deviations in it. This tendency continues in later years so that eventually orthodontic anomalies are usually well masked, though in a younger person the same anomaly would be obtrusive.

12.8 Diagnosis and observation

The dentist should be alert to unfavourable changes in lip position that can present themselves after incisor transition. Changes in lip position can develop particularly in pronounced Class II/1 anomalies. A tendency for the lower lip to be situated behind the maxillary incisors should be recognised early. In this regard a marked distorelation, increased lower face height, steep mandibular plane, retroclined and crowded mandibular incisors, and pointed maxillary arch are all conditions where such a lip position might be expected.

In less serious Class II/1 and Class I anomalies an originally closed mouth can degenerate into an open mouth because there is insufficient lip tissue to cover the teeth in a relaxed state. This scenario is of a temporary character in many instances and changes back to complete lip seal when the "catch-up" in lip growth occurs.

Abnormal lip posture, in which the lip line is excessively high in relation to the maxillary incisors, is exhibited in Class II/2 anomalies and in Class I anomalies with symptoms of Class II/2. A similar situation can occur in the deciduous dentition. It is a matter of concern that this be recognised early.

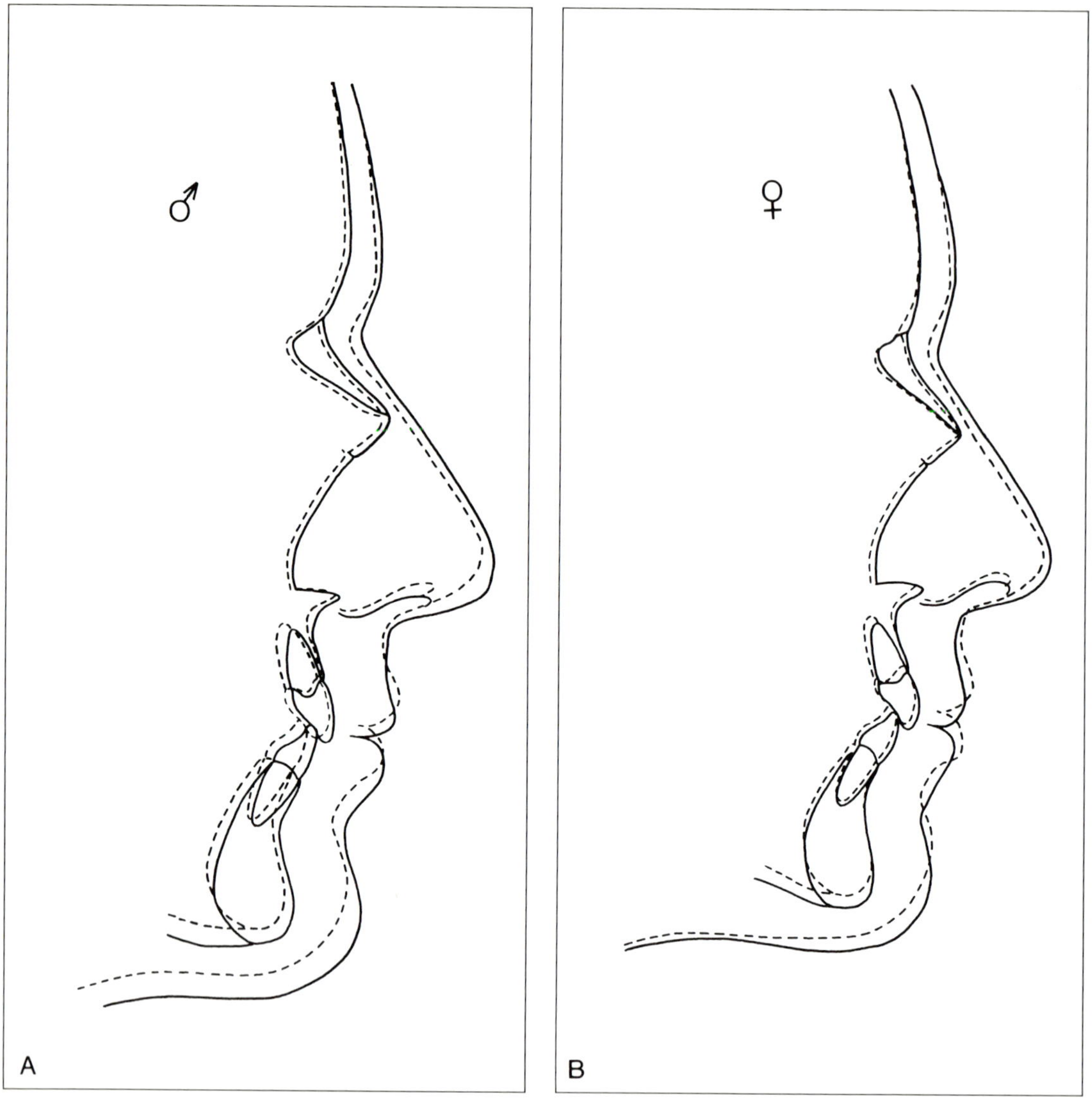

Fig. 12-15 Superimposition of contour changes of anterior skeletal and dental structures and of the profile, such as still occur in adult life. The drawings are based on the mean values of individual changes registered in 113 persons, for whom a lateral cephalogram was taken around the ages of 20 and 50 years.
In females (B) the mandible rotates posteriorly, and the lower face height increases. The face height in males (A) increases also, but the mandible rotates anteriorly, so that the anterior aspect of the mandible moves ventrally. In both sexes the nose becomes larger; the tip of the nose drops and becomes more pointed. The lip line drops and with that the lip position relative to the maxillary incisors descends. The upper lip becomes longer and thinner whereas the lower lip becomes thicker and more prominent. The latter applies also to the soft tissues covering the chin. (From Behrents.[14])

12.9 Prevention and therapy

Abnormal situations affecting the lips, in which the lower lip tends to rest behind the maxillary incisors, can be prevented. Measures to achieve this depend on preventing the development of an excessive overjet.
If thumb-sucking or finger-sucking habits exist, an attempt should be made to break them in a considerate fashion.
In selected cases deciduous canines can be extracted in the maxilla in the expectation that the permanent incisors will then emerge less far labially. In this connection one must take into account the fact that insufficient room will then remain for the permanent canines, so this will need correction at a later date (see 9.8.2).
Impending loss of deciduous canines and molars in the mandible should be prevented. Premature resorption of deciduous canines unfortunately cannot be prevented.
Lip exercises can, at least if performed frequently and over a long period with consistency, achieve a lengthening and improved function of the lips.[90]
The lower lip tends especially to rest behind the maxillary incisors in serious Class II/1 cases. These patients exhibit a marked distorelation of the jaws, abnormal function of the facial musculature, and an increased risk of trauma to the maxillary incisors. This combination of factors calls for a beginning of facial orthopedic therapy at an earlier stage than usual. In this way the jaw relation should be improved, normal functional relationships developed, and the risk of injury to the incisors reduced. Functional appliances (activator and the like) serve this purpose well, which also applies to combinations of functional and extraoral appliances.
When the tendency for the lower lip to fall behind the maxillary incisors is really due to severe retroclination of the mandibular incisors, a lip bumper or 0.045 in. mandibular arch can be used. With these one attempts both to hold the lower lip further forward and to relieve the load on the labial aspect of the mandibular incisors. The mandibular incisors can then move anteriorly under the influence of the tongue.
When confronted with a situation where the lower lip is already located behind the maxillary incisors, then the above therapeutic approaches can still be applied. In so doing one should realise that the maxillary incisors often will have moved into supraposition. This certainly will occur when the deviant lip posture has been adopted for some time. Intrusion of the maxillary incisors is then an essential part of the treatment. If this aspect is disregarded, a situation is created that can lead eventually into a Class I anomaly with symptoms of a Class II/2 anomaly (Fig. 12-16).
If the transition in the posterior segments is already complete, correction of the lip positions becomes a part of the total therapeutic procedure. The correction of abnormal lip positions in Class II/2 anomalies forms a significant component in the complex therapy that such patients demand.
Deviant lip positions in Class III anomalies are usually part of a marked abnormality of the craniofacial skeleton. In such instances it is often not possible to achieve a good result without surgery. Improvement of the lips will occur when a normal overjet is obtained.
Open bites caused by interposition of the tongue, especially when coupled with increased height of the lower face and restricted nasal patency, often cannot be treated to a situation where lip closure is possible without tension. Nevertheless, this objective should be aimed for because the stability of the orthodontic correction

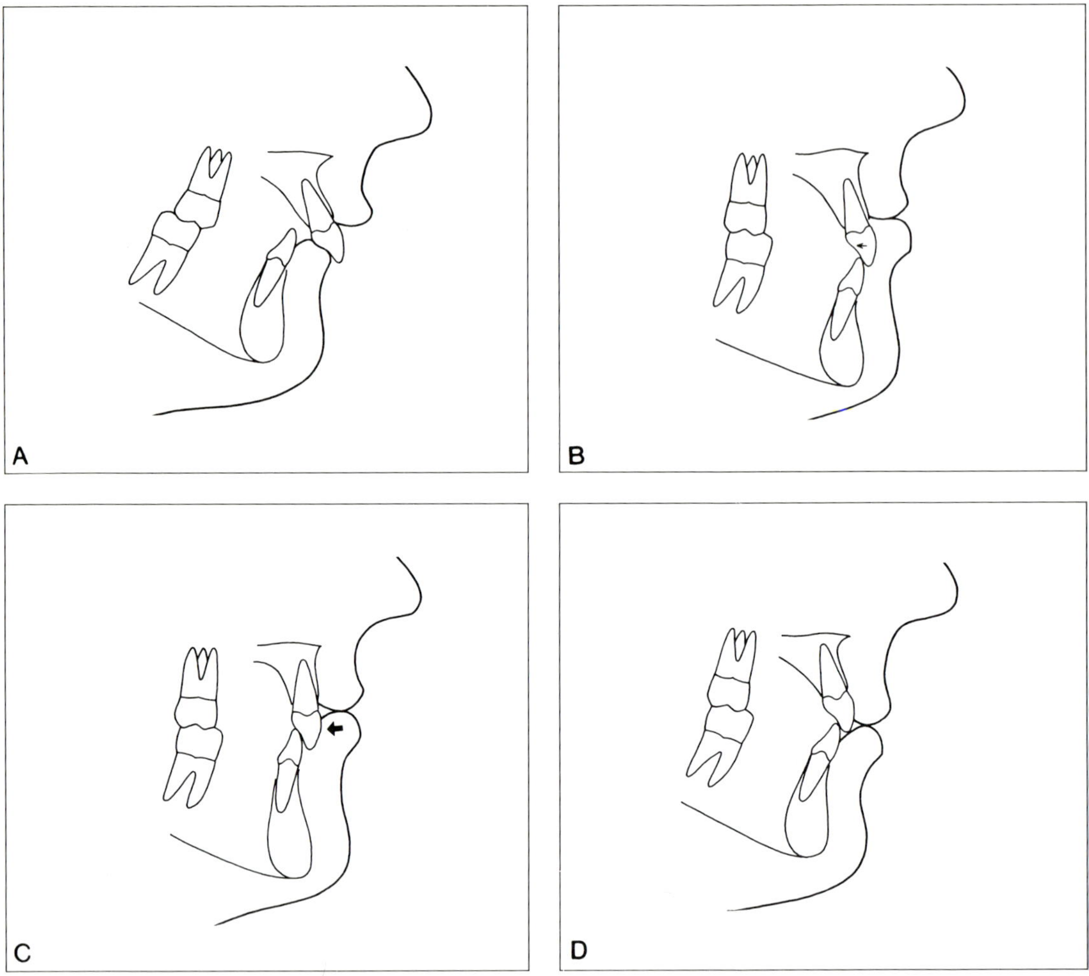

Fig. 12-16 Aspects of lip-tooth relationships in treating Class II/1 anomalies with the lower lip behind overerupted maxillary incisors. (From Van der Linden.[224])

- *A* *Class II/1 situation with lower lip behind the maxillary incisors and with overeruption of these teeth.*
- *B* *Retraction of the maxillary incisors without intrusion of these teeth, but of the mandibular incisors, can lead to a lip-tooth relationship such as is found in Class II/2 anomalies.*
- *C* *After treatment there has been further retroclination and increased overbite. A Class II/2 incisor malalignment has developed.*
- *D* *Alternative treatment has attained a normal lip-tooth relationship by intrusion of the incisors, possibly in combination with stimulated further eruption of the molars. This eliminates the subsequent manifestation of a Class II/2 incisor malalignment.*

depends to a great extent on normal functional relationships and in particular on complete lip seal.

12.10 Supplementary remarks

Normal lip seal demands normal unobstructed nasal breathing. Only if that demand is satisfied can a change from open to closed lip posture be anticipated. If there is inadequate air flow through the nose, consultation and possible treatment by an ear, nose, and throat specialist is indicated.

A separate type of abnormal lip function is the mentalis habit, in which the mentalis muscle is excessively active. This is revealed by pitting of the skin of the chin where the muscle fibres are inserted ("golf ball" effect) and by increased pressure upon the labial surfaces of the mandibular incisors. Those incisors can consequently be tipped lingually. Correction of a mentalis habit can be attempted by lip exercises aimed at relaxation. A lip bumper or functional regulator with labial pads according to Fränkel[59,60] may be used also.

In bringing about a normal lip situation the aim should be to achieve contact between the adhesive zones of the upper and lower lips in a relaxed state.[59] In this regard a good overjet and overbite are of primary importance.

The tone and activity of the lip muscles play a significant role in determining whether or not a closed lip posture is adopted. Frequently children with open mouths exhibit a short upper lip with lack of tone and limited function. The lower lip is usually thick and curled forward. To change over to a closed mouth and normal function the patient must make a conscious effort. In such cases lip exercises can be useful.

Finally, it should be observed that for the best possible conformation of the dentition and face, normal functional relationships are important. Disturbances in this respect require early recognition and treatment and preferably should be prevented from developing.

Chapter 13

Transition Problems in the Posterior Regions

13.1 Introduction

There is great variation in transition in the posterior regions. This variation is described and illustrated for the mandible in Chapter 3 and for the maxilla in Chapter 6 in relation to the size of the middle section of the apical area, the room available in the dental arch for the permanent canines and premolars, and the sequence of emergence. The effect the transition in the posterior regions can have on the position of the incisors is subsequently shown in Chapters 4 and 7.

In this chapter problems that develop during transition in the posterior regions are dealt with according to their clinical manifestations and the possibilities to guide or treat them. Subsequently interceptive measures, rotated canines and premolars, their emergence buccally or lingually, prevention and correction of endo-occlusion and exo-occlusion, lateral open bites, ankylosis of deciduous molars, and impacted canines and premolars are all discussed. A separate chapter (14) has been devoted to premature loss of deciduous molars, and Chapter 15 deals with agenesis of premolars.

13.2 Interceptive measures

Preventing caries of deciduous teeth and timely restoration of carious lesions when they occur will limit the danger of undesired reduction of arch length and of the space available for the permanent canines and premolars.

Deciduous teeth that are retained too long can impede the assumption of correct positions of already emerged permanent canines and premolars. This applies specifically to maxillary canines that emerge high labially and premolars that emerge abnormally far buccally (in danger of developing exo-occlusion). Extraction of persisting deciduous teeth usually results in spontaneous correction of the eruption path of their successors.

Extraction of a maxillary first deciduous molar 6 to 12 months before the time it would normally be expected to exfoliate leads to accelerated eruption and earlier emergence of its successor. In instances where the as yet unemerged permanent canine and first premolar lie in close proximity (small middle section of the apical area), extraction of the first deciduous molar may result in distal movement of the canine crown within the alveolar process. This happens because, after the descent of the relatively broad premolar crown, the narrower premolar roots occupy less space than the crown did. This early distal movement of the canine can result in improved alignment of the lateral incisor.

As has been outlined in earlier chapters, the difference between mesiodistal crown diameters in deciduous and permanent teeth plays an important role in determining whether or not the process of transition progresses optimally. In instances of an unfavourable distribution of these differences, judicious reduction of the mesiodistal diameters of the deciduous crowns will permit a better arrangement of the premolars and permanent canines than would have occurred if nothing had been done. In some circumstances the alignment of the anterior teeth also can improve as a result of such an action. The various situations are outlined in Figs. 13-1 and 13-2. It is often sufficient just to "slice" the mesial surface of the mandibular second deciduous molar, especially when this tooth has a markedly greater mesiodistal diameter than its successor. The advantage of slicing in the maxilla is less than in the mandible and it is consequently less often advocated there.

Finally, it might be noted that overcontoured restorations in first permanent molars can inhibit normal transition; prompt correction of such a situation is essential.

13.3 Rotated canines and premolars

Mandibular permanent canines sometimes emerge rotated. Usually this is a sign of crowding. Should sufficient room become available for them in the dental arch later, natural correction of their position can follow. This usually occurs only partially and certainly not in all cases. The same applies even more strongly to mandibular premolars, which often emerge rotated and improve their position only occasionally because of the influence of occlusion.

The same applies in general to the maxilla, though rotations occur less often there. Rotations of maxillary premolars have more consequences as far as the occlusion is concerned than of mandibular premolars, whose lingual cusps only contact their antagonists to a limited extent or not at all. A correct position of the maxillary premolar palatal cusps is considerably significant, however, in establishing a good interdigitation. Where indicated, rotated premolars should be corrected later.

Fig. 13-1 Transition of the posterior teeth with crowding in the mandibular arch.

A Mandibular incisor crowding is present in the intertransitional period.
B Eruption of the permanent canine with insufficient space in the dental arch.
C The canine overlaps the lateral incisor.
D The first premolar had sufficient space on emergence.
E The canine can profit from the extra space as the second premolar erupts distally.
F The canine has improved its position; crowding of the incisors has increased.

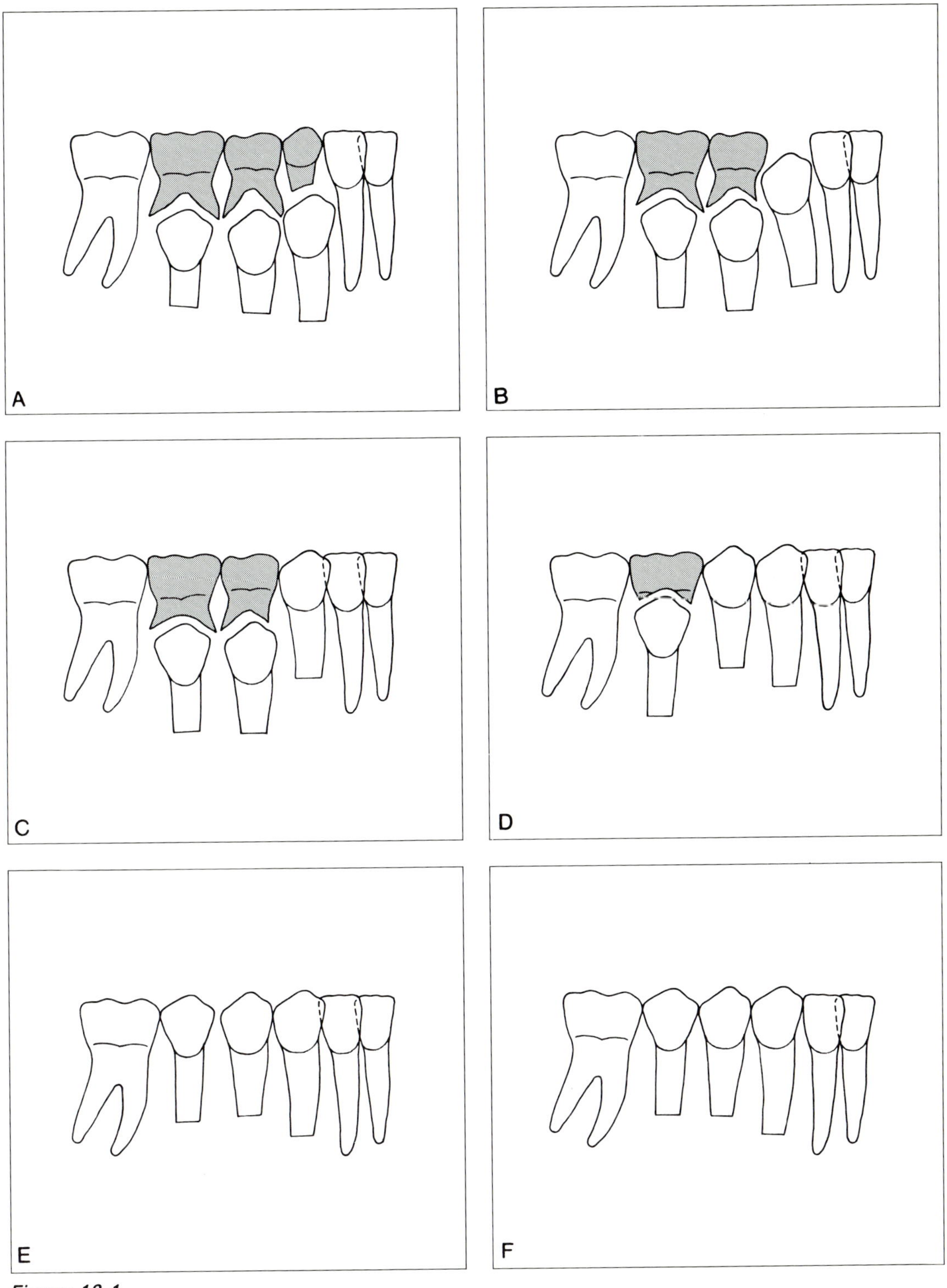

Figure 13-1

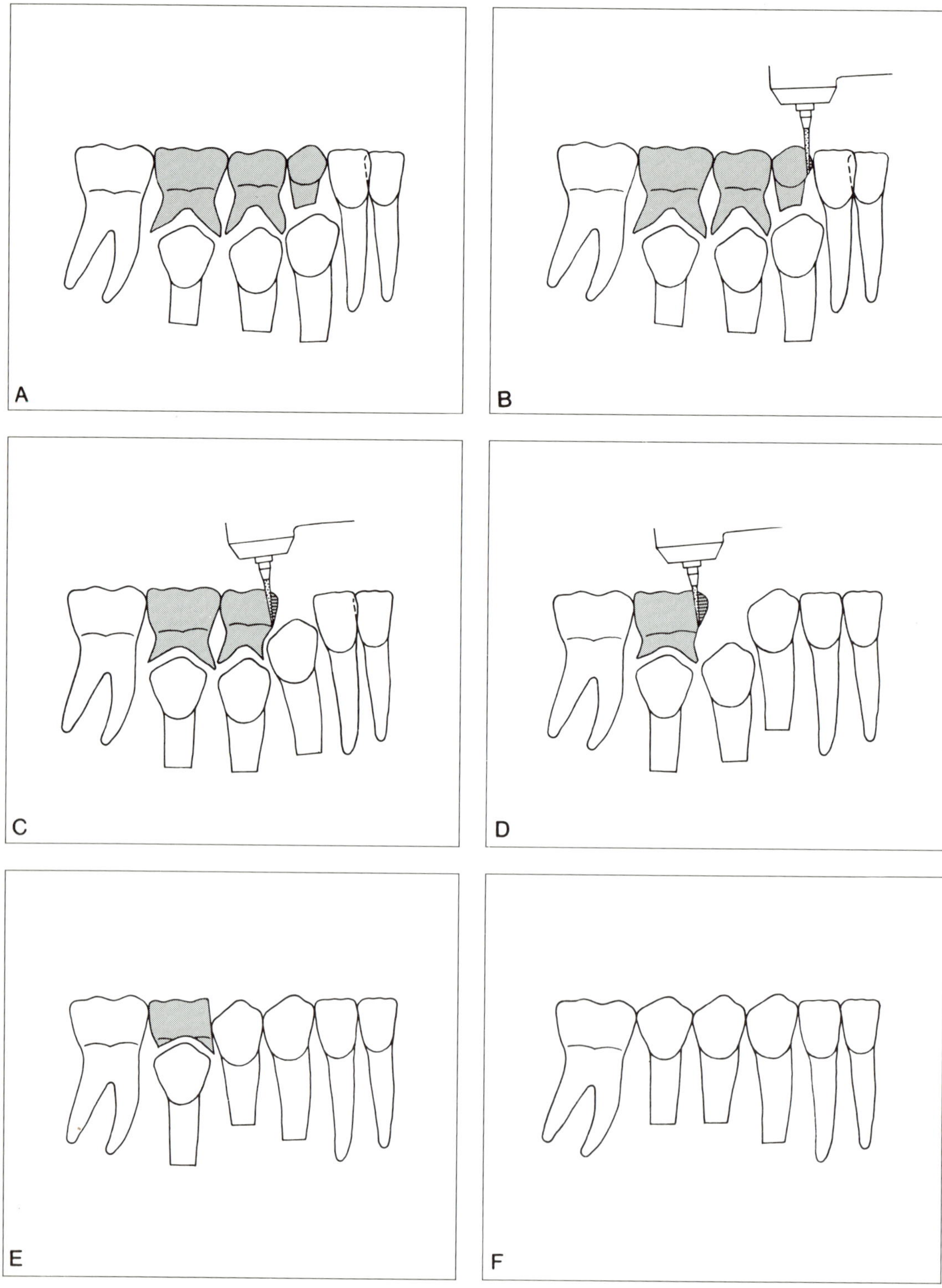

Figure 13-2

Fig. 13-2 The "slicing" procedure, to take advantage of the difference between the mesiodistal crown diameters of the deciduous teeth compared with their successors; this difference may be used to prevent or even correct crowding. The desired effect can often be obtained by slicing only the second deciduous molar at the right time.

A Original situation with mandibular incisor crowding.
B The mesial surface of the deciduous canine is cut back to make extra space for the incisors.
C The first deciduous molar crown is reduced mesially, before the emergence of the permanent canine, in order to provide better conditions for good alignment of the canine.
D The second deciduous molar crown is reduced with the aim of securing a better position for the first premolar.
E The mesiodistal breadth of the second deciduous molar crown after slicing is only slightly greater than that of its successor.
F The leeway is mostly used up; the first permanent molar has moved forward only a little.

13.4 Buccal and lingual emergence of teeth

Emergence of canines and premolars outside the dental arch is usually a consequence of malposition of the tooth germ in a small middle section of the apical area. Anomalous location and emergence do occur on occasion in the absence of crowding. Bringing into the arch a tooth that has emerged outside requires adequate space. In cases of a space deficiency, the necessary room must be provided either by increasing the arch length or by extracting or reducing mesiodistal crown dimensions. Occasionally it will also be necessary to eliminate interference from an opposing tooth.

13.5 Preventing and correcting buccolingual anomalies of occlusion

Deviations in the transverse occlusion of premolars can result from primary crowding, abnormal formation and eruption of premolars, premature loss but also prolonged retention of deciduous molars, a collapse of the mandibular arch, and a combination of these factors.

The only factors that can be influenced are the loss or persistence of deciduous molars and the collapse of the mandibular arch from excessive lip pressure. Where the other factors are concerned it is only possible to make corrections after the faults develop. In those cases, the need for adequate space in the dental arch is also the first requirement.

Depending on the extent of the deviation it will be decided if reciprocal movement of the teeth involved is required, or if independent or differential movement is more appropriate. Elastic bands through the bite are a suitable means of reciprocal movement. These can be attached to cleats or buttons bonded onto the buccal or lingual surfaces of the relevant teeth (Fig. 13-3). When only one or two teeth in the maxilla need to be moved a removable appliance of acrylic resin using suitable springs with a bite plane or an occlusal overlay is simple and effective. This appliance must be

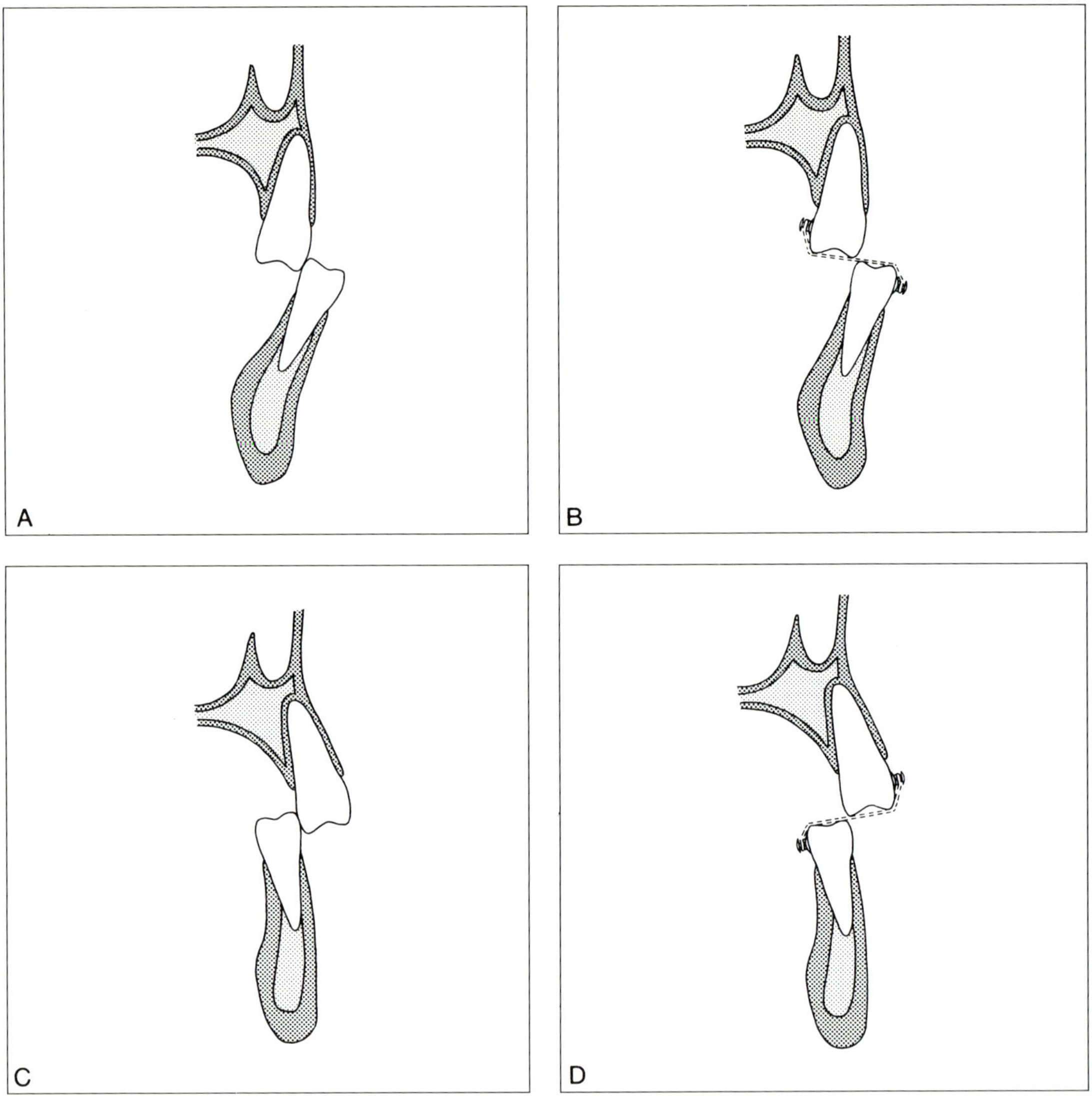

Fig. 13-3 Coronal section of the premolar region showing premolars in buccolingual malocclusions that are corrected with intermaxillary elastic bands through the bite.

A, B *Total crossbite (endo-occlusion of the maxillary premolar) where the elastic band runs from the palatal surface of the maxillary premolar to the buccal surface of the mandibular premolar.*

C, D *Total scissorbite (exo-occlusion of the maxillary premolar) with an elastic band designed to correct it.*

In both situations the elastic band should be worn at all times, because otherwise the tooth is displaced back to its old position by occlusal forces. When a removable acrylic appliance is used instead or as an auxiliary, a bite plane or an occlusal overlay can provide occlusal clearance for the tooth being moved. When it is desired that the two premolars are not moved to equal extents, the anchorage should be designed accordingly. An adjacent tooth can be combined with the one whose movement is to be limited, or an orthodontic appliance can be used that will inhibit or limit the displacement of those teeth it is wished to control.

worn absolutely all the time except when toothbrushing. Otherwise the tooth being moved will be displaced back by the opposing teeth when they occlude.

13.6 Lateral open bites

During the second transitional period it is difficult to determine if lack of vertical contact between premolars is the result of a lateral open bite or is merely a sign of as yet incomplete transition. Only careful observation of the situation (possibly using photography) over a period of 6 months or so can provide a definite answer.
In either case action is not required. If there is a local open bite one cannot evaluate the situation properly until transition is complete in all regions. In by no means every case is it indicated that an attempt must be made to correct a lateral open bite.[226]

13.7 Ankylosis of deciduous molars

A bony connection between alveolar bone and cementum or dentine is evident mainly with deciduous molars and can even be found shortly after emergence. It occurs more often in first than second deciduous molars, and more often in the mandible than in the maxilla. Further, usually more than one tooth is ankylotic (contralateral), and it is seen in some families more often than others. Ankylosis normally occurs during the first transitional period. Depending on the age and origin of the population sample, incidences of 3% to 14% have been reported.[102,106,137,203]
In general, a watchful period of inactivity should be entered into when ankylotic deciduous molars are encountered. There is little sense in extracting such teeth because often they will be lost at the normal time and will have no deleterious effects on further development of the dentition. Early extraction, on the contrary, brings with it the danger of loss of space in the dental arch.[107] Extraction is only desirable in special circumstances. That applies specifically to cases of marked tipping of neighbouring teeth and loss of arch length, a deviant position of the succeeding tooth so that no adequate root resorption is taking place, or a marked infraocclusion. Subsequent to extraction the future development of the dentition needs guidance as it becomes necessary.[108]
If ankylosis of a mandibular second deciduous molar is associated with absence of the successor, the indication for intervention is determined by the agenesis.[109] The ankylotic deciduous molar should preferably be extracted at the beginning of the second transitional period, because then a spontaneous reduction of the extraction space will follow with only limited mesial tipping of the first permanent molar.

There are no research data from which the conclusion can be drawn that ankylosis of deciduous molars is more often associated with agenesis of their successors than with situations in which the premolars are formed than where there is none.

13.8 Impacted canines

After third molars, canines are the teeth next in prevalence of impaction. They are formed furthest from the occlusal plane, and of all teeth their variability of tooth germ location and eruption path is the greatest. Sometimes they emerge palatally; often they do not erupt at all. Considering the importance of the permanent canine in the dentition and for establishing external facial form, bringing an impacted canine into the arch is a necessary objective. If there is little chance of success, preserving the deciduous canine and avoiding orthodontic therapy might be appropriate.

If the permanent canine is located palatally with a fairly normal axial inclination, surgical exposure of the crown followed by packing to establish a permanent opening to the oral cavity will, as a rule, be followed by eruption. It is not necessary in these circumstances to apply an extruding force to the tooth. If one desires to change the eruption path, then during exposure an attachment can be bonded to the crown of the canine in order to apply traction. Such traction can be transmitted by a strong, soft-metal ligature passed through the attachment, with the ends twisted and formed into a hook that can be used to connect it to some form of appliance. A gold chain also can be used, with the advantage of flexibility and easily adjusted length. Using such traction the tooth does not need to be left exposed. By moving the tooth with the mucosa intact, a good gingival attachment will be present later on. Once the canine has erupted sufficiently, the orthodontic attachment can be removed and further correction obtained with a properly located bracket. The ultimate success of such treatment depends partly on providing adequate room in the dental arch for the permanent canine. If there is any doubt about being able to move the canine to its proper place it would be wise not to extract any tooth in that quadrant until it is clear that the treatment is likely to be successful.

A deviating position of a not yet emerged permanent canine can be detected at an early age by palpation. Lack of buccal prominence is a sign of lingual position of the permanent canine. An orthopanthomogram or occlusal radiograph can clarify the situation further. Early diagnosis of a deviating position of an unemerged canine is essential, because extraction of its predecessor generally results in spontaneous correction of the deviating position, at least in the maxilla.[49a]

In palpating, attention also has to be paid to the mesiodistal location of buccally situated maxillary permanent canines, because a deviating eruption pattern may lead to resorption of the root of the adjacent permanent lateral incisor.

The latter is more likely to occur in situations when the permanent canine has a far mesially located crown, a marked mesial angulation, and a relative advanced stage of development of its root.[49b]

Mandibular canines seldom impact. If they do, the same principles are involved as those for maxillary canines, although the narrow alveolar process calls for particular care to maintain satisfactory bone support.

13.9 Supplementary remarks

The sagittal jaw relation and occlusion of the teeth are important aspects of transition of the posterior teeth. A neutrorelation is often associated with an end-to-end occlusion of the first permanent molars during the interval between the two transitional periods. This is particularly the case when the mandibular second deciduous molar crowns have large mesiodistal diameters. In about 70% of cases of a perpendicular terminal plane in the deciduous dentition (i.e., where the distal surfaces of both maxillary and mandibular second deciduous molars are in the same plane when in occlusion) a neutro-occlusion develops after emergence of the second premolars. In about 30% of cases a disto-occlusion of the first permanent molars occurs.[8] Which condition will appear depends largely on the occlusion between the first premolars. In guiding the development of the dentition, it is especially important to keep this in mind. In cases of a deviating jaw relation, facial orthopedic treatment should preferably be instituted before the conclusion of the second transitional period. The premolars and canines can then attain a good interdigitation.

The space available in the dental arch is critical in the transition of the posterior teeth. Problems seldom arise when there is excess space. Quite the opposite happens with a shortage of space; then, besides increasing arch length, the alternative of extracting premolars must be considered (mixed dentition analysis[146]). Sometimes reduction of mesiodistal crown widths can help.

In this chapter only a little has been said about crowding, because this was comprehensively covered in an earlier work.[226] The same applies to abnormal jaw relations.

Some subjects associated with the transition of the posterior teeth are dealt with within another framework in this book, especially premature loss of deciduous canines (Chapter 9), impacted premolars, rotation and tipping of first permanent molars after early loss of deciduous molars (see 14.3) and disturbed emergence of first permanent molars (see 16.2).

Chapter 14

Premature Loss of Deciduous Molars

14.1 Introduction

Deciduous molars can lose all or part of their crowns as the result of caries. Because of pain, the remains of the tooth and roots are often extracted. It can also happen that pulp infection earlier in the course of caries gives rise to inflammatory phenomena that may be dealt with by extraction. Premature loss is found twice as often in the mandible as in the maxilla.[27,84,151,215]

One of the consequences of premature loss can be the migration of adjacent teeth into the space vacated, with the result that the successor to the lost deciduous tooth finds the space intended for it is already partly or fully occupied. This does not by any means always occur. In the majority of cases premature loss has no permanent deleterious effect on the further development and disposition of the permanent dentition.

The results of premature loss of deciduous teeth depend on a number of factors. The following aspects will be dealt with successively: space conditions in the dental arches, occlusion after loss of second deciduous molars, loss of first deciduous molars, stage of development of the dentition at the time of loss, influence of the lips and tongue, effect on the anterior occlusion, regaining lost space, and indications for space maintainers.

14.2 Space conditions in the dental arch

In general, it can be said that in dental arches with excess space the premature loss of deciduous teeth has a negligible effect, if any, on the future development and ultimate arrangement of the permanent teeth. On the other hand, in situations where there is no excess space in the arches, complications in the further development can indeed follow. Premature loss of deciduous teeth in arches with crowding almost always has marked, unfavourable, results. The crowding will, as a rule, increase noticeably.

The space conditions are more favourable in the mandible than in the maxilla, partly because in the mandible the difference between the sum of the mesiodistal crown diameters of the first and second deciduous molars and those of their successors is greater than in the maxilla. A larger amount of space can be lost before it becomes a problem. This applies especially in those situations where much space is available for teeth in the mandibular arch as a whole.

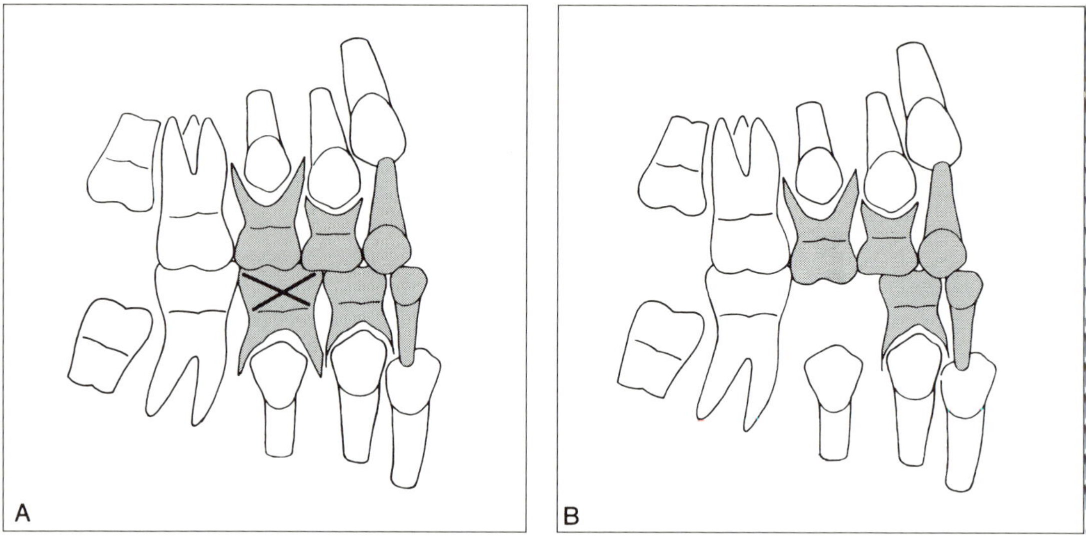

Fig. 14-1 Premature loss of the mandibular second deciduous molar; neutro-occlusion.

A *The mandibular second deciduous molar has a larger mesiodistal crown diameter than the maxillary second deciduous molar. The terminal plane of the deciduous dentition has only a small mesial step.*

B *The maxillary second deciduous molar can overerupt and thereby obstruct the mesial migration of the mandibular first permanent molar. Further development of the dentition shows no deleterious consequences from the premature loss.*

14.3 Occlusion after loss of second deciduous molars

The sagittal occlusion of the individual teeth plays a large part in the effects that result from premature loss of deciduous molars. Overeruption of antagonists can block movement along the arch and may prevent it altogether.

Whether or not an opposing deciduous molar will overerupt after premature loss depends on the occlusion, size of the relevant deciduous molar in relation to the extraction space, and influence of the tongue.

The significance of the occlusion as it affects the results of premature loss of second deciduous molars in both jaws in neutro-, disto-, and mesio-occlusion will be clarified and illustrated. Particularly relevant in this respect is the fact that the mandibular second deciduous molar often has a notably greater mesiodistal crown diameter than the one from the maxilla.

In neutro-occlusion there is usually a flush terminal plane. In these circumstances a maxillary deciduous second molar can overerupt after loss of its antagonist, and by doing so would obstruct the mesial migration of the mandibular first permanent molar

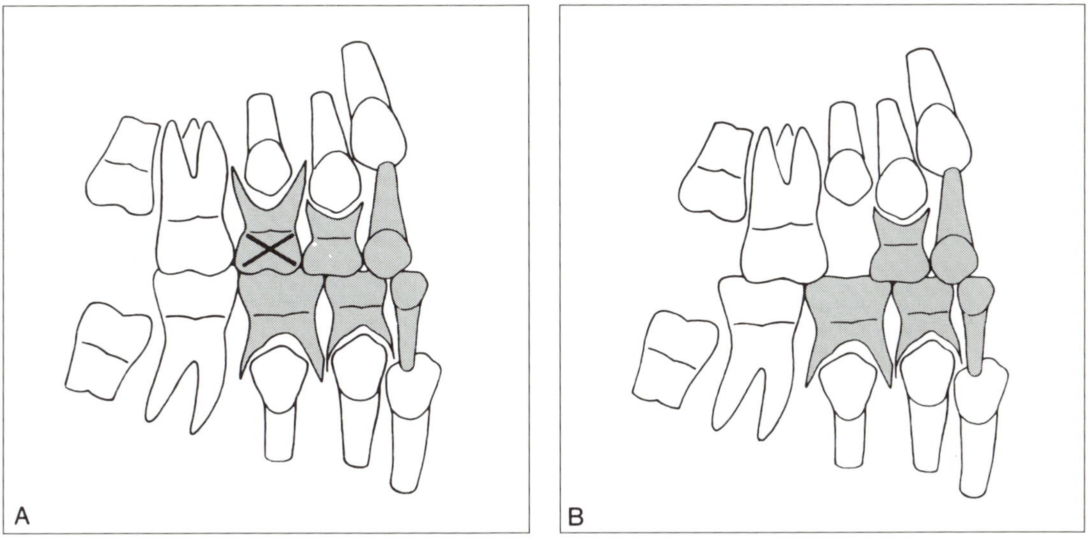

Fig. 14-2 Premature loss of the maxillary second deciduous molar; neutro-occlusion.

A The mandibular second deciduous molar has a broader crown than its antagonist. As a result it occludes with two teeth and when the maxillary second molar is lost, the mandibular molar is still in occlusion with the first deciduous molar in the maxilla.

B The maxillary first permanent molar migrates mesially, and in so doing it rotates around an axis through the mesiopalatal cusp and the palatal root. Consequently, it takes up more room in the dental arch, because the crown has a rhomboid cross section.

(Fig. 14-1). The occlusal relationships determine to what degree migration will occur. More migration will take place in cases of a flush terminal than in those of a mesial step.

When the maxillary second deciduous molar is prematurely lost, the mandibular second deciduous molar will not overerupt because it still has an antagonist: the maxillary first deciduous molar (Fig. 14-2). The maxillary first permanent molar can therefore migrate mesially. However, it does not move bodily but rotates around the axis through the mesiopalatal cusp and the palatal root. The cusp occludes in the central fossa of the mandibular first permanent molar, while the palatal root is the principal, most substantial root of the maxillary first permanent molar.

Loss of the mandibular and the maxillary second deciduous molars on the same side nearly always has an unfortunate effect on further development of the dentition (Fig. 14-3). Mesial migration of the mandibular first permanent molar is no longer inhibited by an overerupted maxillary second deciduous molar. The maxillary molar drifts further than it would have done if the premature loss had been only in the maxillary arch. The occlusion of the mesiopalatal cusp in the central fossa of the mandibular first permanent molar now offers no resistance to mesial migration, because the mandibular molar also moves mesially.

In a case of disto-occlusion it is possible, after premature loss of a mandibular second deciduous molar, that the maxillary deciduous second molar will not overerupt

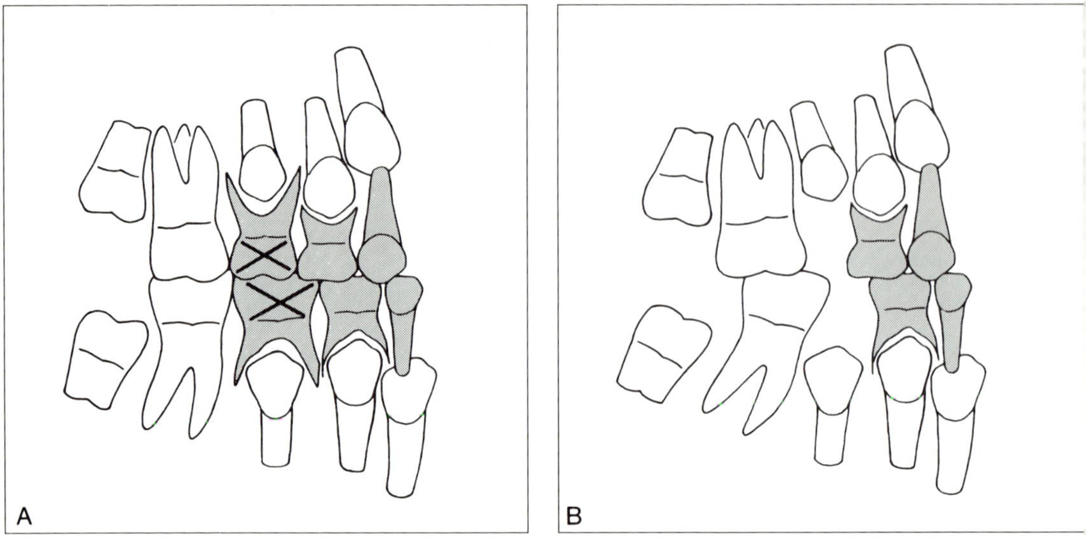

Fig. 14-3 Unilateral premature loss of mandibular and maxillary second deciduous molars; neutro-occlusion.

A After loss of both second deciduous molars there is no obstruction by overeruption of the maxillary second deciduous molar to prevent mesial drift of the mandibular first permanent molar.

B The first permanent molars in both jaws migrate mesially. The maxillary molar does that to a greater degree than it would have if the premature loss had occurred only in the maxilla. The movement of the mandibular first permanent molar frequently takes place in association with a certain degree of mesiolingual rotation. Mesial migration of the first permanent molars after premature loss of deciduous molars can be followed by accelerated eruption and early emergence of the second permanent molars.

because it still occludes with the mandibular first deciduous molar. The mandibular first permanent molar experiences no restraint from the maxillary second deciduous molar in its tendency to migrate mesially (Fig. 14-4).

After loss of a maxillary second deciduous molar, mesial migration and rotation of the maxillary first permanent molar will occur in a case of disto-occlusion comparable to that described for neutro-occlusion (Fig. 14-5).

Should the second deciduous molars be lost in both jaws on one side in disto-occlusion, the first permanent molars in both jaws will migrate mesially (Fig. 14-6). In the mandible this usually is more marked, principally as the result of the greater difference in mesiodistal crown diameters between the teeth that have been lost and those that succeed them.

In unilateral early loss of mandibular first and second deciduous molars in a disto-occlusion, the maxillary second deciduous molar can indeed overerupt. However, the mandibular first permanent molar can migrate a considerable distance mesially, before it is obstructed by the maxillary second deciduous molar that has overerupted (Fig. 14-7).

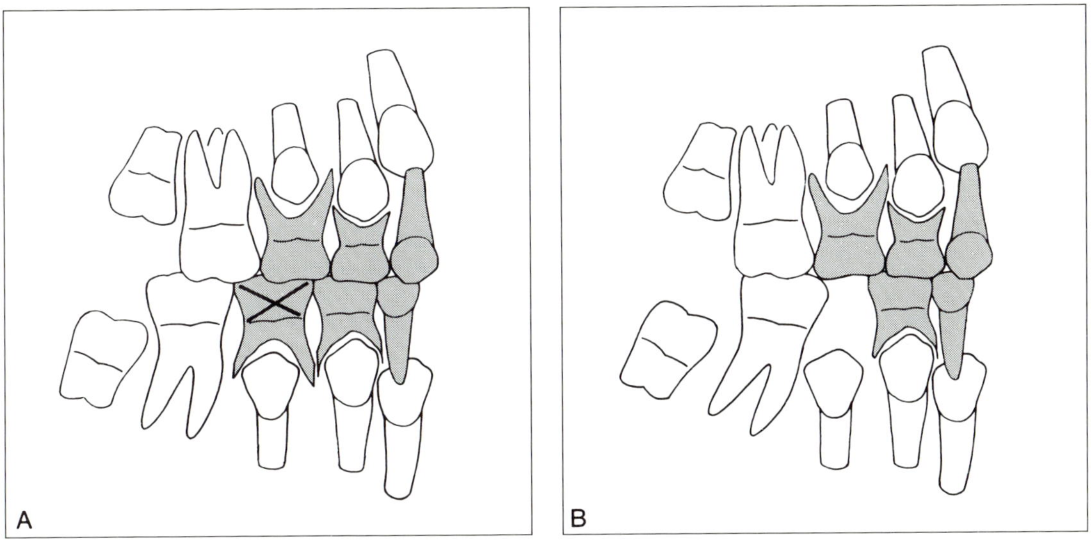

Fig. 14-4 Premature loss of the mandibular second deciduous molar; disto-occlusion.

A The maxillary second deciduous molar occludes not only with the corresponding mandibular one but also with the deciduous first molar.

B Because the maxillary second deciduous molar is unable to overerupt, the mesial migration of the mandibular first permanent molar will not be obstructed. If the lower lip is interposed between the maxillary and mandibular incisors, the existing space in the arch will be lost more from the mesial aspect than would otherwise be the case.

The consequences of early loss of deciduous molars in cases of mesio-occlusion are depicted in Figs. 14-8 to 14-11.

Many cases of early deciduous molar loss have occlusal relations that do not correspond exactly to one of the situations presented before of normal occlusion or a deviation of an entire premolar crown width, but fit somewhere in between. Where the results of premature loss are concerned in relation to the state of the occlusion, each case needs to be assessed individually.

14.4 Loss of first deciduous molars

Only limited consideration is given here to loss of first deciduous molars. The consequences are comparable with those of premature loss of second deciduous molars, though less serious.[27,83,153] The principles that apply to deciding the prognosis

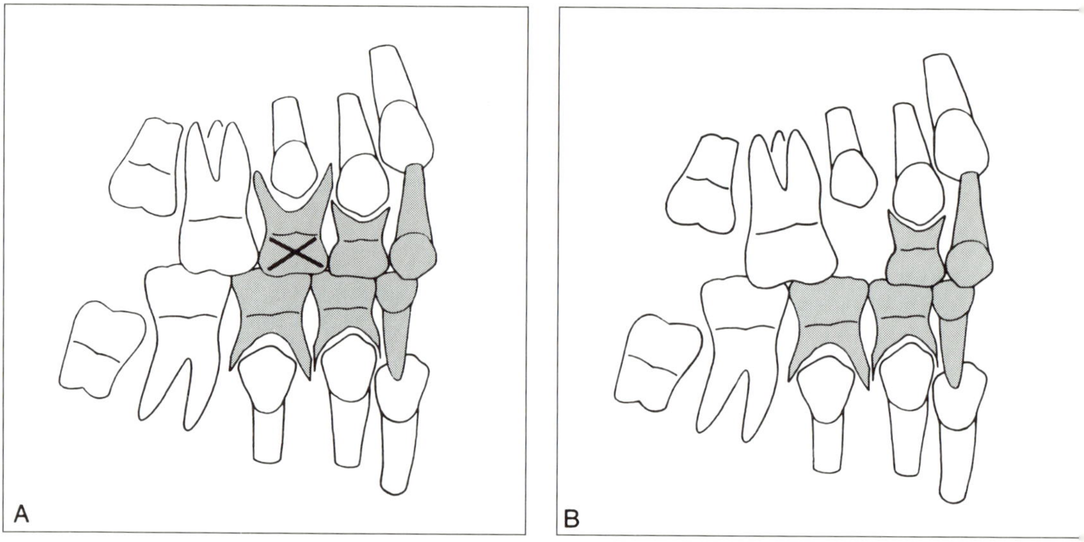

Fig. 14-5 Premature loss of the maxillary second deciduous molar; disto-occlusion.

A The broader mandibular deciduous molar here also is unable to overerupt after loss of its antagonist.

B The maxillary first permanent molar drifts mesially. Its mesiopalatal cusp does not occlude into the central fossa of the mandibular first permanent molar, so that the opposition to mesial migration usually offered by the occlusal interdigitation is reduced.

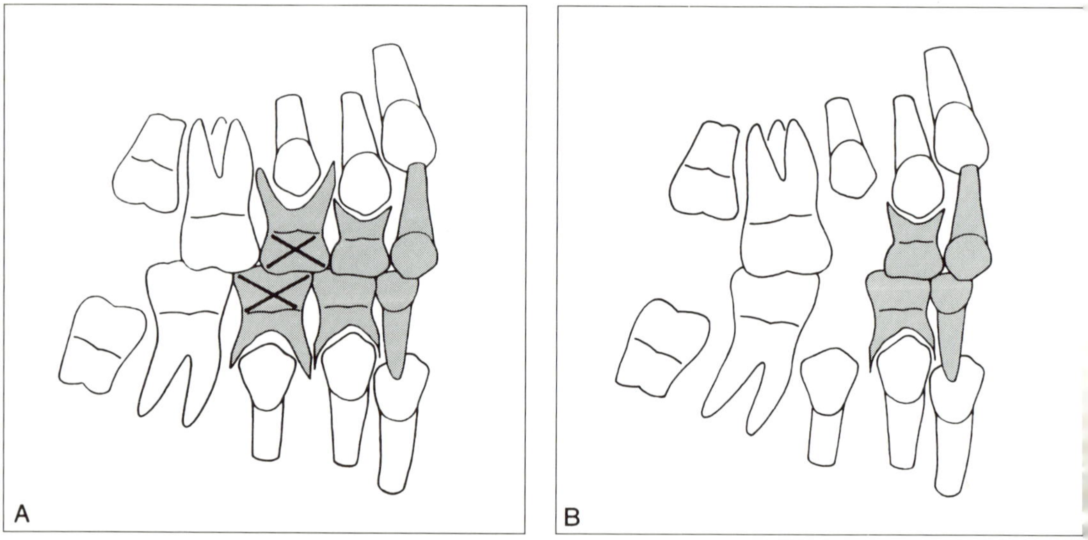

Fig. 14-6 Unilateral premature loss of the second deciduous molar in both jaws; disto-occlusion.

A After loss of both second deciduous molars there is no overeruption of any teeth.

B The first permanent molars in both jaws drift mesially. In the mandible the movement usually is greater because there was a broader deciduous molar there than in the maxilla.

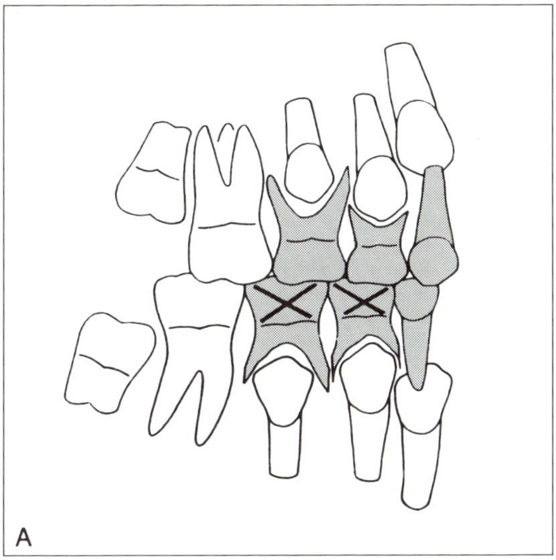

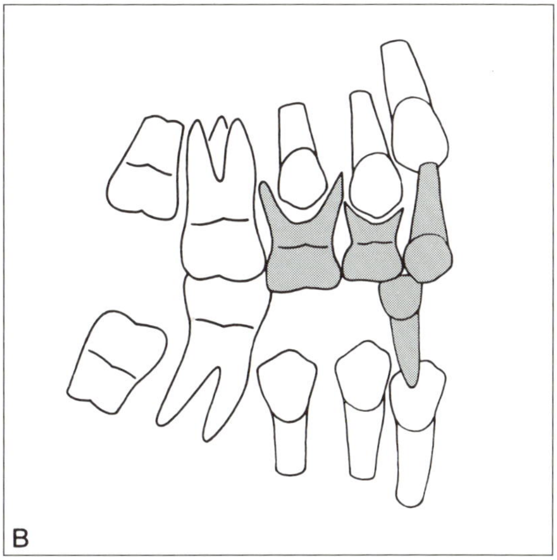

Fig. 14-7 Unilateral premature loss of mandibular first and second deciduous molars; disto-occlusion.

A The maxillary second deciduous molar can overerupt because in the mandible not only the second but also the first deciduous molar has been lost.

B The mandibular first permanent molar moves mesially until it is obstructed by the overerupted second deciduous molar. In addition, space in the mandibular arch has also been reduced by distal movement of the anterior teeth.

after premature loss of deciduous molars, based on the occlusion, are the same for both situations. One distinction is that with loss of first deciduous molars, compared to second deciduous molars, an eventual reduction in the space becoming available will mainly be caused by migration of the mesial teeth distally.

14.5 Stage of development of the dentition at the time of tooth loss

In general, loss of deciduous teeth at an early age has more deleterious effects on the development of the dentition than does premature loss that occurs at a relatively late age.

Premature loss of a second deciduous molar is more undesirable when it occurs before the first permanent molar emerges than when it happens some time afterwards. In the first case the second premolar is still a long way from the occlusal plane and is less of an obstacle to the mesial migration of the first permanent molar than it will be after eruption has placed it more occlusally. Moreover, the first permanent molar drifts sooner and drifts more mesially when the second deciduous molar is missing than

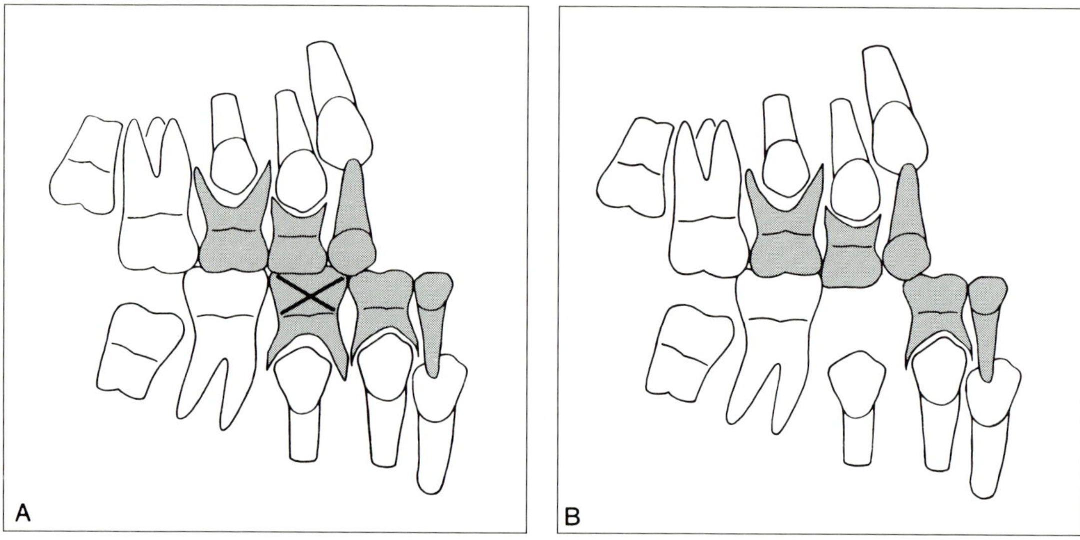

Fig. 14-8 Premature loss of a mandibular second deciduous molar; mesio-occlusion.

A The maxillary first deciduous molar can overerupt into the space existing after loss of the mandibular second deciduous molar.

B The mandibular first permanent molar hardly moves; the overerupted maxillary first deciduous molar has in fact blocked any mesial drifting.

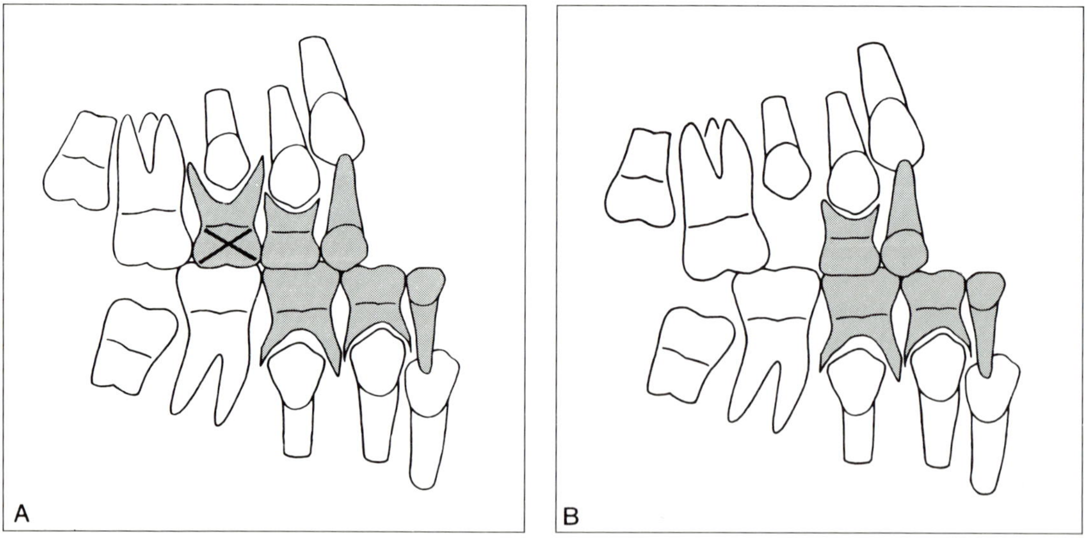

Fig. 14-9 Premature loss of a maxillary second deciduous molar; mesio-occlusion.

A There is no possibility of overeruption of a mandibular molar following premature loss in the maxilla.

B The maxillary first permanent molar migrates mesially in combination with mesial rotation.

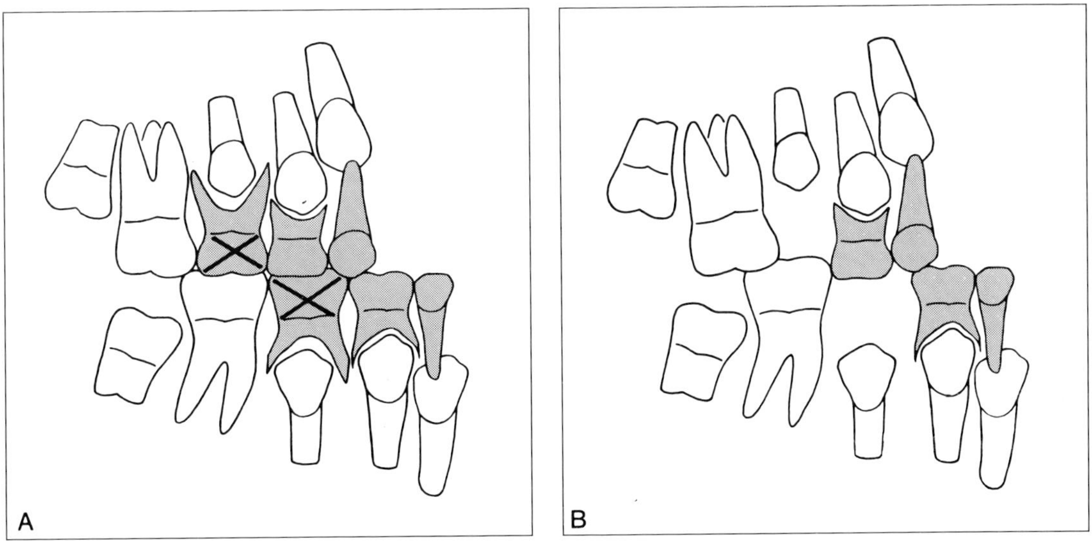

Fig. 14-10 Premature loss of the right second deciduous molars of both jaws; mesio-occlusion.

A Because of the typical occlusal relationships, the maxillary first deciduous molar can overerupt.
B Mesial migration of the mandibular first permanent molar is blocked by the maxillary first deciduous molar, which has overerupted. The maxillary first permanent molar drifts mesially with a mesial rotation.

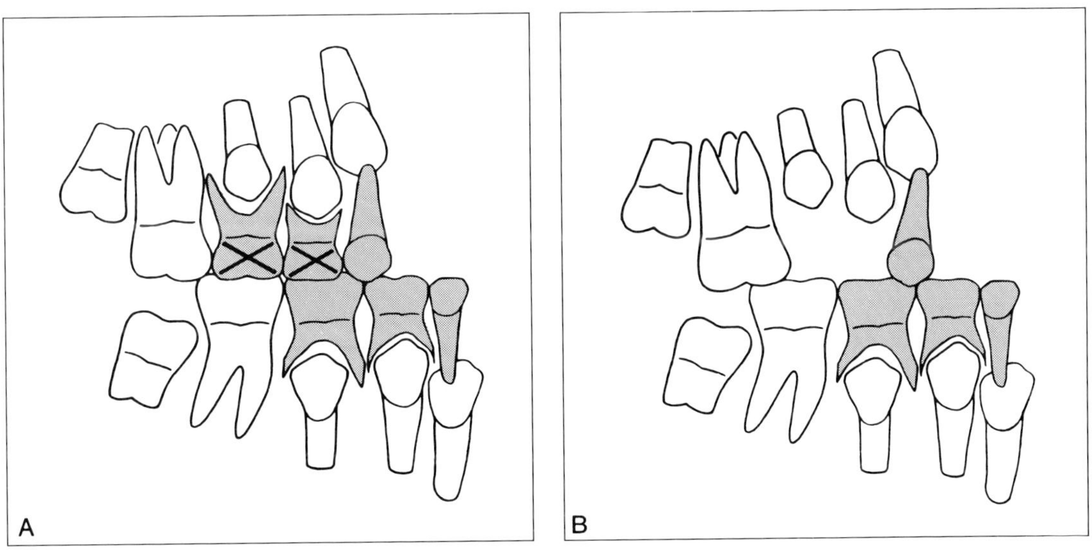

Fig. 14-11 Bilateral premature loss of maxillary first and second deciduous molars; mesio-occlusion.

A Once again there is no overeruption of mandibular teeth.
B The maxillary first permanent molars migrate and rotate mesially. With the reversed overbite, the maxillary incisors can go lingually. The space will be partly reduced from the mesial aspect.

when it is still present.[34,185] If loss of a second deciduous molar occurs before the second permanent molar has emerged, the permanent first molar moves further mesially than it would have done otherwise.[119, 222]
Furthermore, premature early loss of deciduous molars leads to earlier emergence of the second permanent molars.[185]
In addition, the time of premature loss of deciduous molars also influences the moment successors emerge. Loss long before the normal time of emergence of the successor has a retarding effect on its emergence. Loss shortly before the normal emergence time of the successor can, on the contrary, result in acceleration.[33,34,54]
The difference mentioned here in the effect on the time of emergence is probably attributable to the formation of bone and thick and tough gingiva occlusal to the unerupted successor after the loss of the deciduous molar. The effect of the masticatory forces can be to make the gingiva densely fibrous, and the tissue then presents abnormal resistance to tooth emergence. The resultant retarded emergence can be speeded up by surgical exposure of the occlusal surface.[127]

14.6 Influence of lips and tongue

The consequences of premature loss of deciduous molars in Class II/1 anomalies differ from those in a normal dentition, not only because the occlusion is different but also because the soft tissue environment is different. The fact that an abnormal contact exists between the incisors through which relatively more lingual pressure is exerted on the mandibular incisors by the lower lip, and through which the lip can also apply a force on the palatal surfaces of the maxillary incisors to move them labially, is of special importance. The significance of this increases when the lower lip wholly occupies the space between the maxillary and mandibular incisors in rest and in function. Moreover, space in the mandibular arch can be reduced by the extra pressure of the lower lip, the space being lost more from the mesial aspect than otherwise would have been the case.
Premature loss of all four deciduous molars in the mandible in a Class II/1 anomaly is a disaster if the lower lip rests between the mandibular and maxillary incisors. The mandibular incisors will subsequently tip severely lingually. This limits the space remaining for the premolars even more. Particularly when there is mandibular arch crowding, this effect is worse.
In Class II/2 anomalies the high lip position that has produced an abnormal palatal loading on the maxillary incisors gives a relatively greater tendency for distal drifting of those teeth that are located mesial to the position of any premature tooth loss. Premature loss of deciduous molars in the mandible can lead to a more severe retroclination of the maxillary and mandibular incisors. Premature loss of deciduous molars (or canines) in both jaws is especially unfavourable.
In Class III anomalies the lip relation is notably different, and for that reason the influence that the lips have after premature loss of deciduous molars (or canines) is different too.
The tongue can prevent lingual tipping of incisors after premature loss. Further, placing the tongue into the spaces left in the dental arch after loss of two adjacent deciduous molars is credited with a preventive action; drifting should be inhibited or at least limited by this.[27,84]

14.7 Effect on anterior occlusion

Premature loss of deciduous molars can be accompanied by changes in the size of the overjet and the overbite and in the midline relationships of the dental arches.
Premature loss of mandibular deciduous molars leads to increased overjet and overbite in both Class I and Class II/1 situations.
Due to the reversed overbite anteriorly, loss of deciduous molars in a Class III anomaly will produce a tendency not for the anterior part of the mandibular dental arch but for the maxillary dental arch to move lingually. The overjet and overbite will change accordingly.
Premature loss of one or two mandibular deciduous molars on one side, or of two on one side and one on the other, generally leads to a midline displacement in the mandibular arch.

14.8 Regaining lost space

Reduction in available dental arch length resulting from migration after premature loss of deciduous molars can sometimes be regained, at least in part. The conditions are more favourable in the mandible than the maxilla; regaining space seldom occurs in the latter. In the mandible, first permanent molars that have migrated mesially can move distally with the eruption and emergence of the second premolars. Likewise, first premolars that have migrated distally can move mesially. In the maxilla this phenomenon is seldom seen.
The lack of space regaining in the maxilla is partly attributable to the rhombic form of the maxillary first permanent molar. The space between the first premolar that has just emerged and the rotated first permanent molar is trapezoidal, yet the succeeding tooth is more rectangular. The maxillary second premolar will consequently seek the path of least resistance in eruption and emergence and diverge palatally so that the distally directed force fails to be applied to the maxillary first permanent molar. In the mandible this is indeed the case, because the mandibular first permanent molar migrates mesially more or less bodily. Moreover, the mesial surface is nearly straight and thus perpendicular to the line of the dental arch (Figs. 14-12 and 14-13). It is not only on mechanical grounds that a mandibular second premolar can, on eruption and emergence, regain the space originally intended for it; there are also more favourable conditions of bone structure and of jaw form in the mandible than the maxilla. The trapezoid area in the maxilla previously described contains bone that is not compact but cancellous. In the mandible not only are the corresponding bone structures more dense, the limited buccolingual dimension of the jawbone forms an additional restriction for escape.

14.9 Indications for space maintainers

In most instances when deciduous molars are lost early, there is no reason to make a space maintainer because no permanent deleterious effect will occur.

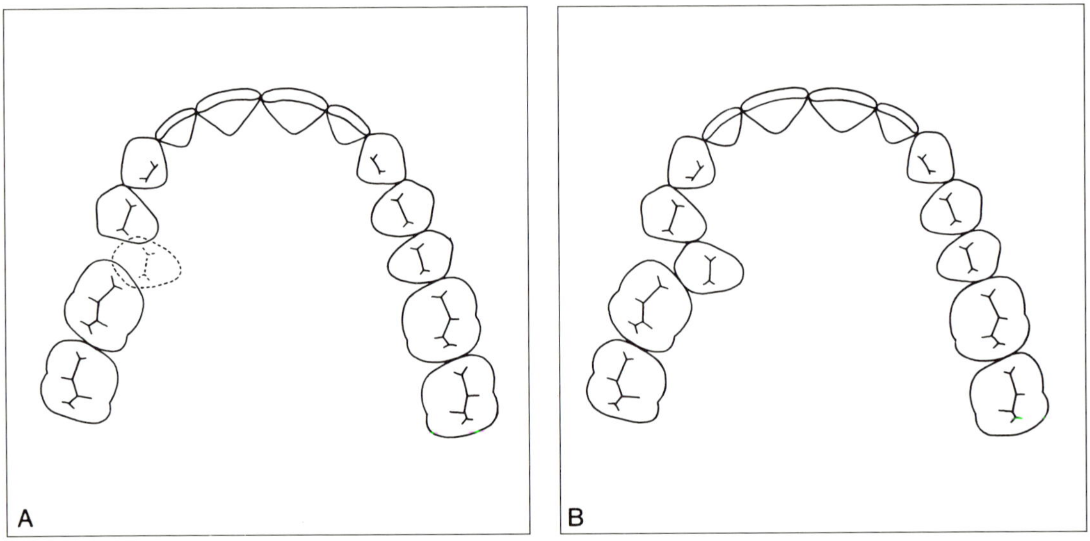

Fig. 14-12 Palatal emergence of a maxillary second premolar after premature loss of its predecessor.

A The first permanent molar is mesially rotated. The space between its mesial surface and the first premolar is trapezoid.

B In eruption and emergence, the second premolar follows the line of least resistance through the cancellous bone of the palate.

As has been said, what determine the result are the space situation in the dental arches, the occlusion, which tooth has been lost, the phase of development of the dentition, and the influence of lips and tongue.

In an arch with excess space and diastemata between all the teeth, including between second deciduous molars and first permanent molars, premature loss of deciduous molars will not affect the development of the dentition. Even premature loss of a maxillary second deciduous molar will have no effect, in contrast with other situations in which loss of that tooth has occurred.

Loss of a mandibular second deciduous molar in circumstances that are otherwise normal usually results in mesial drifting of the first permanent molar. There often remains sufficient space to accomodate the premolars in good positions. Moreover, some of the lost space is often regained.

In disto-occlusion, loss of a mandibular deciduous second molar usually results in substantial reduction in the space available for the premolars; the second premolar fails to emerge or does so only partly, or erupts lingually. If the lower lip is positioned palatal to the maxillary incisors, the results are more serious, certainly when more than one mandibular deciduous molar is lost.

Loss of opposing deciduous second molars mostly has permanent deleterious effects. If many deciduous molars are lost prematurely, considerable drifting can follow. This is particularly so when the loss is at a very early age and where there is crowding.

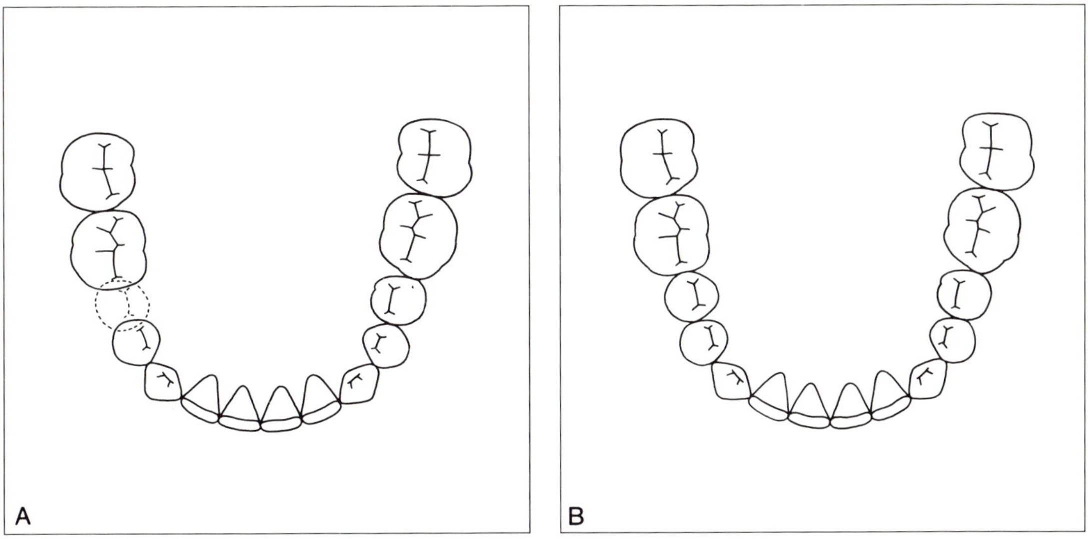

Fig. 14-13 Regaining space in eruption and emergence of a mandibular second premolar after premature loss of its predecessor.

A The first permanent molar has tipped and drifted mesially.
B In eruption and emergence, the second premolar has forced itself between the parallel approximal surfaces of the adjacent teeth and at the same time remained within the cortical walls of the mandible.

To determine if there is an indication for provision of a space maintainer one should first answer the question whether or not drifting would otherwise occur, and if so, how much would there be and would the situation then lead to permanent damage. In that connection eventual regaining of space has to be considered. Then the question must be answered as to whether or not orthodontic treatment will be required and whether the problems resulting from premature loss can be corrected without many difficulties in the course of the major orthodontic treatment when it is undertaken.
Application of space maintainers should be limited to patients who do not have excess space and need no other orthodontic treatment, where maxillary second (and sometimes first) deciduous molars have been lost, or where such loss of deciduous molars occurs that the drifting will be inadequately controlled by overeruption of antagonists.
In patients who will subsequently have orthodontic treatment, placing a space maintainer will only be indicated when the consequences of the premature loss will markedly exacerbate the abnormality. That applies particularly for Class II/1 anomalies, with the lower lip situated in palatal contact with the maxillary incisors or with a disposition to do so at least some of the time.
If it is desired to use a space maintainer, then the type to be used will depend on the location and size of the space that has to be preserved. Generally a space maintainer should be kept as small as is practicable, should be kept free of emerging teeth, and should cause as little damage as possible to the standing teeth and periodontal

structures. Since the development of composite resins, these requirements can more easily be met.
There is no point in making a space maintainer once the space has been lost, and certainly not when a successor is absent. That applies also to cases where it is already clear that extractions will be required in the course of carrying out orthodontic treatment.
Even in patients who otherwise would need no active treatment later on, space can still be regained with little difficulty. The use of a space regainer is often not much more complicated than that of a space maintainer. In doubtful cases one can better adopt a "wait-and-see" attitude.

14.10 Supplementary remarks

The objective of avoiding premature loss of deciduous teeth through prevention of caries takes precedence. When caries does occur it must be handled conservatively, especially in those deciduous teeth whose loss would lead to permanent disadvantage. In this regard, the maxillary second deciduous molar is the most important tooth; its preservation is essential.
Selectively grinding an antagonist of a lost deciduous tooth can result in overeruption and hence lead to obstruction of undesired drifting.
Movements of adjacent teeth principally occur in the first 6 months after loss of a tooth.[172] In the maxilla these movements are larger and quicker than in the mandible.[27,155,184] Further, such migration in the maxilla is limited mainly to mesial drifting (and rotation) of the first permanent molar, while in the mandible those teeth mesial to the space will migrate distally.[155] Nonetheless the loss of space is frequently minimal and of little importance for the further development of the dentition.[26,34,83,119,124,161,195] In many cases the original loss of space has largely been restored by the end of the second transitional period.[126]
Finally, premature loss of deciduous teeth does not always lead to a permanent disadvantage. In cases of adequate space and normal occlusal relations, premature loss of mandibular deciduous second molars seldom leads to difficulty. Against this is the fact that after loss of a maxillary deciduous second molar problems are most likely to arise.

Chapter 15

Agenesis of Premolars

15.1 Introduction

Failure of premolars to form is not expected by patients and parents unless there has been a family history of agenesis. There are no symptoms connected with absence of a premolar that act as a warning until such time as the deciduous molar is seen not to exfoliate. In addition, because the deciduous molars are the last deciduous teeth to be lost, delay in exfoliation may not be noticed, even if the tooth has indeed been recognised by the patient or parent to be a deciduous tooth. Moreover, the agenesis of a premolar does not affect the normal course of events in the transition of the teeth mesial to it.

Agenesis of second premolars is more prevalent in the mandible (approximately 4.4%) than in the maxilla (approximately 1.7%). The clinical consequences of agenesis in the mandible are more significant. Proportionately, agenesis of first premolars is rare (mandibular — about 0.1%; maxillary — about 0.2%).[10]

This chapter starts with a discussion of diagnosis and treatment possibilities. Following this, mandibular agenesis is dealt with, divided into space conditions in the dental arch, dental arch relations and the profile, possibility for guiding the development of the dentition, and unilateral agenesis. Agenesis of the maxillary second premolar is covered similarly. Standard solutions to the problems are presented in tabular form.

15.2 Diagnosing agenesis of premolars

Agenesis has strong genetic origins. In history taking it is essential to enquire about missing teeth in other family members. The lack of mandibular second premolars is often found in several children in a family. Whenever 6 months after the exfoliation of one deciduous molar the contralateral tooth is still present and not loosening, agenesis of the successor should be suspected. An asymmetric sequence of emergence also is suspect. In the mandible, careful palpation of the alveolar process will provide more information. At this stage of development the mandibular premolars that have not yet emerged can be felt within the process unless they are in a markedly abnormal position. In the maxilla this is usually less evident. Palpation of mandibular premolars is frequently possible 2 years earlier, although of course the unerupted teeth are less

easily found then. At that time a plan of action would be formulated if agenesis were suspected, and radiographic confirmation of the situation would then be necessary. With the circumstances fully appraised, it might then be appropriate to design a strategy for guiding the further development of the dentition.
It is a common belief that infraposition of deciduous molars is often associated with agenesis of the successors. However, the literature does not support this proposition with adequate data.[204] A satisfactory basis is lacking for accepting ankylosed deciduous molars as a specific symptom of agenesis.

15.3 Therapeutic possibilities

There are three possible options:

1. Preserve the deciduous molar as long as possible
2. Orthodontically close the spaces that are caused by the absence of the premolar and its predecessor by guiding the development of the dentition and/or use of appliances
3. Replace the missing tooth with a prosthesis

The pros and cons of these alternative treatment modes will be considered in the following paragraphs.

15.4 Agenesis of premolars in the mandible

No other teeth are so often absent as the mandibular second premolars. Bilateral agenesis occurs regularly. Mandibular first premolars are very seldom absent; consequently that condition will not be dealt with specifically.

15.4.1 Space conditions in the mandibular dental arch

In situations of crowding in the mandibular dental arch, removing the deciduous molars and using the existing space to relieve the crowding is the obvious solution. This applies especially to bilateral agenesis and severe anterior crowding. The intended orthodontic space closure does not necessarily involve use of appliances. In cases of agenesis of a second premolar, timely extraction of the second deciduous molar can, in favourable conditions, secure spontaneous correction of the situation without active therapy being needed later (see 15.4.3).
Agenesis frequently is associated with relatively smaller mesiodistal crown diameters of the teeth that do form. That being so, crowding occurs less often, with spacing being more common.
In cases of crowding in the mandibular dental arch and no other need for orthodontic therapy, the first indication is to preserve the deciduous molar. A mandibular second deciduous molar that does not become ankylotic can function well for a long period, sometimes until old age.[125] In particular, if there has been minimal root resorption the

prognosis for prolonged retention is good. An intact crown is also important because indirect pulp changes resulting from caries appear to encourage root resorption. Deciduous teeth with good caries resistance may also exhibit less tendency toward root resorption in the absence of successors.
In situations where regardless of agenesis there would be some need for orthodontic treatment, absence of premolars would be an extra indication for treatment. In this regard, orthodontic closure of any spaces would form a part of the total therapy.

15.4.2 Dental arch relation and profile

The sagittal arch relations and the profile also play an important part in making treatment decisions.
Class I anomalies with mandibular crowding often also exhibit maxillary crowding. Agenesis of a mandibular premolar in such cases calls for extraction of two maxillary premolars (and usually one mandibular premolar from the side opposite to where the agenesis is). A contraindication for this approach is a profile showing a sunken mouth, or where there is a danger of such a profile developing after extractions.
Absence of mandibular premolars, whether because of agenesis or extraction, makes treatment of Class II anomalies significantly more complicated. It makes extraction of maxillary teeth almost unavoidable. Subsequently, treatment with fixed appliances is essential, particularly because bodily movement of the teeth bounding the spaces in the arch will be required. The maxillary incisors often have to be moved bodily palatally.
In Class II/1 anomalies with marked crowding in both dental arches the most likely solution involves finishing each quadrant with just one premolar. When there is no crowding this approach contains the considerable risk of undesirable retrusion of the mandibular incisors, because mandibular premolars and canines tend to drift distally if space is present there. This risk especially prevails in Class II/1 anomalies of a full premolar crown width, and even more so when the lower lip is interposed between maxillary and mandibular incisors or if that becomes possible as the mandibular incisors tilt lingually. The lingual tipping is even more likely when thumb or fingers are still being sucked. In such cases, depending on the seriousness of the abnormality, there may be an indication for a relatively early start with treatment. Timely referral to an orthodontist is always desirable.
In Class II/1 anomalies with a normal mandibular arch and a deciduous second molar in good condition, retention of that tooth can be the most suitable action when agenesis of its successor is apparent. This is particularly so when, as a result, simple orthodontic treatment restricted to the maxillary complex can secure the desired improvement.
With Class II/2 anomalies it is generally undesirable to reduce the amount of tooth material in the mandible. To conserve a good deciduous second molar for as long as possible is of great importance when no orthodontic treatment is to be instituted. However, if orthodontic treatment is planned, whether or not a second deciduous molar is conserved must be considered in connection with the total, usually complex, treatment plan. Transplantation of a maxillary premolar to the site of the agenesis certainly comes into view.
Class III anomalies are less of a problem when agenesis of a mandibular premolar occurs. Closing diastemata can be associated with correction of the reversed overjet.

15.4.3 Guiding the development of the dentition

Attention was previously drawn to the fact that it usually is not necessary to verify with radiographs any suspected agenesis of a premolar prior to 1 year before the beginning of the transition of the posterior teeth and the emergence of the second permanent molar. Extraction of a second deciduous molar (and/or a first) can, at that stage, still result in good natural space closure in the mandibular arch. The first permanent molar then drifts mesially almost bodily; the first premolar drifts distally. Also, originally unfavourable mesiodistal inclinations of the first premolars can spontaneously correct themselves, particularly when they have not yet emerged. Good contact between the marginal ridges usually is established and triangular interproximal areas that would give rise to food impaction do not develop.[95]

Mesial migration of the mandibular first permanent molar can be enhanced by extracting only the distal root of the second deciduous molar and leaving the mesial root in place for some time. Of course, the hemisection and extraction should be preceded by endodontic treatment. When the deciduous molar is ankylosed the effect is optimal. In a corresponding manner one can remove the mesial root and retain the distal root if one seeks maximum distal displacement of the first premolar and canine. However, there is seldom a need for that (Fig. 15-1).

Less demanding but also less effective is the mesial or distal slicing of the deciduous molars. If this procedure is adopted it is essential to guard against pulp exposure.

15.4.4 Unilateral agenesis of a mandibular second premolar

In general, solutions that lead to a missing tooth on one side of the mandible should be avoided. A deviation of the midline of the mandibular dental arch, an increased overjet, and overbite and problems with interdigitation are difficult to control. When agenesis is unilateral the retention of a good second deciduous molar, as advocated previously, is more likely to be required than in cases of bilateral agenesis.

Sometimes it will not be possible or indicated to preserve the second deciduous molar, while extraction of a premolar on the other side would not be sensible. Then a good solution will in general only be obtained by moving the permanent molars mesially on the side of the agenesis. In doing this the other teeth on that side may not move distally more than a limited amount, if at all. Generally this calls for use of fixed appliances.

15.5 Agenesis of maxillary premolars

In the maxilla, agenesis of premolars is seen about as frequently as that of lateral incisors.[10] Second premolars are absent less than half as often in the maxilla as in the mandible. Agenesis of maxillary first premolars is rare.

15.5.1 Space conditions in the maxillary dental arch

In cases of crowding in the maxilla and agenesis of second premolars, removing deciduous molars without successors is a possible remedy. Diastemata corresponding with the missing second premolars close more from the distal aspect than do those

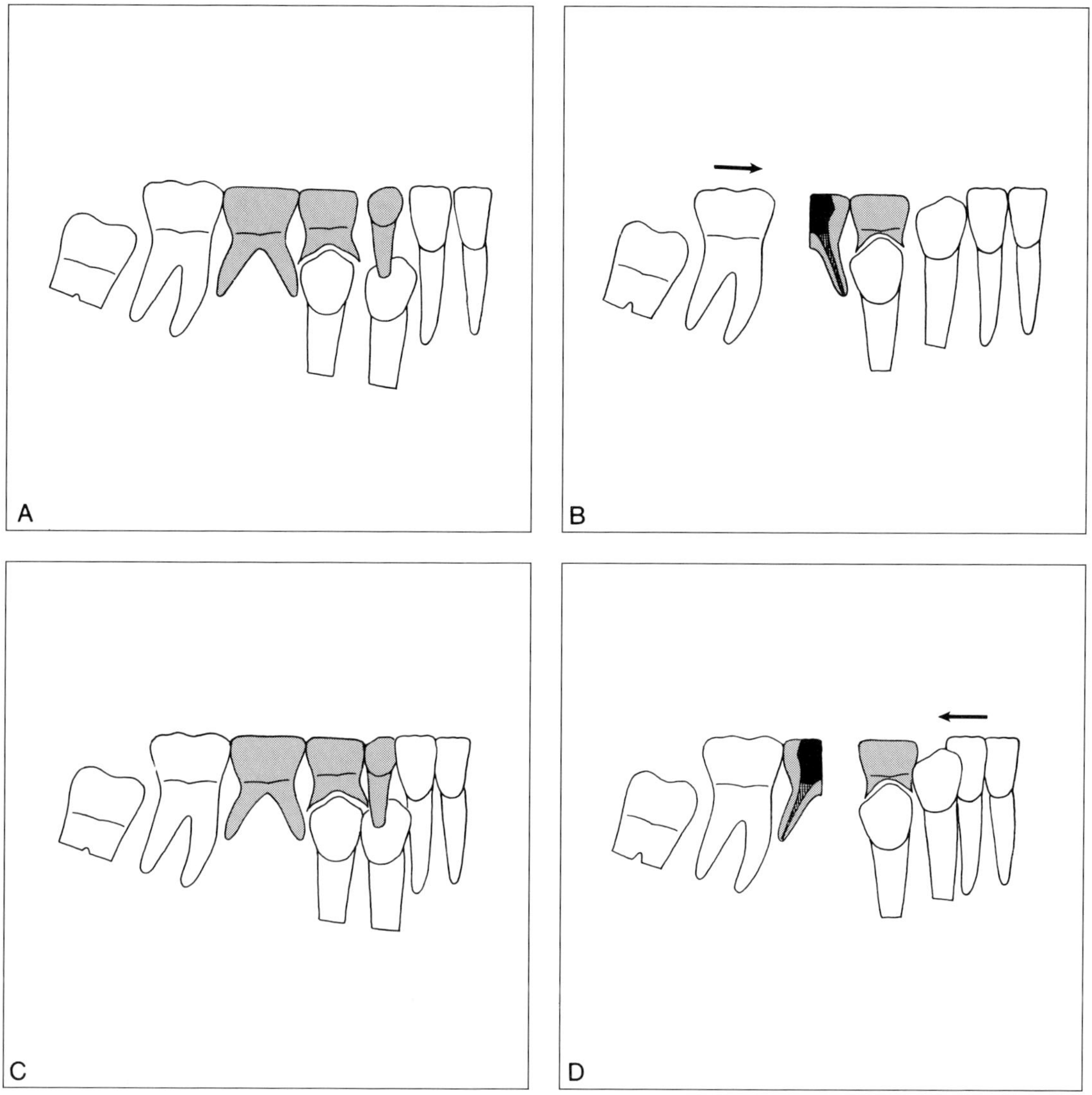

Fig. 15-1 Hemisectioning of the (ankylosed) mandibular second deciduous molar after endodontic treatment in cases of agenesis of its successor.

A Excess space in the dental arch, where maximal mesial movement of the mandibular first permanent molar is aimed for.
B After removing the distal half of the second deciduous molar the first permanent molar is free to move mesially.
C Severe overlapping of teeth can disappear markedly when the teeth anterior to the second deciduous molar can move distally.
D After removing the mesial half of the second deciduous molar, favourable conditions are created for relief of the anterior crowding.

Hemisectioning of deciduous molars is particulary effective in cases of ankylosis when the remaining half serves as an absolute anchorage device when orthodontic appliances are inserted. For example, in the situation illustrated in B, the permanent first molar can be moved mesially until contact is established with the remaining half of the deciduous second molar that subsequently has to be extracted. In the situation given in D, maximal use can be made of the space created by the extraction of the mesial half of the deciduous molar when the teeth anterior to it are aligned.

in the mandible. It is true, however, that the permanent first molars rotate mesiopalatally in the process and the occlusion worsens. Nonetheless, the diastemata will close entirely, without significant mesial tipping; triangular interproximal spaces will not develop.
If there is marked crowding in the incisor-canine region, the "agenesis space" can be fully used only in conjunction with orthodontic appliances.
In instances of no crowding or only minor crowding, orthodontic appliances might not be required unless needed for other reasons.
Preservation of deciduous second molars in the maxilla is, contrary to the indications in the mandible, seldom required. The maxillary arch has little tendency to collapse. In addition, there is the fact that deciduous second molars in the maxilla have a smaller mesiodistal crown diameter than those in the mandible. Space conditions in the dental arch, functional factors, and the direction of emergence of the permanent molars are more favourable in this respect in the maxilla than in the mandible.

15.5.2 Dental arch relation and profile

In Class I anomalies with marked crowding in both jaws, extraction of two mandibular premolars (and if necessary a maxillary premolar on the side without agenesis) is an obvious remedy. Of course, it is necessary to bear in mind the danger of the profile collapsing. In cases of little or no crowding it is usually preferable not to extract in the mandible, and to restrict the treatment (whether or not using appliances) to the maxilla alone.
With Class II/1 anomalies the agenesis space can be used to move the teeth positioned mesially to it distally and to retrude the maxillary incisors (with unilateral agenesis it is necessary to extract a first or second premolar from the maxilla on the other side). If a good result is sought, orthodontic appliances will be required. Specifically this is necessary to avoid the maxillary molars moving too far mesially. The disto-occlusion of the molars must remain as it is, although if there was not a full disto-occlusion in the beginning, the molar relation should be allowed to move to a full premolar crown width of disto-occlusion. If there is significant crowding in the mandibular arch, extraction of mandibular teeth should be considered. In that case the arch relations need to be corrected. This treatment would be complex, and comprehensive appliance therapy would be required.
In Class III anomalies agenesis in the maxilla is particularly unfavourable. The reversed overjet will generally worsen as deciduous molars are lost without a successor. If the Class III anomaly is moderate and normally there would be no indication for orthodontic therapy, it can be desirable to conserve for as long as possible any deciduous molars without successors. In severe Class III anomalies with agenesis in the maxilla, any orthodontic therapy without surgery will normally require extractions in the mandible and no space closure in the maxilla.

15.5.3 Guiding the development of the dentition

It is not necessary to verify suspected agenesis until a year before the beginning of the second transitional period. Extraction of a second deciduous molar can still be done in good time.
Hemisection and slicing are seldom indicated in the maxilla. The morphology of the crown and the configuration of the roots do not lend themselves well to that approach. In this connection it should be noted again that the form and condition of the roots of deciduous molars are better seen on radiographs of the deciduous molars in the mandible than in the maxilla.

15.5.4 Unilateral agenesis of a maxillary second premolar

Except in pronounced crowding and Class II anomalies, extraction of a maxillary premolar on the other side from the agenesis is not indicated. Only the deciduous molar that has no successor is usually considered for extraction. The effect of unilateral lack of a second premolar is more limited in the maxilla than the mandible. That applies as much to the displacement of the arch midline as to the labiolingual position of the anterior teeth and the overjet and overbite.

15.6 Standard solutions

In Table 15-1 and Fig. 15-2 some standard solutions are presented, primarily for bilateral agenesis. Only the right hand side is mentioned and illustrated. Most of the solutions are applicable to unilateral agenesis as well. It is essential to carefully weigh the advantages and disadvantages of different approaches for each patient. The standard solutions given here are intended as guidelines for the decision-making process.

15.7 Supplementary remarks

In considering eliminating spacing resulting from agenesis, the vertical aspect of the occlusion in that region also plays a part. The danger involved in the absence of a premolar is that the antagonist will overerupt. This does not always happen and even when it does is not a justification alone for space closure.
Occasionally a second premolar does form much later than usual. At the age of 10 years a radiograph can reveal a developing premolar even when 2 years previously it was not visible. Second premolars that develop abnormally late frequently are deficient in form, size, and substance.
When both premolars in a quadrant are agenetic, consideration of transplantating a premolar (preferably as yet unerupted) from a quadrant without agenesis is merited. Transplantation of a premolar from the maxilla into a space caused by agenesis in the mandible in Class II/1 and especially in Class II/2 anomalies would be a good remedy.[105,112,199]

TABLE 15-1
Standard solutions for treating patients with premolar agenesis (Fig. 15-2, pages 293 and 294)

Tooth	Anomaly	Standard treatment
45	Class I	*(1)* Conserve tooth 85 (Fig. 15-2A); *(2)* extract tooth 85 and move tooth mesially, secure mesio-occlusion of molars (Fig. 15-2B); *(3)* extract tooth 85 and replace with prosthesis (Fig. 15-2C); *(4)* extract teeth 85 and 15 (or 14) (Fig. 15-2D).
45	Class II	*(1)* Conserve tooth 85 and secure neutro-occlusion of molars (Fig. 15-2A); *(2)* extract teeth 85 and 15 (or 14) and secure neutro-occlusion of molars (Fig. 15-2D).
45	Class III	*(1)* Extract tooth 85 and preserve mesio-occlusion of molars (Fig. 15-2B); *(2)* extract teeth 85 and 15 (or 14) and secure neutro-occlusion of molars (Fig. 15-2D).
15	Class I	*(1)* Conserve tooth 55 and preserve neutro-occlusion of molars (Fig. 15-2E); *(2)* extract tooth 55 and replace with prosthesis (Fig 15-2G).
15	Class II	*(1)* Extract teeth 55 and 25 and preserve disto-occlusion of molars (Fig. 15-2F); *(2)* extract teeth 55 and 45 and secure neutro-occlusion of molars (Fig. 15-2D).
15	Class III	*(1)* Conserve tooth 55 and secure neutro-occlusion of molars (Fig. 15-2E); *(2)* extract teeth 55 and 45 and secure neutro-occlusion of molars (Fig. 15-2H).

It is more or less impossible to predict the durability of a good second deciduous molar. Information regarding comparable situations in family members may give an indication. If retention has been decided upon, the tooth must be conserved as well as possible. Then hope for the best. The longer it remains in place, the shorter the period during which a possible prosthetic appliance might be required.
Second deciduous molars normally do not occlude well with premolars. Occlusal grinding to improve interdigitation is best avoided rather than risk root resorption. The same applies to interproximal reduction of enamel, despite indications derived from analysis of tooth size discrepancy (TSD) that it be done.

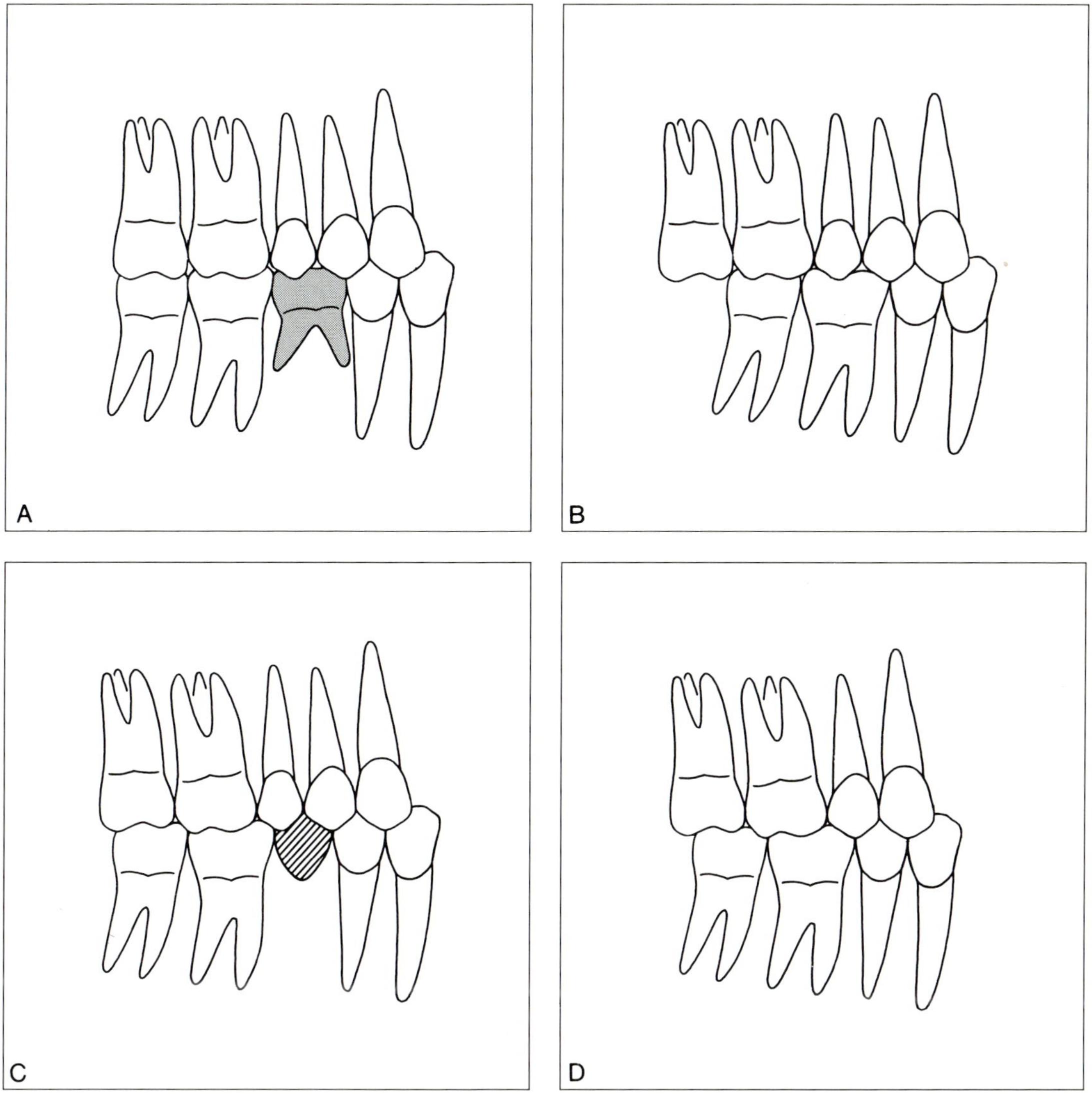

Fig. 15-2 Standard solutions for treating cases of premolar agenesis (Table 15-1, page 292).

A The mandibular second deciduous molar has been conserved; there is a mild disto-occlusion of the molars because the second deciduous molar is about 2.5 mm broader than a second premolar.

B After extraction of the mandibular second deciduous molar the molars have been moved mesially into a mesio-occlusion of one premolar crown width.

C After loss of the mandibular second deciduous molar a prosthetic replacement has been provided; the molars are in neutro-occlusion.

D The mandibular second deciduous molar and the second (or first) premolar in the maxilla have been extracted; the molars are in neutro-occlusion.

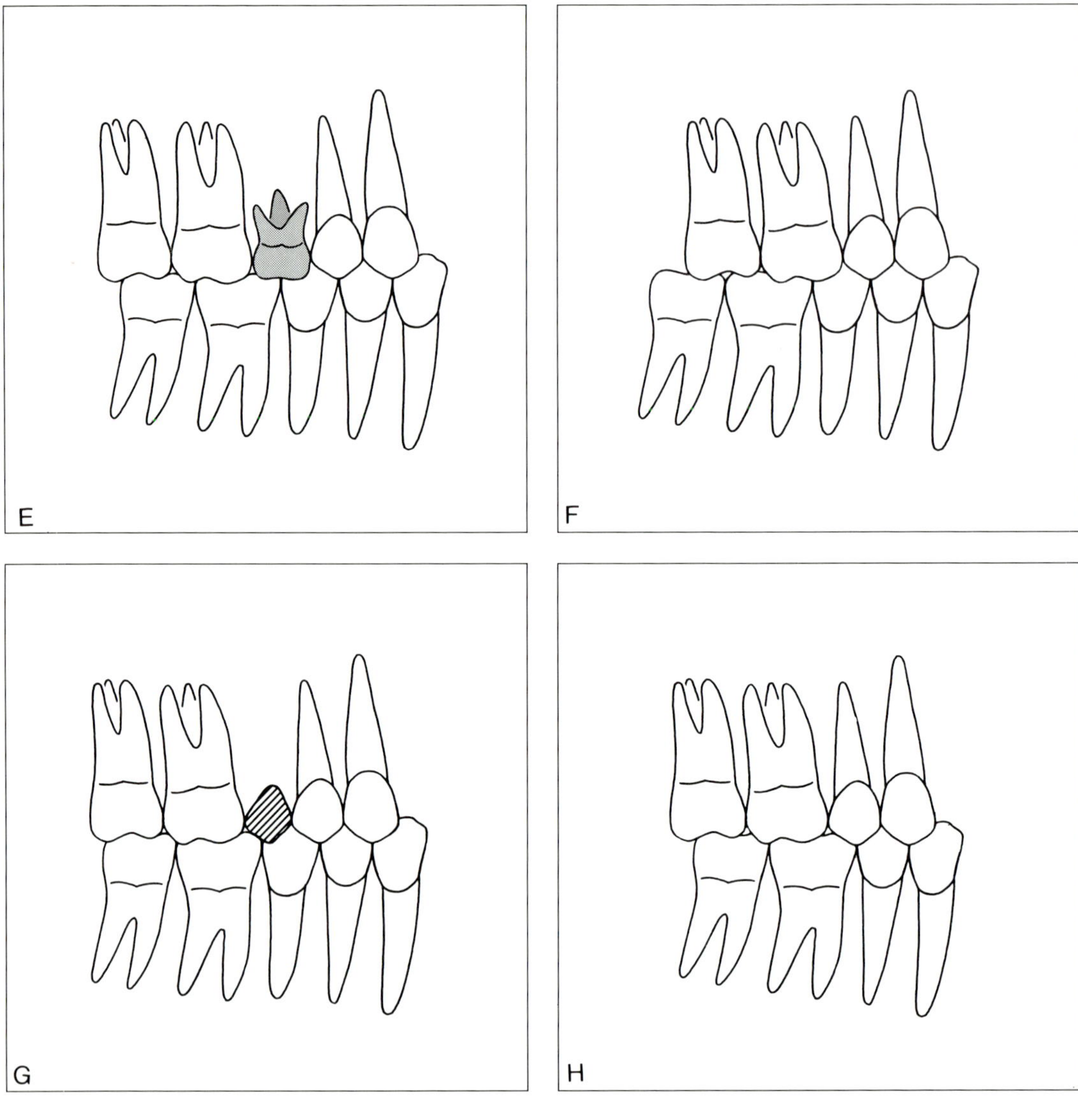

(Legend 15-2 continued)

E The maxillary second deciduous molar has been conserved; the molars are in neutro-occlusion.

F Extraction of the maxillary second deciduous molar; the molars are in disto-occlusion.

G After loss of the maxillary second deciduous molar it has been replaced prosthodontically; the molars are in neutro-occlusion.

H Extraction of the maxillary second deciduous molar and the opposing mandibular second (or first) premolar; the molars are in neutro-occlusion.

When a retained second deciduous molar eventually is lost, it must be decided whether or not a prosthodontic replacement is necessary. If it is clear that overeruption of the antagonist will not occur, for example, then doing nothing is an obvious solution. It is always possible to decide on orthodontic treatment for space closure at this stage, or later.

Occasionally, after orthodontic treatment has procured closure of an agenesis space in the mandible, the diastema re-opens. It is usually unwise to re-treat it because there will remain a risk of relapse unless permanent retention is employed.

In considering the advantages and disadvantages of orthodontic space closure, the presence or absence of third molars has some bearing. Absence of a premolar increases the chance of adequate space being available distally for good emergence of the third molar in that quadrant.

When in a Class I anomaly the space caused by agenesis of a mandibular premolar is closed by mesial movement of the permanent molars, allowance should be made for the fact that the last maxillary molar will probably have no antagonist later. Such a tooth can then overerupt and give rise to occlusal disturbances. In such cases it is appropriate to recall the patient over several years to check developments in that area. Such examples indicate the need for long-term thinking and planning.

Finally, it should be repeated that the danger of development of a dished-in face as a result of treatment to close diastemata caused by agenesis should not be underestimated. Usually the decision to initiate such treatment, and its subsequent execution, take place before facial growth is complete. Marked development of the nose and chin can follow, which, combined with an overretracted dentition, can lead to an ugly, prematurely aged profile and reduction of facial animation. Examining the profiles of parents or other relatives can supply a hint of what is to come in the development of the young patient.

Chapter 16

Problems in Eruption of First and Second Permanent Molars

16.1 Introduction

The dentition in the molar region develops over a long period of time. The formation of the first permanent molars begins before birth; on average they emerge at about age 6 years. The second and third molars follow at about 12 and 18 years, respectively. Duration of development of this region is connected with the relatively slow increase in size of the related tooth-bearing parts of the jaws.

Compared with the regions of the dentition mesial to the permanent molars, the development is simple. There are no deciduous teeth that must exfoliate, and the eruption sequence does not vary. Problems in the molar region are thus limited principally to anomalies of position, eruption, and crowding.

The aspects dealt with in this chapter are: ectopic eruption of first permanent molars, submerged second deciduous molars, agenesis of permanent molars, and ankylosis, impaction, and crowding in the molar region.

16.2 Ectopic eruption of first permanent molars

In approximately 3% of children the first permanent molar erupts too far mesially. It usually contacts the roots of the adjacent second deciduous molar via its mesio-occlusal marginal ridge. This results in atypical resorption of the deciduous molar root.[17] Ectopic eruption occurs mainly in the maxilla, seldom in the mandible. Ectopic eruption of the maxillary first permanent molars is associated with mesial angulation and sometimes with a relatively large crown. Spatial relationships within the jaws and arches appear to have only a limited importance.[18]

Ectopic eruption can be diagnosed clinically on the basis of partial or total failure to emerge. The picture on radiographs is explicit: the mesio-occlusal marginal ridge of the permanent molar is located apical to the crown of the second deciduous molar and is trapped under it.

In the maxilla about half the cases of ectopic eruption appear to correct themselves spontaneously. The first permanent molar ceases to be restrained by the deciduous molar and resumes eruption. In the remainder (and those usually have relatively large

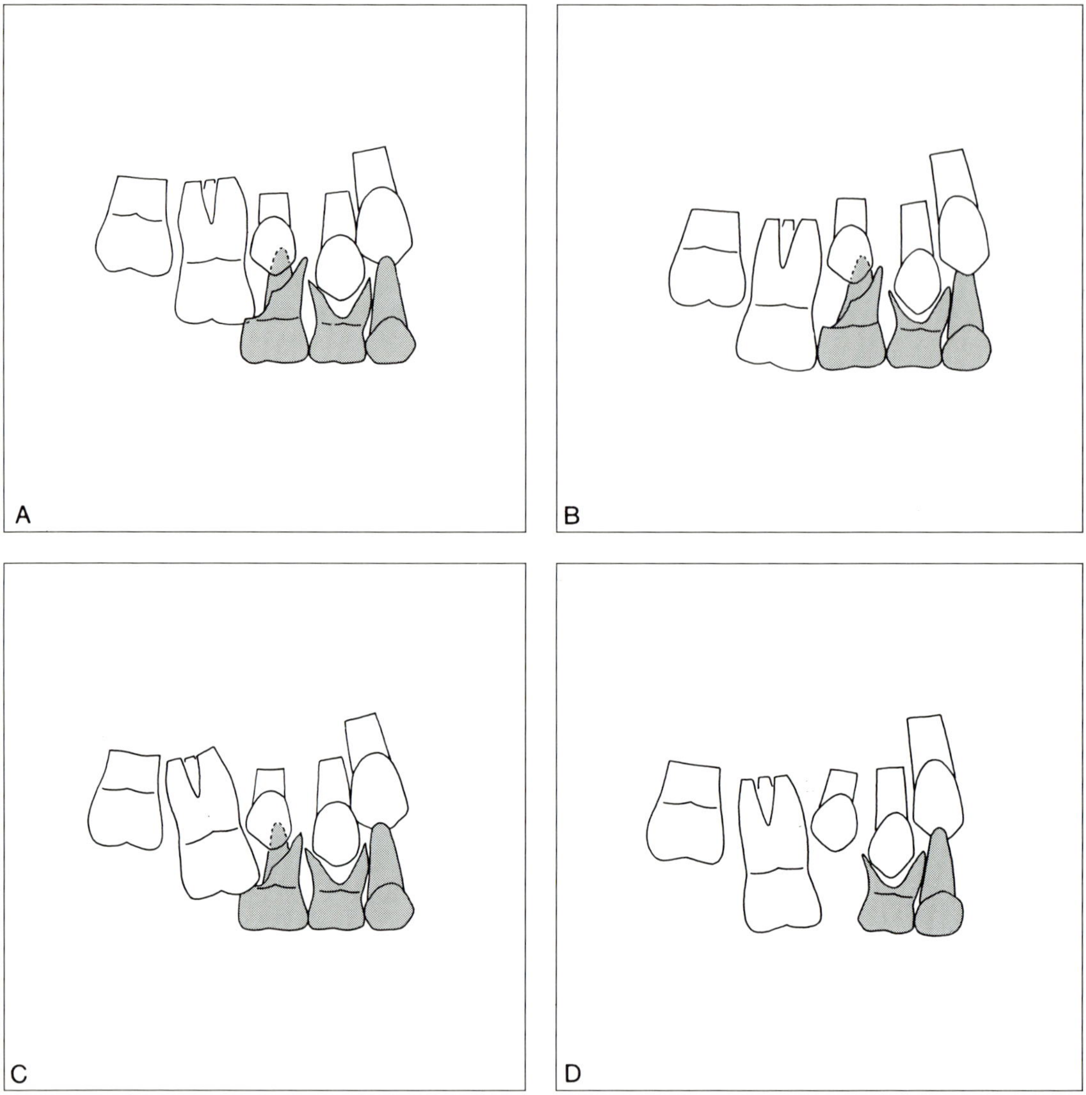

Fig. 16-1 Ectopic eruption of maxillary first permanent molars. (Drawings based on radiographs from Bjerklin and Kurol.[18])

A The mesio-occlusal marginal ridge of the maxillary first permanent molar is located apical to the crown of the second deciduous molar, the roots of which show atypical resorption.

B Spontaneous correction of the situation in A, a year later. The limited obstruction has been overcome by movement of the first permanent molar.

C Marked mesial angulation with resorption of the second deciduous molar; spontaneous correction cannot be expected.

D After exfoliation of the second deciduous molar, the first permanent molar has emerged along its mesially directed path; the space available for the second premolar is significantly reduced.

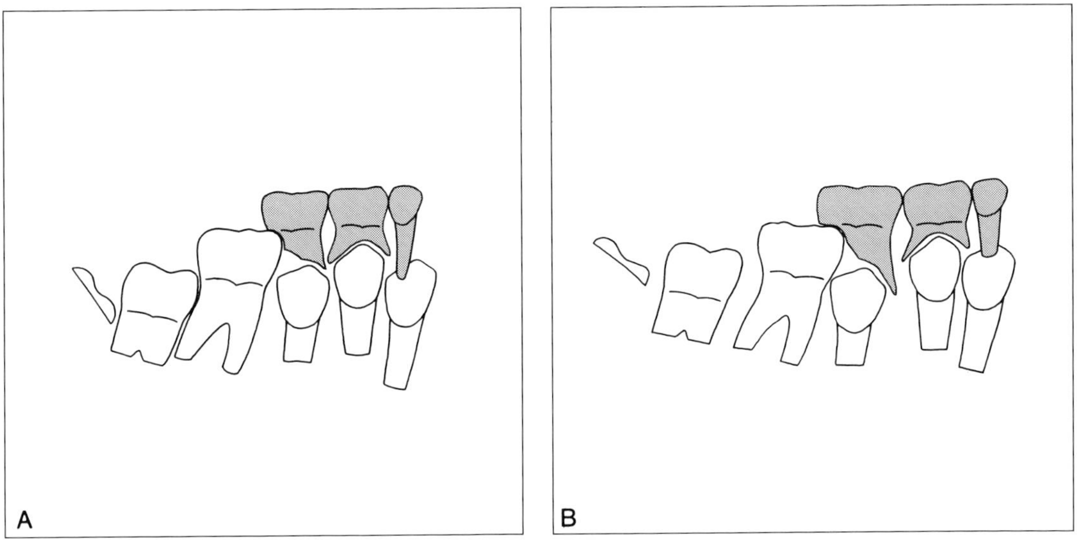

Fig. 16-2 Ectopic eruption of the mandibular first permanent molar, where the phenomenon seldom occurs.

A Because the limited obstruction is associated with crowding in the molar region, spontaneous corrective movement is not possible. The second deciduous molar will only exfoliate when the roots have resorbed.

B Marked obstruction that does not correct itself despite ample space dorsal to the first permanent molar (large posterior section of the apical area).

first permanent molar crowns) the obstruction remains and the first permanent molar does not erupt farther until the deciduous molar exfoliates or is extracted (Figs. 16-1 and 16-2).

When ectopic eruption of a first permanent molar is found, an estimate should be made of the likelihood that emergence will happen spontaneously or not occur until after the second deciduous molar has been lost. If it has not fully emerged by the age of 7, most likely no natural correction will take place.[18] The best way to judge the situation is by comparing the tooth in question with the corresponding one on the other side. If that had emerged a year or more previously, prognosis for normal eruption will be poor. Radiographs will provide positive information; the extent of the obstruction by the deciduous tooth and the degree of its root resorption are immediately obvious. The approach to follow depends mainly on these conditions.[242]

If spontaneous correction is not expected, the obstruction should be eliminated. When resorption of the deciduous second molar that is caused by the first permanent molar is only slight, the first molar often can be displaced sufficiently distally by inserting a brass ligature between it and the deciduous molar and tightening it every few days. If the contact point is accessible enough, self-locking separating springs or plastic separating rings can be inserted.

Where the atypical resorption is extensive, extraction of the deciduous molar can be considered. A removable orthodontic appliance can be used to move the permanent molar distally once it has emerged sufficiently. Subsequently a space maintainer should be employed to hold the space that was regained, until the second premolar has emerged (Fig. 16-3).

One can also conserve the second deciduous molar and use it as anchorage for a force uprighting the first permanent molar and moving it distally. An advantage of this approach is that no retention is necessary afterwards if the deciduous tooth remains (Fig. 16-4).

Distal slicing of the deciduous second molar is not recommended. Indeed, the first permanent molar may emerge, but too far mesially. Above all, there is a danger that the crown of the permanent molar may be damaged by the slicing.

In many cases of ectopic eruption it will be desirable to intervene and move the first permanent molar distally. Obviously, distal movement is not indicated when the second premolar or other teeth from the same quadrant are congenitally absent. That applies often also when the overall orthodontic treatment plan requires removal of a permanent tooth later in that region.

16.3 Submerged second deciduous molars

Second deciduous molars that ankylose early can become separated so far from the occlusal plane that emerged first permanent molars may tilt mesially across them. The ankylotic deciduous molars become overlapped and more or less trapped. The periodontal membrane on the mesial surface of the permanent molar can be damaged. Submerged second deciduous molars can even become fully engulfed in the mucosa (Fig. 16-5).

Depending on the occlusion, the antagonists of submerged deciduous molars can overerupt and cause occlusal disturbance as a result of their supraposition.

Occurrences such as those above need to be prevented. The development of the dentition and the vertical growth of the lower face should be observed critically at regular intervals. Extraction of ankylosed deciduous molars should be accomplished in good time (see 13.7).

16.4 Agenesis of permanent molars

First and second permanent molars are seldom congenitally absent; if they are absent, other teeth are usually missing as well. Depending on several aspects of the state of the dentition and facial morphology, various procedures can be employed. Active space closure, autotransplantation of suitable other (third) molars, or provision of prosthodontic replacements are possibilities. On the whole, sometimes it is better to leave things alone.

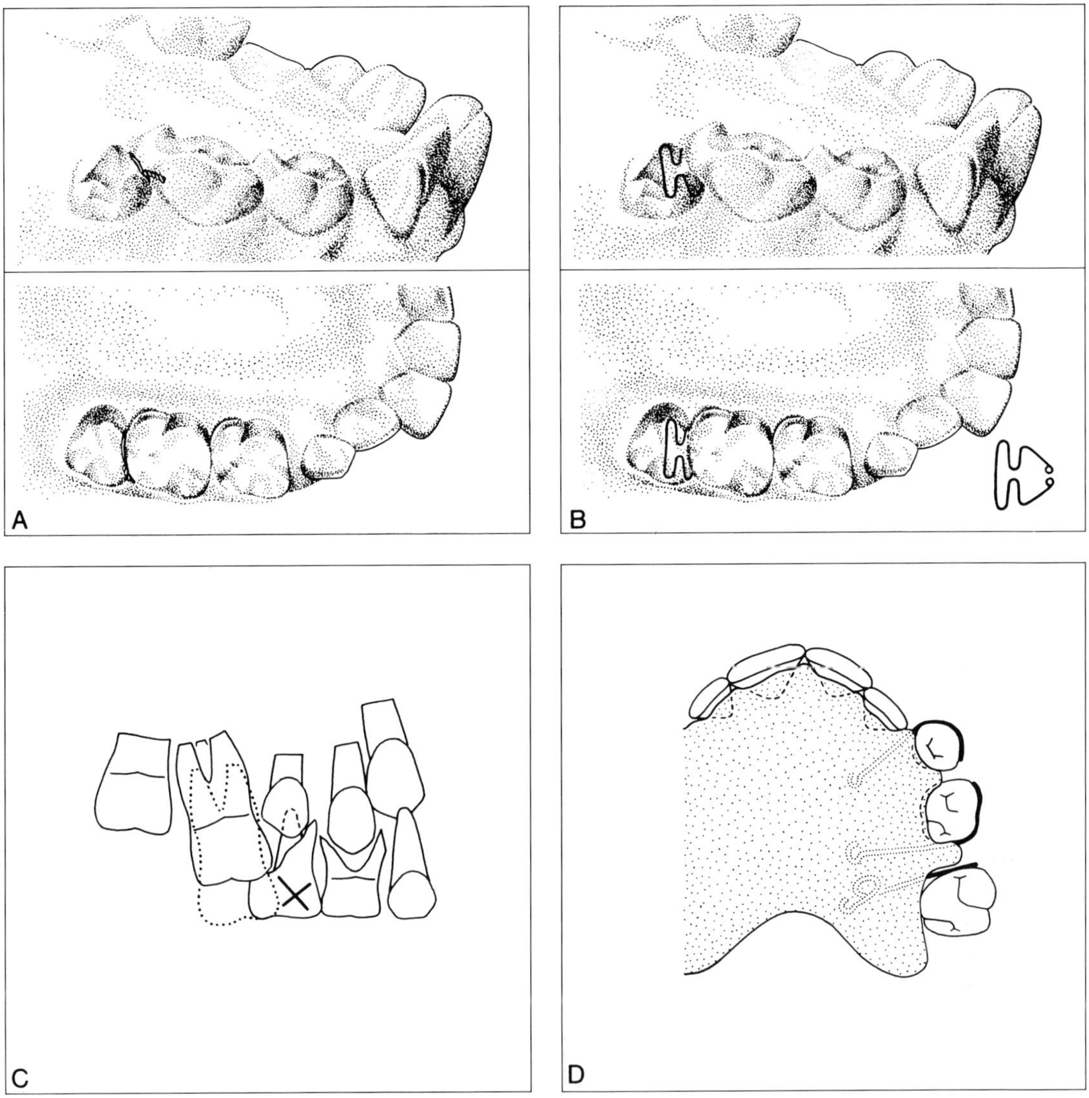

Fig. 16-3 Methods for correcting ectopic eruption of maxillary first permanent molars.

A Where the atypical resorption of the second deciduous molar is limited, a soft brass ligature (0.4 to 0.6 mm in diameter) can be used to clear the obstruction. The wire should be tightened every few days.

B The necessary space can also be gained using self-locking separating springs or plastic separating rings.[232]

C Where the obstruction is considerable, removal of the second deciduous molar should be considered. Subsequently, the first permanent molar will arrive too far mesially in the dental arch.

D For distal movement of the first permanent molar an acrylic resin removable appliance can be used. In certain cases, a simple lip bumper (.045-inch arch) or a headgear placed on the first permanent molars can serve well.

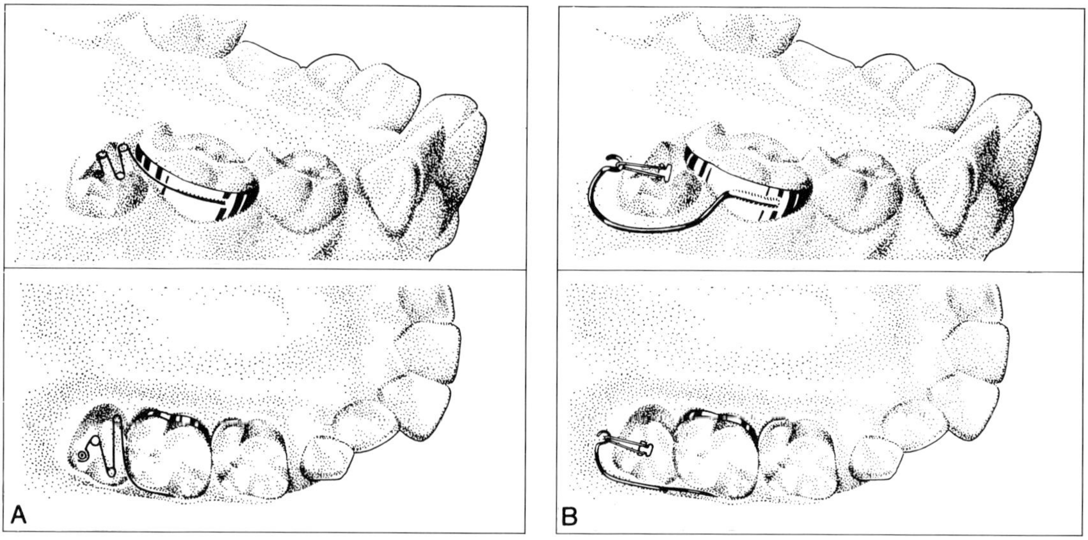

Fig. 16-4 Techniques for obtaining distal movement of a severely obstructed ectopic erupting first permanent molar, when removal of the second deciduous molar is not desired.

A A spring is soldered to a band fitted to the second deciduous molar. After the band has been cemented, the spring is hooked under a button bonded on the occlusal surface of the first permanent molar.[79,163]

B A strong extension of orthodontic wire is fixed to the band on the second deciduous molar. A hook has been bonded to the first permanent molar and an elastic band is stretched between the two.[114]

A first permanent molar can also be uprighted and moved distally by use of two bonded brackets between which a wire is attached that exerts the required force.

16.5 Ankylosis of permanent molars

The consequences of ankylosis are closely related to the degree to which the development of the dentition and growth of the face had progressed at the time the ankylosis occurred. If ankylosis takes place after all the permanent teeth have reached occlusion, then little or no infraocclusion will occur. If transition is incomplete and the face not fully developed, ankylosed permanent teeth (particularly first molars) can give rise to gross disturbances. The natural movement of adjacent teeth is inhibited; antagonists can overerupt.
An attempt can be made to correct ankylosis of permanent teeth by using extraction forceps after local anaesthesia and carefully moving the tooth. After achieving some mobility, the tooth can be moved slightly up and down its long axis. A day later an extruding force must be applied. This force can be generated by using elastic bands through a wire guide (fork) mounted on a removable appliance bearing a hook to which

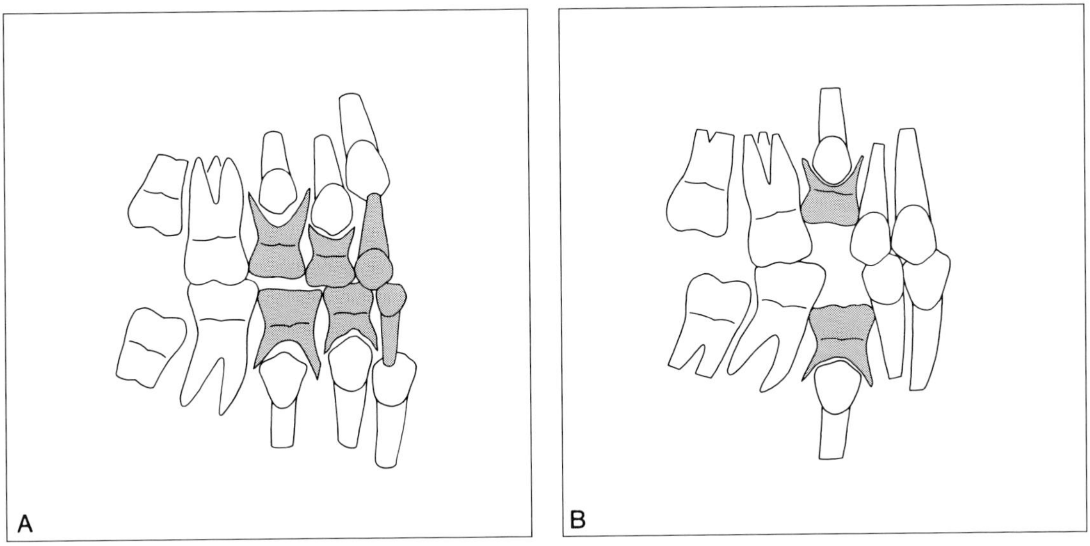

A B

Fig. 16-5 Disturbance of the eruption and emergence of first permanent molars caused by early ankylosis of second deciduous molars.

A The situation shortly after mandibular and maxillary second deciduous molars have become ankylosed.
B With considerable vertical development of the lower face the second deciduous molars can become separated quite a distance from the occlusal plane. First permanent molars can tip markedly mesially.

one end of the elastic band is attached. Suitable cleats or buttons to attach the other end of the elastic band can be bonded to the crown of the tooth (Fig. 16-6).
Another approach is to provide an appliance on the opposing dental arch to which a vertical intermaxillary elastic band can be attached. A single tooth that is not in occlusion and is not ankylosed is unsuitable for that purpose because it would be extruded into supraposition by the traction. What is required is more than one tooth so that the reaction to the force is better distributed. The force applied to the previously ankylosed tooth should be greater than that normally used on such a tooth for orthodontic movement. After some weeks the tooth can have reached the desired level. Should ankylosis return later, one might consider repeating the procedure.
The prognosis for permanently breaking the ankylosis of a tooth with one root is fair and for one with more than one root is dubious. Nevertheless, an attempt to displace the tooth might be justified in view of the consequences of the ankylosed condition. If such an attempt is not undertaken or turns out to be unsuccessful, the choice has to be made between preserving the tooth concerned, with such restorative heightening of the crown as might be required, or extracting it. In this choice one should realise that the chance of keeping an ankylosed tooth over a long period is limited. They often are lost due to root resorption.

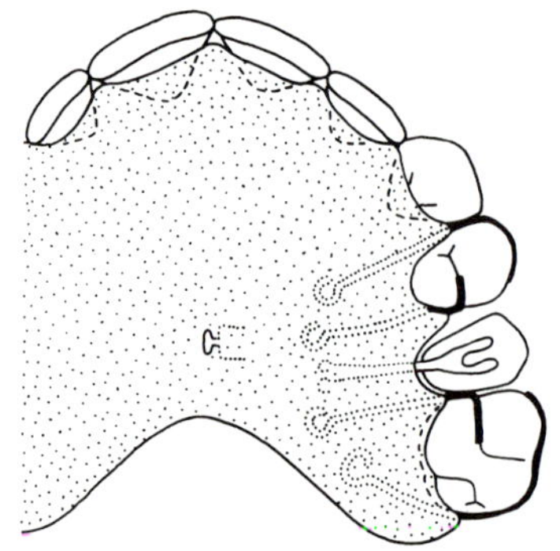
A

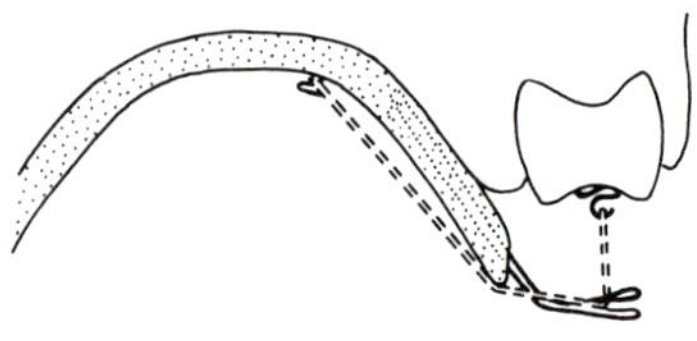
B

Fig. 16-6 Method to attempt to move a tooth occlusally after breaking down its ankylosis.

A One day after the ankylosis has been forcibly disrupted an extruding force is applied using a removable plate and an elastic band.
B The force is delivered by an elastic band hooked onto a cleat or similar attachment bonded to the crown. Note the occlusal rests employed to prevent apical displacement of the plate and the forked extension through which the elastic band operates.

Extraction of first permanent molars should usually be followed by closure of the space created. Extraction is an obvious solution when crowding is a problem and there are other grounds for undertaking orthodontic treatment.
Moreover, another possibility that should be considered after extraction is to retain the first molar space (space maintainer), and later to transplant a developing third molar to that location when the roots have developed sufficiently. Before undertaking transplantation the space available in the dental arch should be increased because some excess space is required to improve the prognosis.
Extraction has few disadvantages when it concerns an ankylosed second permanent molar, particularly when the third molar might assume an acceptable position in the dental arch after removal of the second molar. In the maxilla, no additional treatment is usually required; in the mandible the angulation and position of the third molar later may often be unsatisfactory (see 16.6).

16.6 Impacted first and second permanent molars

Unlike the third molars, the first and second permanent molars are seldom impacted. Occasionally a clear reason for impaction can be seen, such as an odontoma, osteoma,

follicular cyst, or a supernumerary tooth. In such cases removal of the obstacle will usually result in emergence of the impacted tooth.
In most cases, however, a clear cause of the failure to erupt cannot be indicated, except when it may form part of a syndrome such as cleidocranial dysostosis. The tooth can fail to erupt fully or can have moved toward the occlusal plane to a limited extent only.[191]
The vertical development of impacted first permanent molars remains behind that of their neighbouring teeth and the vertical development of the alveolar process. The adjacent second premolar and second permanent molar tilt together across the impacted molar, introducing a danger of periodontal damage. Generally the third molar in these cases does not emerge.
The consequences of impacted second permanent molars are less serious. Distal tilting of the first permanent molar is rarely or never observed. However, the third molar usually does impact. Depending on the occlusion the antagonist of the second molar can overerupt and initiate occlusal interference.
Treatment involves surgical exposure of the crown with subsequent packing to prevent regeneration of the mucosal cover. Regular observation will show if eruption is proceeding. Adequate space must be available in the dental arch or be provided first by active appliance therapy. If eruption does not follow, an attachment can be bonded to the occlusal enamel through which traction can be applied, which often means a second surgical intervention in order to get adequate access. Traction on the tooth can be applied with a removable appliance using an elastic band through a fork-shaped guide, particularly in the maxilla. In the mandibular arch a partial fixed appliance is usually preferred.[217]
If a tooth remains impacted for a long time, a follicular cyst can develop, which may eventually give rise to chronic or acute inflammation.

16.7 Crowding in the molar region

The space condition in the molar region is determined by the sum of the mesiodistal diameters of the molar crowns, the size of the region of the jaw in which they are invested, the size increase of that region as the result of growth of the face, and by the mesial migration of the first permanent molar during transition in the posterior segments. Extraction of teeth mesial to that region may provide additional space for the molars.
The presence of third molars is an essential factor. Their absence is seldom associated with crowding in the molar region. Further, the crowns of the rest of the teeth are on average smaller in such cases than in those where the third molars are indeed present.[69]
Crowding in the molar region is judged clinically by considering the position of the permanent molars that have emerged and the space available dorsally for the remainder of the dentition. In the maxilla this space can be determined accurately as the posterior limit, which is clearly demarcated by the tuberosity. In the mandible it is necessary to estimate with the aid of palpation the extent of the region into which teeth can emerge.

In growing individuals, the size of the posterior section of the apical area in both jaws increases dorsally by about 1 mm per year.[177,178] The amount of growth that is still available is the decisive factor, and it should be greater for males than females of the same ages. Girls are usually a little ahead of boys in the development of their dentitions; growth of their faces, however, ceases significantly earlier. Many girls have already achieved their adult size by the age of 14 or 15 years. However, many boys exhibit substantial jaw growth after that age.

Relatively late emergence of second permanent molars is a symptom of crowding in the molar region. However, crowding is usually not obvious until it is clear that the third molars cannot emerge. In extreme cases crowding in the molar region is already evident as the second permanent molars emerge, those in the maxilla being distally angulated and lying buccal to the dental arch and those in the mandible being unable to emerge fully or at all.

Whether or not the third molars are present can usually only be determined radiologically. Third molars are absent in approximately 16% of the population.[70]

Without radiological information, one should begin with the assumption that the third molars are formed.

In a growing person it is possible to guess fairly accurately whether or not adequate space will develop in the maxilla. Such an estimation is based on the existing situation and the growth that can be expected in the region of the tuberosities. Facial orthopedic procedures acting on the maxillary complex affect growth in the tuberosity regions. Extraoral traction with a dorsally acting force is likely to result in less growth in the tuberosity region. Further, the first permanent molars can become displaced distally. Applying ventral traction to the maxillary complex will have the opposite effect and encourages the development of a larger posterior section of the apical area in the maxilla. In addition, the first permanent molars will usually move mesially.[224]

In the mandible future development is difficult to forecast. The variation in the extent of the growth of the relevant regions is probably greater in the mandible than in the maxilla. The space seen between the second and third molars on a radiograph cannot always be taken as an indication of absence of crowding. The angulation of the third molars also is not a reliable indication of crowding; a pronounced mesial angulation can be associated with either a shortage or an excess of room.[177]

In general, a reliable prognosis can be derived from combining radiological and clinical data. Palpation of the lingual aspect of the mandible gives an indication of the cross section and extension of the part in which teeth can position themselves upon emergence. Distobuccal rotation of mandibular second permanent molars indicates that space will be limited. A radiograph showing space between the three molars indicates a large posterior section of the apical area; severe overlapping vertically and transversely is a sign of a small section.

Crowding in the maxillary molar region presents few problems for patients. If a second permanent molar emerges buccally and a crossbite (exo-occlusion) develops, an adequate transverse occlusion can generally be realised by easy means (elastic bands through the bite). Of course, account has to be taken of the fact that the third molar will have inadequate space. When that tooth emerges it can easily be extracted if necessary. The antagonist in such cases will usually be impacted. Indeed it seldom happens that there is no space for a maxillary third molar and yet adequate room in the mandible. The reverse, however, is often encountered.

Extraction of the second permanent molars is often a good solution for relief of crowding in the maxillary molar region, provided that the third molars are normally positioned with well-formed crowns and roots of normal size (not too small). After extraction of the maxillary second permanent molars, the third molars move mesially, upright themselves, and emerge in such a way as to take up a good position in the dental arch, contacting the first molars. Particularly in instances when second permanent molars emerge buccally or are carious, hypoplastic, or heavily restored, their removal has distinct advantages.[31] After extraction of the maxillary second permanent molars, the teeth mesial to them can be displaced distally. Crowding in the anterior or posterior segments may be reduced or eliminated in that fashion.
Although mandibular second molar extractions have been advised,[239] the results obtained from that procedure are considerably less favourable in the mandible than in the maxilla. An optimal occlusion usually does not come about. Uprighting of third molars and improvement of interproximal contacts with the first molars are often desirable.
When the conclusion is reached that the mandibular second permanent molars should be extracted, this removal should be executed preferably before the roots of the third molars are formed. This does not apply in the maxilla where extraction at a later stage does not affect the prognosis for angulation and occlusion of the third molars.
Crowding in the molar region can also be relieved by removing first permanent molars (Chapter 17).
In the mandible, removal of the third molar tooth germs at an early age (germectomy) may be a useful procedure (Chapter 18).

16.8 Supplementary remarks

Establishing a good sagittal occlusion between the permanent molars depends primarily on the sagittal jaw relation and the occlusion of the second molars and first deciduous premolars. Development of a neutro-occlusion can be influenced through selective interproximal reduction of deciduous molars during the second transitional period.
Nevertheless, a good occlusion in the molar region does not always result, even when the relations within and between the jaws are optimal. The most important cause inhibiting development of a solid interdigitation is interposition of the tongue. The cone-funnel mechanism and the rail mechanism are then inactive and usually the maxillary arch will be too narrow in relation to the mandibular arch.
Before extracting a permanent molar for local reasons it is essential to view the circumstances regarding the effect the extraction might have on the entire dentition. In this respect, lack of an antagonist for the most posterior molar, and the implications of possible hypoplasia or other abnormalities of the involved molars, should be considered. In general, early extraction is preferred to later extraction, but it does require a serious attempt to be made to predict the outcome of the intervention.

Chapter 17

Whether or not to Extract Defective First Permanent Molars at an Early Age

17.1 Introduction

In children between 6 and 10 years of age, defective first molars can be an indication of inferior quality of all the permanent teeth. This inferior quality can be caused by imperfect formation of the dental tissues, an oral environment providing greater caries susceptibility, or both. In such cases the dentition can be maintained in a healthy state for a long period only if much care is taken of the teeth from an early age. Application of measures for caries prevention (sensible eating habits, good oral hygiene, and use of fluoride) and optimal professional dental care are of considerable importance. Procedures that might encourage caries and gingival disorders, such as use of orthodontic appliances, call for some restraint in their employment.

Besides inferior quality of all permanent teeth, isolated defective crown formation in first permanent molars can occur. Use of orthodontic appliances in such cases is less of a problem than where the deficiencies are general. The latter situation is usually seen when hypoplastic enamel occurs in the first permanent molars and in the incisors because of influences affecting these teeth when their formation is proceeding in more or less the same period.

When a child has very bad first permanent molars, consideration should be given to removing those teeth at an early age with the aim of obtaining the most satisfactory space closure. Extraction of the first permanent molars is then based primarily on the possibilities to influence the development of the dentition in such a way as to limit unfavourable effects. In that regard it is not only the time of the extraction that is important, but also the sequence used in removing first permanent molars in the two jaws.

This chapter begins by indicating the importance of the first permanent molars. After that follows discussion of the consequences of extraction and of some abnormal conditions, indications for and implications of extractions, and procedures involved in choosing the sequence of extractions. In addition, general guidelines are given.

17.2 The importance of first permanent molars

The first permanent molars are the teeth with the largest crowns and the largest root surface area. They are the principal teeth used in mastication. Moreover, they are essential in the development of the dentition and the coordination of facial growth.

They support the occlusion in a vertical direction and determine lower face height; during the second transitional period they are sometimes the only teeth that are in function. Further, their location largely determines the position that the premolars and other permanent molars will take up in sagittal direction after emerging. On top of this, the first permanent molars fulfill a significant role in the adjustment of the width of the maxillary dental arch to that of the mandibular one. Matching the transverse growth of the maxilla with the dimensions of the mandible is achieved by the good interdigitation of the first permanent molars together with other posterior teeth that solidly interdigitate in a buccolingual direction. A comparable situation exists in the coordination of anteroposterior growth of mandible and maxilla, in which the mesiodistal interdigitation is the important factor.[223,224] For these reasons, preservation of the first permanent molars is clearly desirable and from the above it may be seen that their early loss does not just affect the ability to chew.

One of the objectives to be considered in choosing the least unfavourable moment for extraction of the first permanent molars is to limit if not entirely eliminate the period during which interdigitation is inadequate. Thus, extraction of the first permanent molars at the age of 7 years in a case of marked attrition of the deciduous molars leads to a significant period of inadequate interaction between the jaws of the kind mentioned above.

17.3 Consequences of extracting first permanent molars

It occasionally happens in orthodontics that expectations are not fulfilled, and that applies also to the consequences of extracting first permanent molars at an early age. In this discussion, however, it will be assumed for didactic purposes that the original expectations should be achieved.

At every patient visit one should check to what extent the development conforms to expectations. The situation in the mouth should be compared with the initial conditions, which preferably have been recorded with good plaster models. Systematic examination of and thought about the changes in both dental arches and the occlusion, in particular bearing on the second permanent molars, will provide the information needed to show whether or not everything is going as planned. If not, intervention can be undertaken according to what is necessary for that patient.

17.3.1 Migration, tipping, and rotation of adjacent teeth

Extracting teeth results in migration of adjacent teeth. Migration in this context refers to movement within the jaw before emergence as well as movement of teeth in the dental arch after emergence. Migration often is associated with tipping and sometimes with rotation around the long axis of the tooth.

Extraction of the first permanent molars leads to mesial (and occlusal) migration of the second permanent molar and distal migration of the premolars (Fig. 17-1). The second permanent molars not only tip mesially, they rotate mesiolingually as well.

There is a difference between mandibular and maxillary teeth in the degree of migration, tipping, and rotation that follows extraction of first permanent molars. This

difference is related to the diversity in development of the molar regions in both jaws. In the mandible, before the second and third molars emerge they are oriented with their crowns mesially and lingually inclined. In the maxilla, however, the second and third molars before emergence have their crowns inclined distally and buccally.
After extraction of a maxillary first permanent molar, the adjacent erupting second permanent molar performs a tipping movement in which the crown moves more mesially than the apices. This movement corresponds more or less with the normal changes in mesiodistal angulation that an erupting second permanent molar would experience if the first one had not been extracted at an early age. The tipping movement is, however, a little greater.
A considerably more unfavourable situation exists in that respect in the mandible. Under normal circumstances a second permanent molar that originally was mesially inclined would upright itself on eruption. Extracting the first permanent molar affects the eruption path of the not yet emerged second molar, which subsequently will display little or no uprighting movement, or even will tip more mesially. This last movement is the opposite to what is required to achieve an acceptable angulation after emergence.
In contrast to the mandibular teeth, the maxillary second permanent molars in the absence of the first permanent molars show only a slight abnormality in mesiodistal angulation. To reach a good mesiodistal angulation the root apices of the maxillary molars do not need to move so far mesially as those in the mandible.[12,192] It also makes a difference how far the eruption of the second permanent molars has progressed at the time the first permanent molars are extracted. A second permanent molar that has not yet emerged will migrate mesially in the jaw when the adjacent first molar is removed. It will then emerge farther mesially than it otherwise would have done. The degree to which it emerges mesially will depend on the time span between extraction of the first permanent molar and the moment of emergence of the second molar. The longer the interval the greater the mesial drifting will be. The extent to which the second permanent molar will tip after extraction of the first depends on the spatial conditions in the jaw, the original orientation of the second molar, and its pattern of eruption. For both jaws, if one waits until the second permanent molar has emerged before extracting the first molar, the second molar subsequently will end up in a more mesially tilted position than it would have if the extraction had been executed a year earlier.
The mesiolingual rotation of the second permanent molar after extraction of the first molar is more pronounced in the maxilla than the mandible. Maxillary second permanent molars rotate about an axis more or less through the mesiopalatal cusp and the palatal root. Mandibular second molars also rotate mesiolingually, but less so. This distinction can be attributed to the conformation of the roots and the morphology of the investing structures of the respective jaws.

17.3.2 Closing spaces and changes in occlusion

After extracting the first permanent molars the adjacent second molars drift more mesially in the maxilla than in the mandible. The space resulting from the removal of the maxillary first permanent molar is eliminated more or less completely by this reaction. The maxillary premolars move distally only slightly so that the larger part of

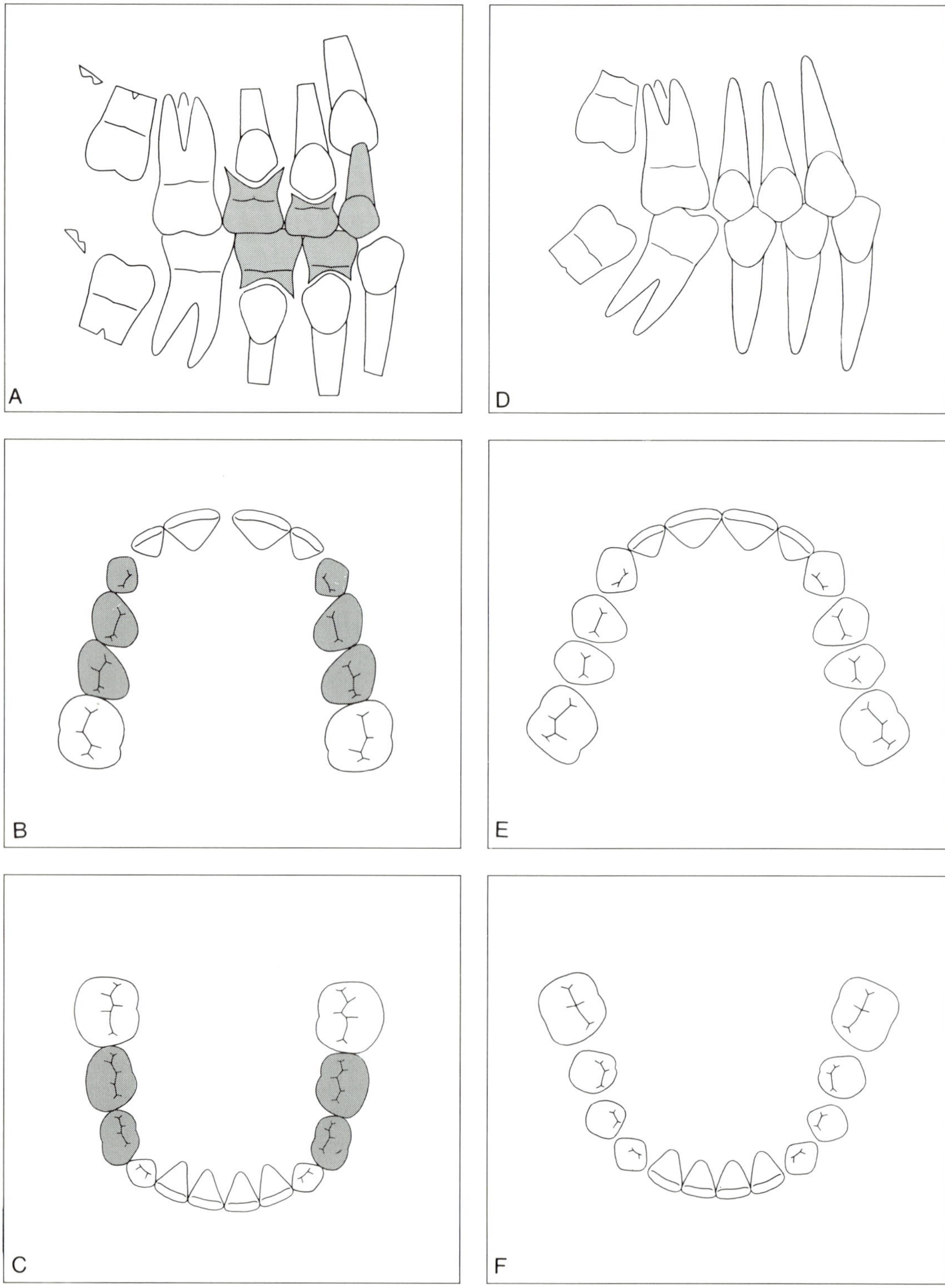

Figure 17-1

Fig. 17-1 Development of the dentition when first permanent molars in both jaws are extracted in otherwise normal cases. The drawings A, B, and C reproduce the situation shortly before extraction. In the adjacent drawings D, E, and F, the conditions are shown as they would be expected to exist some years later.

A At age approximately 10 years, the occlusal marginal ridges of the second molars are still about one crown height away from the occlusal plane. Their bifurcations have already formed. When the third molars are present the crown formation is already proceeding.

B Spacing is present between the maxillary incisors. The buccal surfaces of the first permanent molars are farther buccally than those of the second deciduous molars.

C No spaces are present in the mandible. The teeth are positioned harmoniously in the line of the arch.

D Some years after extraction of the first permanent molars the mandibular second permanent molars have tipped mesially and only the distal part of their occlusal surfaces contacts the maxillary molars. The latter are also tipped mesially, though to a lesser extent. The third molars have moved mesially within the jaws and will probably emerge without problems. This is fairly certain for the maxilla but not for the mandible. Sometimes the mandibular premolars, and particularly the second premolars, are tipped distally. Diastemata are present in the posterior regions; these are larger in the mandible than in the maxilla.

E In the maxilla the second permanent molars not only have migrated mesially, they have also rotated markedly mesiopalatally more or less around an imaginary axis through the palatal root and the mesiopalatal cusp. The second premolars have drifted distally and moreover have rotated distopalatally. The first premolar has also been displaced distally, usually without significant rotation.

F In the mandible the second permanent molar has been displaced less mesially than in the maxilla. The rotation that has occurred is more limited. In the mandible the premolars move more distally after extraction of first permanent molars than in the maxilla. There is also more distolingual rotation by the mandibular second premolars than by the maxillary ones. Further, a similar rotation can be seen in the mandibular first premolars, though to a lesser extent than in the mandibular second premolars.

the space reduction is accomplished by mesial migration of the maxillary second permanent molar. In the mandible diastemata often remain, even though the mandibular premolars migrate more distally than those in the maxilla.[158,159] Further, the mandibular premolars rotate more distolingually than the maxillary premolars, whereas in both jaws this rotation is more marked for the second premolars than for the first premolars.

Extraction of first permanent molars at a young age leads to an earlier emergence of the second and third permanent molars.[55] The effect on the overjet is only minor. The mandibular and maxillary incisors become a little more upright, the interincisal angle increases a little. The effect on the facial profile is also limited; the lips usually only fall back insignificantly.[131,212]

The mesial tipping of the second permanent molars (especially in the mandible), their mesial drifting and rotation (especially in the maxilla), and the distal tipping and rotation of the premolars (especially in the mandible), lead to a ramshackle occlusion. Both transversely and sagittally, good interdigitation is lacking. Normally the situation improves over the years and a more favourable occlusion develops. A really good occlusion, however, is almost never achieved, essentially because the mandibular

second molar seldom uprights sufficiently. From a periodontal point of view the situation between the second premolar and the second permanent molar (particularly in the mandible) usually remains unsatisfactory because of that lack of uprighting.
The changes indicated above that result from the loss of a first permanent molar at an early age apply to otherwise normal circumstances (Fig. 17-1, page 312). If there is crowding or spacing, a non-Class I situation, no normal lip relationship, and/or a deviating function, the changes will often present themselves in a different form.

Fig. 17-2 Development of the dentition when all first permanent molars are extracted at an early age in a patient with crowding in both jaws. The drawings A, B, and C reproduce the situation after the second deciduous molars have already been lost prematurely and shortly before the first permanent molars are to be removed. In the adjacent drawings D, E, and F, the conditions are shown as they would be expected to exist after a few years.

A Because of the earlier premature loss of the second deciduous molars the first permanent molars have already drifted and tilted mesially, more in the mandible than in the maxilla. Also, the second permanent molars, which are still within the alveolar processes, have moved slightly mesially. The premolars and permanent canines are closer to each other than when there is more space available in both jaws (compare with Fig. 17-1).

B Crowding in the maxilla is partly caused by premature loss of the deciduous molars. The first permanent molars have migrated and rotated mesially.

C Some crowding also exists in the mandibular arch. The first permanent molars have migrated mesially.

D Some years after extraction of the first permanent molars and completion of the transition, the second permanent molars have reached a reasonable sagittal occlusion. The interdigitation is not optimal. The mesial cusps of the opposing second permanent molars do not occlude adequately. Both second molars, mandibular more than maxillary, are tilted mesially. In accordance with the initial crowding, all spaces in both arches are now closed. The premolars interdigitate reasonably well. They exhibit no abnormal mesiodistal inclination.

E The limited distal migration of the premolars provided some extra room for improvement of the positions of the incisors. The second permanent molars have drifted mesially and rotated mesiopalatally. The contacts with the second premolars are not located in the proper place.

F In the mandible the second permanent molars have moved mesially, with a little rotation to mesial too. The second premolars that have migrated distally are a little rotated, but in a distolingual direction. The contacts between the second premolars and the second molars are not well placed. This is also the case with the contacts between first and second premolars. The mandibular incisors have been able to profit from the space provided by the distal migration of the premolars: the irregular alignment of the mandibular incisors has spontaneously corrected itself.

The review given in this figure also applies in broad outline to situations in which the crowding has not been contributed to by premature loss of deciduous molars. Also, when the crowding is entirely attributable to a discrepancy between the mesiodistal dimensions of the crowns and the available dental arch length of both jaws (arch length discrepancy, ALD), early extraction of first permanent molars can result in an important improvement. That particularly concerns the alignment of incisors and canines, especially in the mandible. Taken overall, the extraction of first permanent molars has fewer detrimental consequences in arches with crowding than in those with ample or excess space.

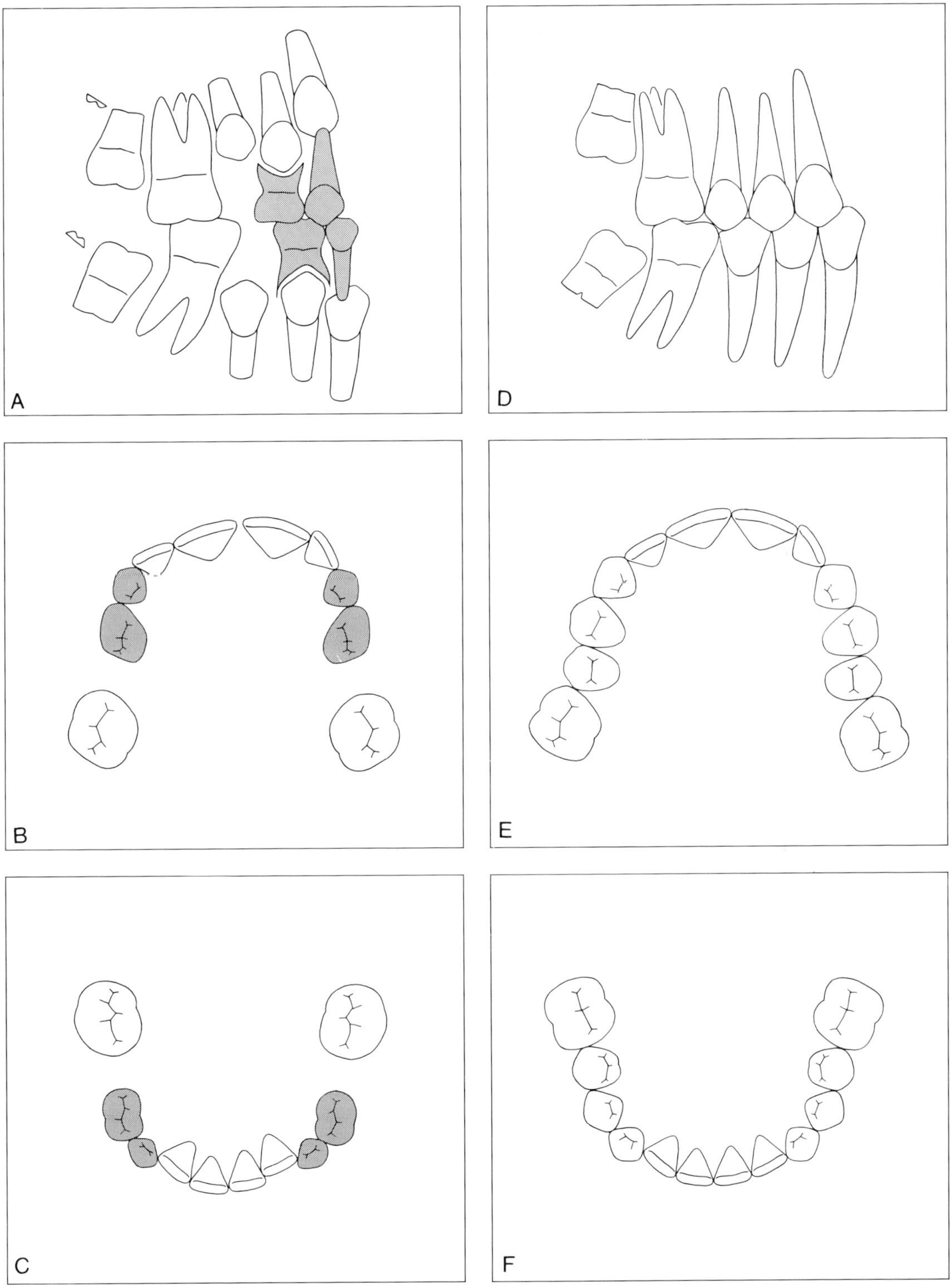

Figure 17-2

17.4 Consequences of anomalous conditions

After outlining the consequences of extracting the first permanent molars in a normal dental situation, consideration will follow of the results of such extractions in anomalous conditions. In addition, a number of side effects will be detailed.

17.4.1 Crowding and spacing

Consequences of early loss of the four first permanent molars are not as bad in situations of crowding as in those of spacing (Fig. 17-2).[81,211] Where crowding is concerned, it is noted that especially in the mandible more space becomes available for rotated or overlapping incisors and canines, as a result of distal drifting of premolars. In the maxilla this is less evident. Extraction of a maxillary permanent molar provides only limited space gain for a permanent canine that is emerging labially.

17.4.2 Abnormal sagittal dental arch relations

Extraction of a mandibular first permanent molar in Class II/1 anomalies involves the danger that the disto-occlusion of the premolars and canines will be increased. The overjet and overbite can become significantly greater and the mandibular incisors can tip lingually. The activity of the lower lip can aggravate this tipping, particularly if the lower lip is or becomes positioned between the maxillary and mandibular incisors.
In Class II/2 anomalies it is unfavourable to extract any permanent teeth in the mandible, and this of course includes first permanent molars. The force of the lower lip, which is transferred to the mandibular incisors via the maxillary incisors, will lead to still greater retroclination of the mandibular incisors.
For Class III anomalies, a situation corresponding to that of Class II exists, though inverted. Extraction of maxillary molars is particularly undesirable. The diminished maxillary dental arch makes it difficult to correct a reversed overbite.

17.4.3 Asymmetrical extraction

When in both jaws the first permanent molars are extracted on one side only, the changes described above will be limited chiefly to that side. The midlines will become displaced toward the extraction side. This deviation is limited in extent and is seldom recognised as an esthetic disorder. Of course the dental arch midlines often cease to correspond because the mandibular incisors migrate more than the maxillary incisors. Pronounced asymmetries and disturbed occlusions develop when on one side a mandibular molar is extracted and a maxillary molar is removed from the other side.

17.4.4 Extracting molars from one arch only

Extracting only two mandibular first molars will result in a smaller mandibular dental arch that will not fit properly against the maxillary arch. The overjet and overbite increase undesirably. The occlusion in the posterior segments becomes disordered. As has been pointed out before, the effects of extracting mandibular first permanent

molars are particularly far-reaching in Class II/1 and Class II/2 anomalies. To arrive at a good result, extraction of maxillary teeth is required to match that of the mandibular first molars, especially in Class II anomalies. Subsequently, complex orthodontic treatment must be undertaken.
Extracting only maxillary first permanent molars generally has less serious consequences than when only mandibular molars are extracted (except in Class III anomalies). This applies both for unilateral and bilateral extractions. Unfortunately it happens that carious lesions of first permanent molars are more frequent and severe in the mandible than in the maxilla.[186] This is even more regrettable since loss of a mandibular first permanent molar almost always needs to be compensated for by extraction in the maxilla. The distinction mentioned here between the caries susceptibility of mandibular and maxillary first permanent molars does not apply to hypoplasia. There is no evidence that more mandibular than maxillary molars are lost because of hypoplasia.

17.5 Indications for and implications of extracting first permanent molars

Definite contraindications prevail against extracting first permanent molars, as has been pointed out in the explanation of the importance of first permanent molars (see 17.2).
Indications to extract one or more first permanent molars for orthodontic reasons alone are seldom, if ever, encountered. If extraction therapy is required, preference for removal goes to premolars or occasionally second permanent molars. Only when first permanent molars are so defective that there can be no hope of keeping them intact despite the best of care, and the premolars are sound, would the molars be sacrificed rather than the premolars. It should be realised that such cases will require orthodontic therapy that is considerably more complex than usual. It will demand the use of full fixed appliances for a long period. This certainly is undesirable in a situation where defective first molars are a symptom of a generally weak dentition with a high caries susceptibility.
The only actual indication for extracting first permanent molars is the impossibility of conserving them for the greater part of the life of the patient. Schwarz[192] stated that when first permanent molars appeared likely to be lost as a result of caries before the age of 30 years, removal at an early age is indicated. This applies even more strongly if the prognosis is worse still. In such circumstances it is better to perform the indicated extraction of first permanent molars at a properly chosen time rather than be forced to extract because of pain or other reason at an inappropriate moment. The resultant spontaneous corrections will then usually lead to a more favourable situation than when the extraction is performed regardless of the development of the dentition and the progress of facial growth.
In conclusion, a purely orthodontic indication is rarely found for extracting first permanent molars. Nonetheless, these teeth are sometimes extracted in the context of orthodontic therapy. Two circumstances justify this approach. The first is when removal of a qualitatively worthless first molar takes the place of extracting, for example, a sound premolar. The second is when orthodontic treatment required for

other reasons can be employed to correct most of the undesirable effects of extracting defective first molars. In these cases extraction would not be contemplated as part of orthodontic treatment if the molars were at all reasonable in quality.

17.5.1 Extractions in normal and abnormal occlusions; compensating extractions

In the indications for extracting first permanent molars a distinction can be drawn between patients with and without an orthodontic abnormality.

In patients with a normally developing dentition, in which a mandibular first permanent molar cannot be conserved over a long term, its removal at an early age should be seriously considered. The extraction should be performed before the emergence of the adjacent second permanent molar. Some time later the maxillary first molar has to be removed also, otherwise a less satisfactory result will be obtained with one tooth too many in the maxilla (unless the third molar does not form). Eventually the maxillary third molar without an antagonist would overerupt and require extraction. In a Class I situation the extraction of both mandibular and maxillary first permanent molars results in a better interdigitation with a less disturbed occlusion than when just the mandibular first molar is removed.[85] As already has been indicated above, when it is not possible to preserve a mandibular first permanent molar on one side, extracting the first molar on the other side is usually neither necessary nor desirable. However, when in Class I patients both mandibular first permanent molars have been removed, both maxillary first molars should also be extracted.

In patients with a deviating occlusion, another maxillary tooth than the first permanent molar might be more suited for compensatory extraction. In situations with crowding in the canine or incisor regions, removal of a first premolar might be more appropriate. Extracting a maxillary first permanent molar does not automatically imply that compensation by extraction in the mandible is required. That particularly applies for Class II anomalies with no crowding in the mandibular arch. In a Class I situation with crowding in the mandible it is often sensible to remove a mandibular premolar to compensate for the loss of a maxillary first permanent molar. Nonetheless, in these cases the existing occlusion and the expected development of the dentition with and without compensating extractions are the most essential criteria.

If one decides to remove first permanent molars, it is absolutely imperative to verify the presence of second premolars. This applies also, but less strictly, to the presence of third molars. Occasionally, extraction of a first permanent molar will be unavoidable despite knowing that the third molar is congenitally absent. As a rule this is unfavourable, especially in cases of marked spacing. Naturally one would not carry out a compensatory extraction of a conservable tooth in a quadrant in which there were agenesis of a tooth.

Holm[86] has composed the following rules of thumb for compensatory extractions:

Compensatory Extraction in the Other Jaw

- When 46 (36) are lost, always also extract 16 (26)
  — if 13 (23) are excluded labially, consider extracting 14 (24) instead of 16 (26).
- When 16 (26) are lost: do not always extract in the mandible.
- Essential stipulation: no agenesis.

The loss of a mandibular first permanent molar can be compensated for by extracting any tooth in the opposing posterior region. The choice depends on the quality and position of the teeth under consideration. The fact that maxillary first permanent molars exhibit notably less caries than mandibular molars often makes it possible, when a mandibular first molar could not be conserved, to use a different tooth from the maxillary first permanent molar when performing the compensatory extraction. This can simplify the use of orthodontic appliances or render them unnecessary. It is also not essential to compensate bilateral extractions of mandibular first permanent molars with removal of the corresponding maxillary teeth. Most essential in the choice of which tooth is going to be extracted for compensatory reasons is the quality of the occlusion that can be realised in that quadrant with the least trouble. To make responsible decisions in this respect a good insight into normal development of the dentition is required, as is a knowledge of the changes that follow extraction of a permanent tooth.

In situations of a normal sagittal jaw relation and crowding in both dental arches, an unavoidable extraction in the mandible may relieve the crowding and improve the overall condition, certainly when compensatory extraction in the maxilla is also undertaken.

Concerning patients who require orthodontic treatment at a later time, the person responsible for such treatment should be consulted regarding possible extractions of permanent teeth before they are executed.

17.5.2 Extractions in Class II/1 anomalies

In Class II/1 anomalies, as explained earlier, the conservation of mandibular molars, and every other mandibular tooth, is of utmost importance when there is no or only limited crowding in the mandibular arch. When extraction of mandibular molars cannot be avoided, initiation of early orthodontic treatment should be considered, at least to prevent a deterioration of the anomaly.

Most suited for that purpose is a facial orthopedic appliance that corrects the disto-occlusion, prevents lingual tipping of the mandibular incisors, and does not encourage caries. By using an activator an attempt can also be made to improve the angulation of the second permanent molars. For this purpose the acrylic resin placed occlusally must be ground in such a way that the distal cusps of the four first permanent molars bite upon it. The mesial cusps must not touch the acrylic resin.

Where compensatory extractions are concerned in the maxilla, the same principles apply as were suggested above for a Class I situation. Indeed, sometimes one is more likely to extract a maxillary first premolar in Class II/1 anomalies to facilitate retrusion of the maxillary incisors.

The orthodontic treatment of Class II/1 anomalies in which first permanent molars have been removed is complex and cannot be done satisfactorily without fixed appliances. Correction of a sagittal discrepancy is more difficult to achieve if the four first molars have been lost. Retrusion of the maxillary incisors is more troublesome when the maxillary first molars are missing. Orthopedic measures appear to work less well. Moreover, there are no good substitutes for the maxillary first permanent molars as attachment points for extraoral traction.

17.5.3 Extractions in Class II/2 anomalies

In Class II/2 anomalies removal of mandibular first permanent molars has particularly adverse effects. Not only will both the dental arches collapse, but the overbite will increase further. This will increase the likelihood of biting on the gingiva palatal to the maxillary incisors and labial to the mandibular incisors. In addition, the profile will change for the worse. The nose and chin become more prominent. The collapse of the mouth will produce an impression of a prematurely old face. Only with complex and lengthy orthodontic therapy can the unfavourable consequences be countered but usually not be completely eliminated. In conclusion, in Class II/2 anomalies with high caries predisposition every possible means of preventing caries should be employed to avoid loss of permanent teeth.

17.5.4 Extractions in Class III anomalies

For Class III anomalies much the same applies as for Class II cases except in an inverted fashion. Extractions in the maxilla are usually undesirable; subsequent orthodontic treatment is difficult and lengthy with a dubious prognosis.

17.6 Decision-making procedures for extracting mandibular and maxillary first permanent molars

For a sensible decision as to whether or not first permanent molar extractions are indicated it is essential to be certain whether or not second premolars are present. To a lesser extent this also applies to third molars. A third molar can be reckoned to be absent when no radiographic evidence of its formation can be noticed by the time the bifurcation of the adjacent second permanent molars is formed. There is no use in taking a radiograph for confirmation before the age of 9 years, especially because extraction of first permanent molars before that age is normally not desirable.
The mandibular first permanent molar should preferably be removed shortly (about 1 year) before emergence of the adjacent second permanent molar.[12,66,193] By that time the bifurcation of the second permanent molar is formed and presence or absence of the third molar can be determined with sufficient certainty. It would also have been obvious for some time whether or not the premolars had formed. The best results are obtained if the extraction of the mandibular first permanent molar is undertaken when the occlusal surface of the second permanent molar is at the level of the first molar's cervical margin. The mandibular second molar can then move not only horizontally but also vertically in the course of its eruption to emergence, which results in less mesial tilting[86] (Fig. 17-3). The maxillary second molar migrates mesially faster than does the mandibular second molar after extraction of the adjacent first molar. The uprighting of the mesial angulation of the opposing second molars is assisted whenever their distal cusps occlude. To promote this action the mandibular first permanent molar should be extracted before the maxillary first molar. Then the mandibular second permanent molar has time to move sufficiently mesially to obtain the desired occlusal contact with the maxillary molar after emergence. Because normally the maxillary first permanent molar applies an uprighting movement to the already somewhat mesially migrated

mandibular second molar through its occlusal contact, it is not so important when the maxillary first permanent molar is extracted. Moreover, extraction of the maxillary first permanent molar later than that of the mandibular first molar is favourable for attaining as good a sagittal interdigitation as possible between the second permanent molars.

On the basis of the above considerations it is best if extraction of the maxillary first permanent molar takes place a year or more after that of the mandibular first molar. Proportionately less horizontal movement and more marked tipping will occur if extraction of the first permanent molars is delayed until the second molars have emerged. This applies more to the mandible than the maxilla. The untoward effects of late extraction of maxillary first permanent molars (rotation and tipping of the second permanent molars) are usually moderate. When a definite crowding exists in the maxillary arch and in particular when room for the permanent canines is lacking, it is wise to delay extraction of the first permanent molars until the second molars have fully emerged.[86] In such cases the extraction of the first premolars is often to be preferred.

Holm[86] has set up some further rules of thumb for extracting the first permanent molars:

Extracting First Permanent Molars

- Extract 46 (36) shortly before emergence of 47 (37)
  — watch position and eruption path of 45 (35).
- Extract 16 (26) much later than 46 (36)
  — extraction can wait until emergence of 17 (27)
  — wait until emergence of 17 (27) if 13 (23) are crowded out.

Mandibular premolars as yet unerupted and having a distal inclination can migrate distally and also tip distally after extraction of adjacent first permanent molars. The prognosis is more favourable when all the premolars are more or less perpendicular to the occlusal plane. In cases of a lot of room within the jaws, the end result generally will show more inadequacies than in cases of crowding to begin with.

The presence of mandibular third molars is no guarantee for closing spaces. However, the prognosis is better when the radiographs show some contact between the mandibular second and third molars.[81] In the mandible, the position of the third molar can change in connection with the mesial migration of the second molar after extraction of a first permanent molar. It can tip mesially and come to lie more horizontally. Instead of emerging normally, the occlusal surface can finish up against the distal surface of the second molar. Unfortunately, extraction of the third molar would then be indicated.

A final judgement of the effect of the early extraction of first permanent molars can only be given after the third molars have emerged and the development of the dentition is complete. Only then will it be seen if the third molars have attained a good place in the dental arch. Moreover, it is only then that it can be evaluated how well the inclination of the second molars, the interdigitation in transverse and sagittal directions, and the closing of spaces has improved. Fortunately, in the 10 years after extraction of first permanent molars improvements still can occur. Occlusal contacts have an important part to play in that respect.

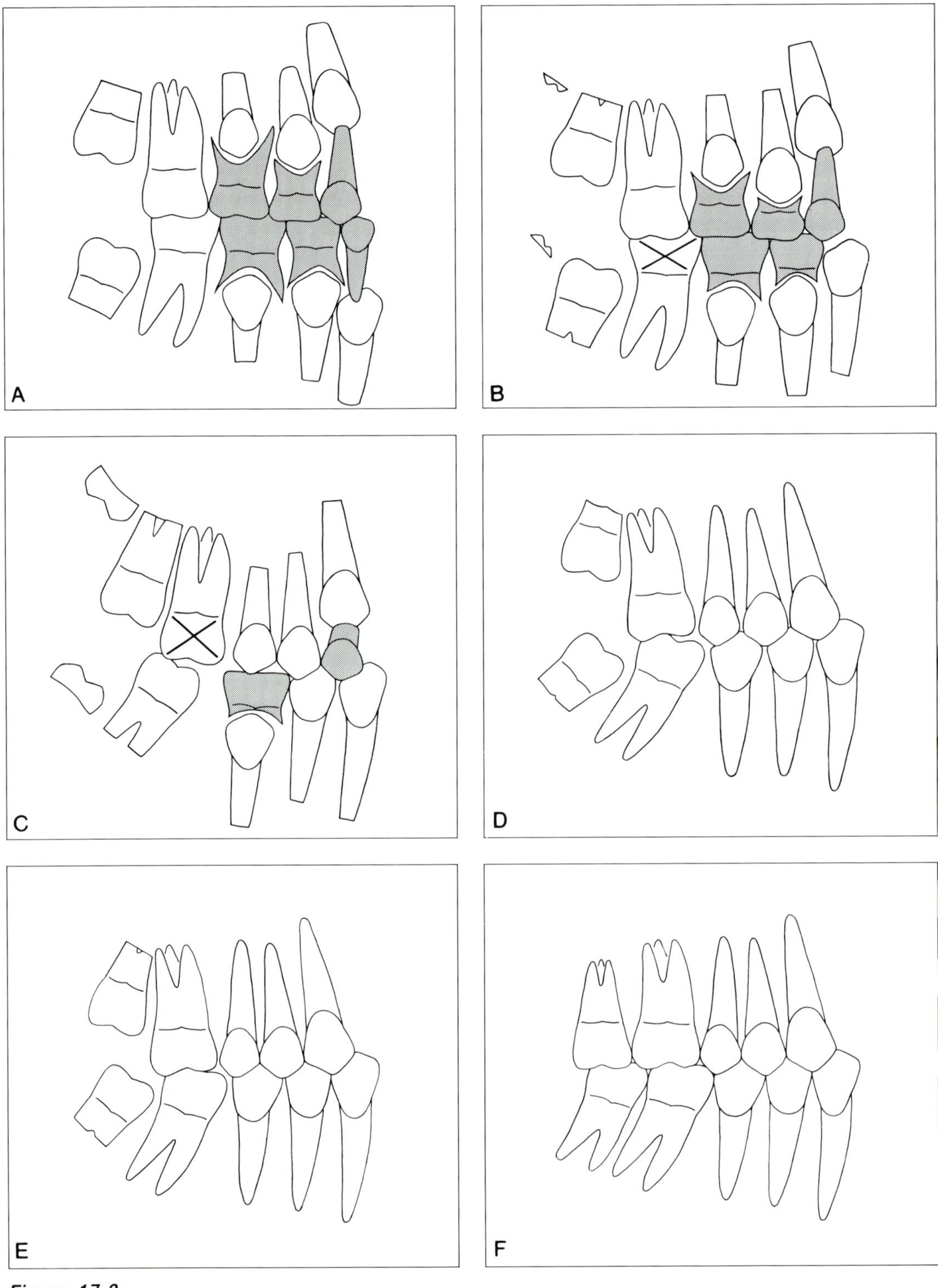

Figure 17-3

Fig. 17-3 The factors involved in the decision-making procedures for early extraction of mandibular and maxillary first permanent molars. In addition, the situations that generally would be seen after 5 (E) and 10 (F) years are displayed.

A At about age 8 years the second premolars are still an appreciable distance away from the occlusal plane. Extraction of first permanent molars at this stage may lead to abnormal eruption of the second premolars. Occasionally, the mandibular second premolar especially has a tendency to tilt distally. Moreover, there is still uncertainty as to whether or not the third molars are forming. The bifurcation of the second permanent molar is as yet not realised.

B Extraction of the mandibular first permanent molar should not be executed before the stage of development depicted here. One has to wait until the second premolars are closer to the occlusal plane, the bifurcation of the second molars has been realised, and the third molars are likely to be forming. The mandibular first permanent molar should be extracted when the second molar is still about one crown height away from the occlusal plane. To wait longer with the extraction is undesirable. Timely extraction allows the second molar to move horizontally and vertically. Both movements will improve the later mesiodistal angulation.

C After emergence of the mandibular second permanent molar, it erupts to contact the maxillary first permanent molar with its distobuccal cusp. As a result it uprights itself somewhat, also when it migrates more mesially. The time of extraction of a maxillary first permanent molar is less critical than that of a mandibular first molar; the maxillary first molar can be removed a year or more after removing the mandibular molar. The maxillary second permanent molar moves mesially far more quickly than the mandibular molar. Moreover, less undesirable mesial tipping occurs as the normal path of eruption is already in that direction. Shortly after emergence it will come into contact with the mandibular second molar.

D After full emergence of the maxillary second molar, occlusal contact between the distal cusps of the second molars comes about. The uprighting effect on the mandibular molar becomes reestablished. The maxillary second molar also is favourably loaded for such a movement. In both jaws spaces are present between the first and second premolars, being larger in the mandible than in the maxilla. To a large extent the third molars have accompanied the second molars in their movement.

E The diastemata in both arches have reduced in size. The mandibular second molar has uprighted farther and has moved mesially. A better occlusion with the maxillary molar has developed. The third molars have migrated farther mesially and approached closer to the occlusal plane than they would have if the permanent molars had not been extracted early. They will also emerge about 1 1/2 years sooner.

F The third molars have taken up good positions and occlude well. The inclination of the maxillary second permanent molar is nearly normal. The mandibular molar is still tilted mesially and will not upright anymore. In the mandible the interdental space between the second premolar and the second molar remains periodontally unfavourable. The occlusion of the second molars is not optimal. This applies also, though to a lesser extent, to the premolars with their rotations that do not correct spontaneously. The spaces in both dental arches have closed. In the maxilla this almost always happens. However, in the mandible spaces will occasionally remain.

17.7 General rules

In a dental practice one is occasionally confronted with the question as to whether or not extraction of first permanent molars would be justified. If the patients involved have only defective first molars in an otherwise good dentition (e.g., only hypoplasia of the crowns of all first permanent molars), the decision is less difficult. If there is no agenesis, the decision to extract will meet few reservations if orthodontic treatment can be instituted to eliminate undesirable consequences. In such patients the rest of the dentition is of sufficiently good quality to be able to tolerate the treatment without harm. The latter does not apply when poor general dental conditions exist. Then it is necessary to carefully weigh the pros and cons of deliberate and timely extraction of first permanent molars. In doing so, the conditions to be expected 15 or 20 years later should have considerable influence. In general it can be said that the dental health of a

GENERAL RULES FOR EXTRACTING DEFECTIVE FIRST PERMANENT MOLARS

Quality of dentition / Orthodontic conditions	Very poor dentition	Poor dention; limited orthodontic treatment possible	Poor first molars but other teeth good
No marked orthodontic anomalies	Early extraction 46 (36), with subsequent extraction 16 (26)	or ← or →	Early extraction (later fixed appliance therapy)
Moderate Class II/1 anomaly	Early extraction 46 (36), with subsequent extraction 16 (26) (watch lower lip) as necessary ↓	or ← or →	Early extraction; activator (later fixed appliance therapy)
Marked Class II/1 Any Class II/2 anomaly	No extractions 46 (36) before facial growth complete	Early extraction 46 (36), then 16 (26); activator or similar appliance	Early extraction; activator: later fixed appliance therapy
Class III anomaly	No extractions 16 (26) before facial growth complete	Early extraction 46 (36), then 16 (26); Delaire appliance	Early extraction; Delaire appliance: later fixed appliance therapy

25-year-old would be better if the first permanent molars had been removed at age 10 or 12 years than if they had been removed about 5 or 10 years later. That holds particularly true in patients with a normal jaw relation, lip position, and soft tissue activity.
However, in dealing with a pronounced Class II/1 or a Class II/2 anomaly, in which orthodontic treatment is not indicated or possible, the situation will be otherwise. Extraction of the mandibular first permanent molars at the age of 10 to 12 years would have such a detrimental effect on the subsequent development of the dentition and the facial growth that a much worse situation would come to pass by age 25 than would have developed if the extractions had been left until completion of facial growth and the development of the dentition. In marked Class II/1 anomalies every attempt to conserve first permanent molars in the mandible should be made regardless of the effort necessary. If they must be lost it should not be before the age of 15 for girls and 18 for boys. If conservation of these teeth until those ages cannot be achieved, an improvement in jaw relationships should be aimed for using facial orthopedic therapy. Class III anomalies require conservation of permanent teeth in the maxilla in a corresponding though inverted way. A similar train of thought is applicable as that concerning Class II/1 anomalies outlined above.
In the table-like survey presented here an attempt has been made to summarise the important aspects that need to be considered regarding early extraction of first permanent molars.
Finally, it should be pointed out that when considering the guidelines given for the time when extraction of first permanent molars should be performed, they should not be used too rigidly. In particular cases it will be impossible to avoid extraction earlier than it should be done, yet it is sensible to go through with it. Extracting earlier than considered desirable does not always turn out to be a disaster. The individual situation affects the outcome. In this regard, as in other decision-making processes, one should make one's decisions only after carefully weighing all the factors involved. It is essential to realise that great individual variation exists in development of the dentition and this makes it impossible to dictate absolute rules.

17.8 Supplementary remarks

Holm[86] has properly declared that every extraction of a first permanent molar is a compromise. It remains a matter of balancing interests that usually are not compatible. One is obliged to choose the lesser of two evils. Each case will be different. General rules such as were given above have to be fitted to the existing situation every time they are used. In each case it is necessary to take note of the occlusion and its changes; the anticipated development of the dentition and growth of the face should be estimated as well as possible and the actual changes accurately monitored.
Despite the fact that in the 10 years after extraction of first permanent molars quite noteworthy improvements can occur, there is practically never a good occlusion without active intervention. Mandibular molars seldom upright themselves adequately. Rotations of maxillary molars and premolars remain and can prevent the

development of a good transverse and sagittal interdigitation. These limitations, above all, are not susceptible to correction by simple orthodontic procedures. The use of fixed appliances is mandatory.

Nevertheless, early extraction of first permanent molars is sometimes indicated, even when no orthodontic treatment will follow. In considering whether or not to follow this procedure, all of the many aspects should be reviewed carefully. An incorrect decision could lead to permanent damage to the dentition and face of the unfortunate patient.

Chapter 18

Problems Concerning Third Molars

18.1 Introduction

Third molars can cause much trouble, especially in the mandible. Often the problem is not revealed until the teeth themselves fail to appear on time. In many cases the dentist can make a diagnosis at a much earlier stage. On the basis of clinical observation and radiographs he or she can determine if intervention is called for.
The subject will be dealt with as follows: development and eruption of third molars, frequency of agenesis and impaction, morphology and growth of the jaws, third molars and incisor crowding, prediction of the chance of normal emergence, and age at removal.

18.2 Development and eruption of third molars

The bony crypts of third molars are present at an average age of 8 years, and root formation begins about age 14. However, significant variation exists in this respect, and the same applies to the speed at which the crown and roots form.
Before age 7 the third molars cannot be detected radiologically. Third molars can be considered absent if there is no image on a radiograph taken after age 14.[44]
The late development of third molars is associated with the slow and gradual expansion of the region of the jaws in which they must emerge. Third molars are laid down in the mandible cranial to the level of the occlusal plane; in the maxilla they are close to the occlusal plane (Fig. 18-1).[41]
Mandibular third molars are laid down with a mesial angulation and a lingual inclination. They erupt from this position, accompanied by an uprighting movement. This change in orientation is essential for proper emergence (Fig. 18-2). They become more upright after puberty than before.[80] Between 14 and 16 years normally erupting mandibular third molars move toward a position from which they can emerge normally.[171,174] Significant changes in inclination over a relatively short period can also occur between the ages of 18 and 20 years.[188]
Maxillary third molars are laid down facing distally and buccally. Their orientation also changes slowly and evenly. After occlusal contact is established the mandibular molars provide guidance by the cone-funnel mechanism (Fig. 18-3).

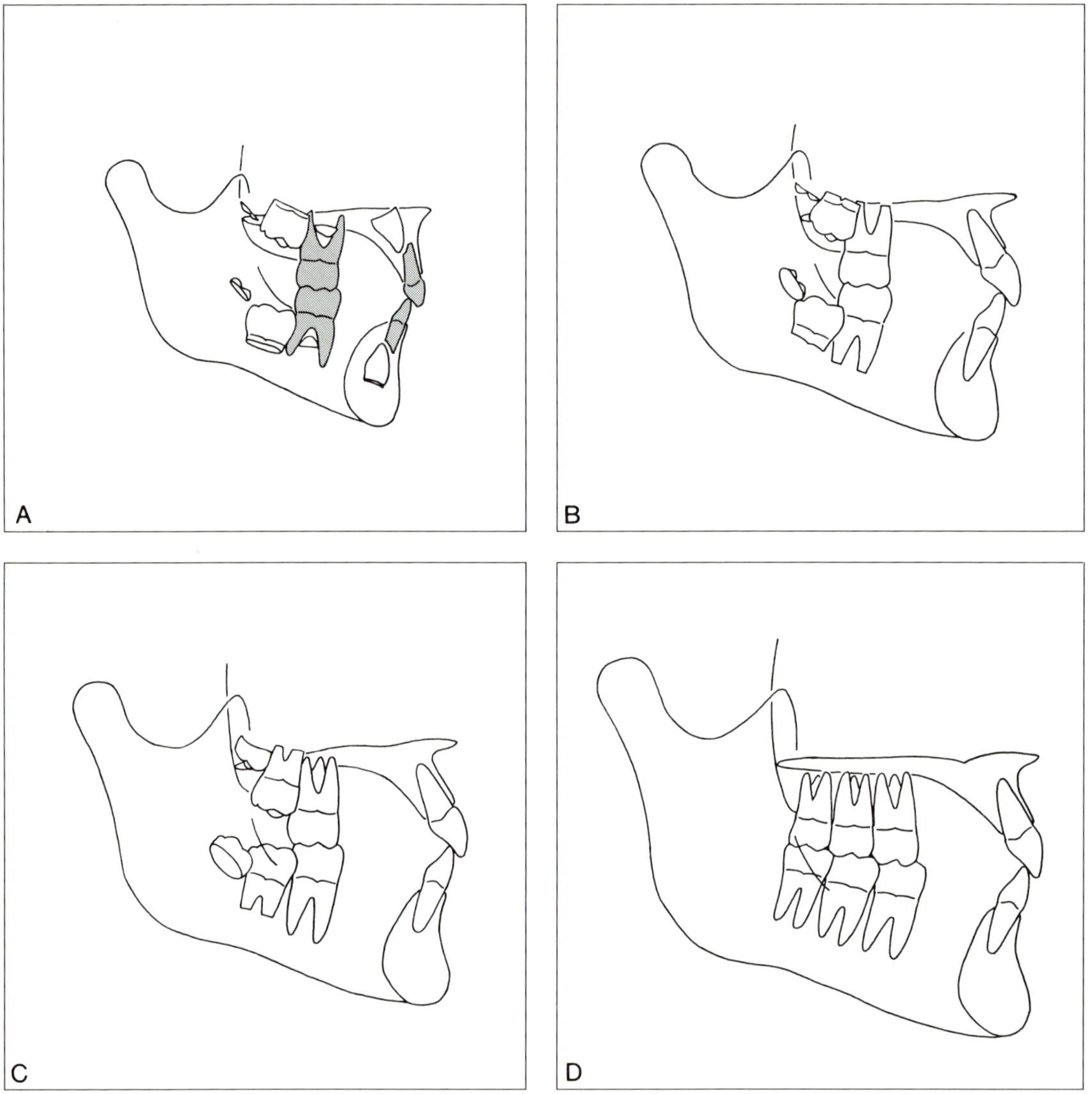

Fig. 18-1 Positions of the permanent molars at different ages. (From Van der Linden.[224])

A *At age 4 years, the germ of the mandibular second permanent molar is located in the ramus and lies more cranially than the occlusal surface of the crown of the mandibular first permanent molar. In the maxilla, the occlusal surface of the germ of the second permanent molar lies only slightly more cranially than that of the first permanent molar. Before calcification commences, the germ of the maxillary second permanent molar is located even more caudally than the occlusal surface of the first molar.[41]*

B *At age 9 years, the mandibular third molar is located in the ramus; its occlusal surface is at about the level of the occlusal plane.[100] The maxillary third molar is situated with the occlusal surface at about the level of the neck of the second permanent molar.*

C *At age 12 years, the crown of the mandibular third molar has not followed the vertical displacement of the other teeth and has come to lie caudally to the occlusal plane, and*

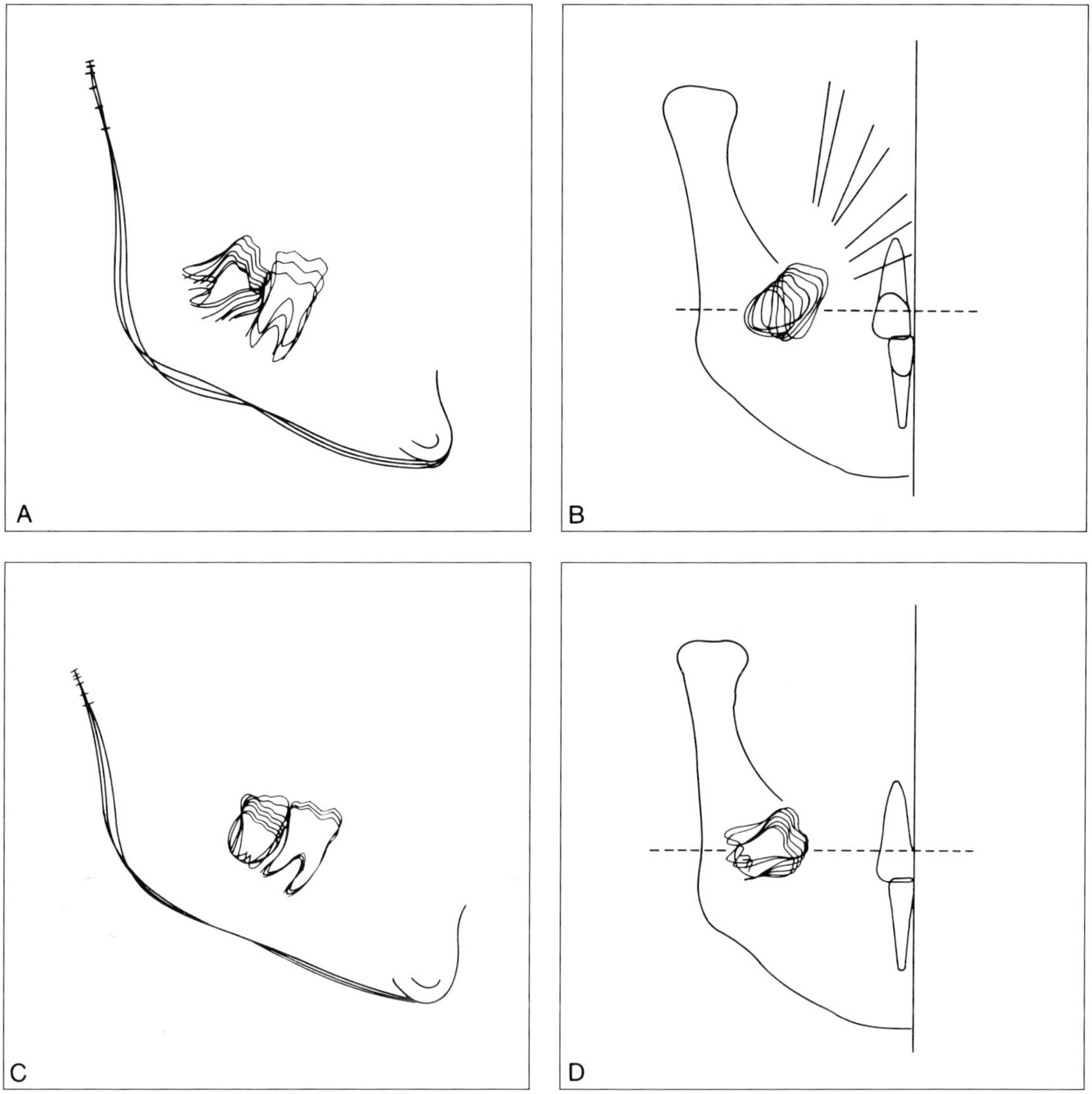

Fig. 18-2 Examples of changes in position and orientation of mandibular third molars, illustrated with superimposed tracings from lateral and frontal cephalometric radiographs. (Figures in mirror image from Svendsen et al.[206])

A, B Development from 12 to 18 years in a girl. The third molar has uprighted, both sagittally and transversely (lines in B indicate axial changes).

C, D Development from 13 to 19 years in a boy. The angulation and orientation of the third molar have changed little; the tooth is impacted.

particularly to the mandibular second molar, which has partly erupted. The maxillary third molar is still placed high.

D At the age of 21 years the mandibular and maxillary third molars are harmoniously added to the dental arches.

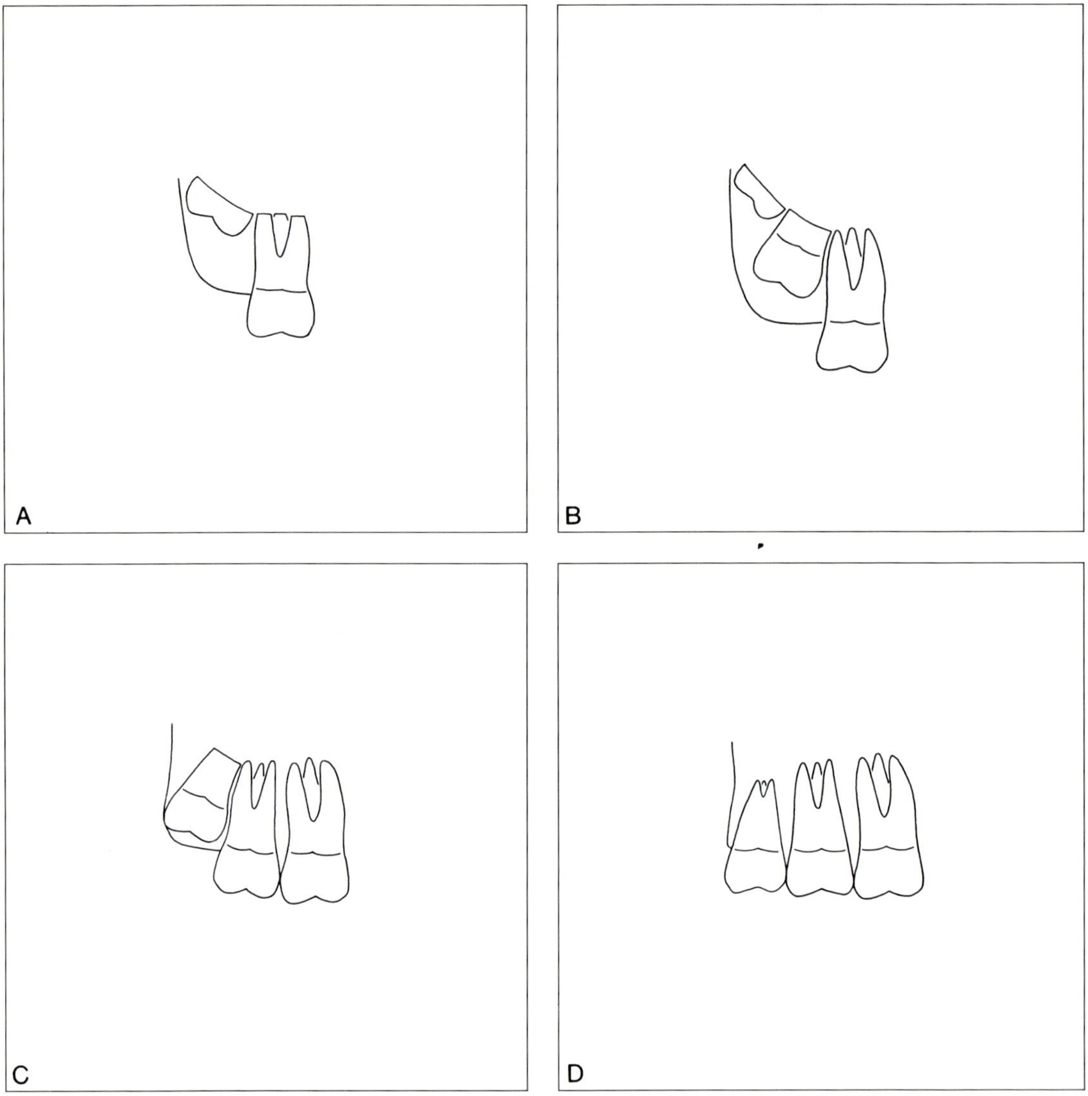

Fig. 18-3 Changes in inclination and angulation of maxillary molars.

A to D *Maxillary second and third molars are laid down with distal angulation, and as sufficient room becomes available in the jaw they gradually upright themselves from that position until, long after reaching occlusion, they assume a mesial angulation.*

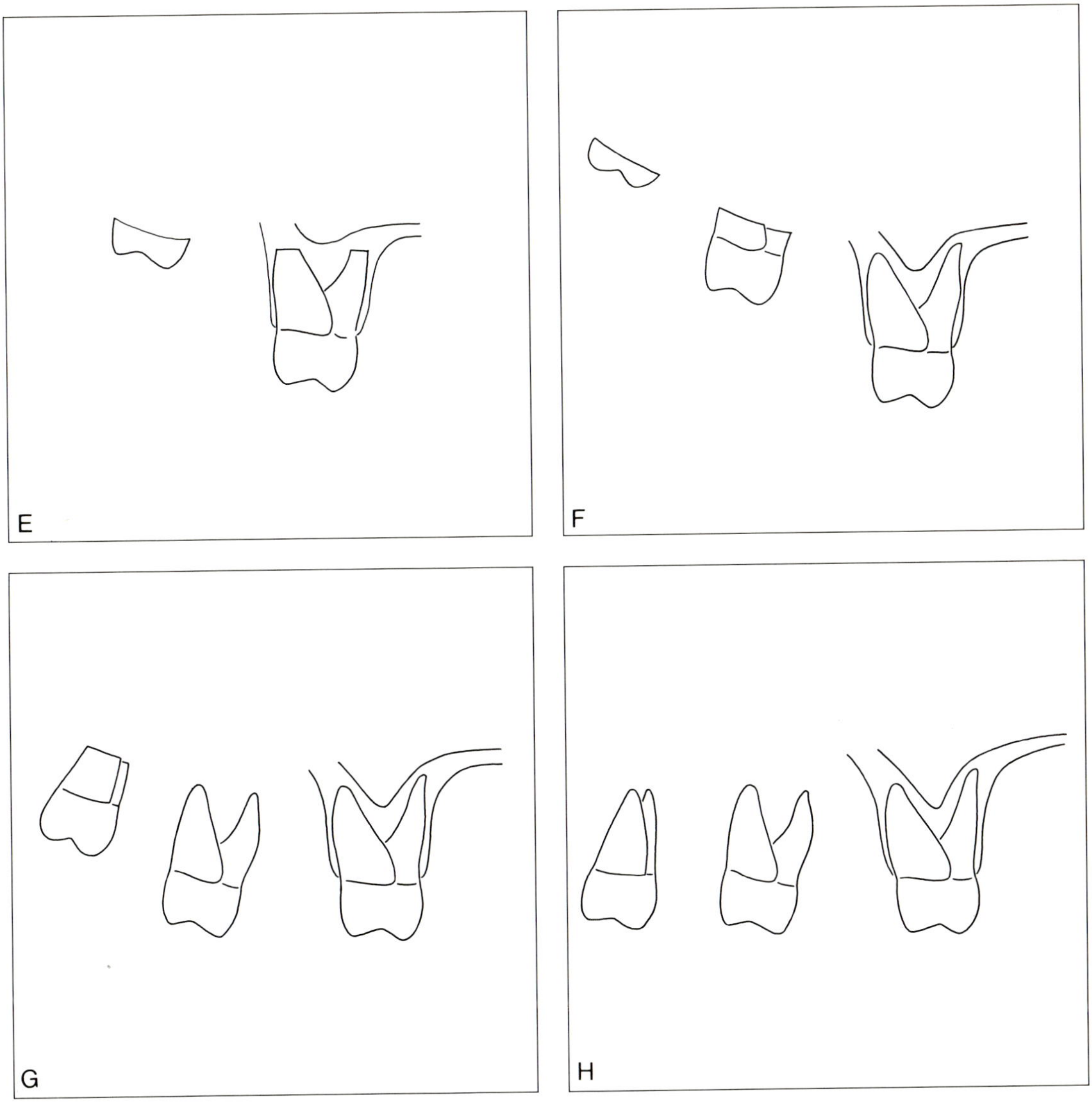

E to H *Maxillary molars are laid down with a buccal inclination and gradually become upright. They keep the buccal angulation after emergence. The apical area is built out buccally only to a limited extent.*

molars erupt normally.[176] But impacted third molars are one manifestation of crowding and cannot be considered a cause of it.

18.6 Predicting the chance of normal emergence

Though some connection exists between the space that is available or becomes available for the mandibular third molars and the distance between the ventral border of the ramus and the distal surface of the mandibular second molar,[19,174] it is not possible to forecast the chance of proper emergence on that basis alone. As already stated, some particular morphological features, although significant, cannot be assessed from either panoramic or cephalometric radiographs. Hence, from that source no satisfactorily reliable indication can be obtained of the space that is available or becomes available for emergence of the mandibular third molars.[96] That applies also to cephalometric analyses even where very large data bases are available.[179,190]

The size of the posterior section of the apical area in the mandible, the buccolingual dimension of the relevant region, the breadth of the buccinator groove, and the size of the plateau are best judged clinically by palpation.

As far as the space for the maxillary molars is concerned, a lateral skull radiograph provides only limited information. The dorsal border of the tuberosity is not directly anterior to the pterygoid process, nor does it lie in contact with it. The maxilla grows dorsally in the sphenomaxillary space and the tuberosities are located lateral and posterior to the pterygoid processes.[36]

Clinically, the size of the posterior section of the apical area of the maxilla can be well determined by visual inspection and palpation. It is also possible to give a reliable estimate of the situation by using a good study model that is well extended and includes the entire tuberosity.

The way in which the molars are positioned in the jaws can only be ascertained with satisfactory reliability by using radiographs, of course. However, without clinical inspection and palpation, supplemented by use of study models, it is difficult to obtain a three-dimensional picture of the situation.

The combination of the different observations makes it possible to predict what space is or will be available for the third molars. The criteria to be used are to be found in the section dealing with crowding in the molar region (see 16.7). Appraisal of the buccolingual dimensions of the pertinent region of the mandible should be included in those criteria.

18.7 Age at removal

The third molars are usually removed when development of the dentition and facial growth are complete.

Complaints about wisdom teeth are limited mostly to the mandible and usually concern incomplete emergence. Removal often requires surgery, and inconvenience and aftereffects are associated with that procedure. Moreover, there is the danger of

damaging the periodontal membrane of the second molar distally, resulting in a distal pocket.
In the maxilla adequate space usually is available for the third molars, even when the mandibular counterparts are unable to emerge. If they are impacted however, they seldom cause complaints. Even where there is insufficient space they will emerge, probably buccally. They can subsequently be extracted easily if that is indicated. Moreover, the procedure for surgical removal of maxillary third molars is relatively simple and implies less inconvenience than that in the mandible.
There are advantages to removing mandibular third molars at an earlier stage, when the roots are as yet incomplete and it can be determined that they cannot emerge properly. Usually that is the case at age 16; the uprighting must by then have been completed. Extraction at that stage, when the roots are one half to one third formed, can be carried out with less inconvenience, complications, and sequelae. There will also be less aftereffect on the second molar than when the roots are fully formed.[170]
Moreover, the first permanent molars appear to drift less mesially.[194] Further, it is also suggested that less mandibular incisor crowding develops than would be the case with later removal, although it is not possible to predict whether or not there will indeed be a reduction in that crowding.[120]
When at about age 8 or 9 years it is evident that mandibular third molars will not have sufficient room to take up a good position in the dental arch, "germectomy" can be considered if the calcification of the crown has not yet begun, or if the crown is still in the initial stage. The germ is located at the level of the occlusal plane on the lingual aspect of the junction of the body and ramus and is not yet covered by bone. After administering local anaesthetic and making a small incision, the germ can be sucked out or curetted. The dental sac must be totally removed. This procedure is relatively simple, gives little trouble to the patient, and avoids damage to second molars.[180]
Germectomy at an early age is justified in patients where there is sufficient certainty that the teeth involved will never be functional. By its means a more extensive intervention later will be avoided and a more favourable situation for the dentition will be established. Naturally one weighs against this the possible psychic trauma associated with surgery at a young age.

18.8 Supplementary remarks

Impacted third molars can lead to periodontal destruction at the distal aspect of the second molar in the mandible and to a lesser extent in the maxilla. Pocket formation and root resorption may occur. Further, follicular cysts can develop.
Third molars that have emerged into the mouth are often difficult to clean, resulting in caries, periodontal pockets, and pericoronitis. If that occurs, it often is unwise to indulge in extensive therapy, but extraction is indicated. This is especially so when there is no antagonist.
In itself lack of occlusal contact is not a reason to extract. Only when overeruption leads to supraocclusion and associated disturbances of the articulation is there a clear indication for it. A third molar can remain intact for years without any problems. Conservation can be warranted when at a later age some form of prosthesis is required and the third molar can be utilised.

Chapter 19

Adult Orthodontic Treatment

19.1 Introduction

Adults are seeking orthodontic treatment more often. The proportion of older patients being treated in a specialist practice has become greater and will continue to increase. There are special aspects of treatment of this kind that justify devoting a separate chapter to its discussion.

Adults for whom orthodontic treatment is contemplated can be divided into four types according to periodontal conditions: *(1)* patients with healthy intact periodontal tissues, *(2)* patients with inflammation and intact periodontal tissues, *(3)* patients with healthy tissues that have receded, and *(4)* patients with inflamed periodontal tissues that have receded.

In this chapter the subjects dealt with are general aspects such as psychological factors, oral hygiene and cooperation, the structure of bone and collagen, and magnitude and direction of forces. Specific aspects concerning the periodontal tissues such as preparatory treatment, periodontal therapy, appliances and tooth movements that conserve the periodontal structures, and regeneration potential are dealt with separately.

Therapy is divided into late treatment of orthodontic anomalies, treatment as it applies to restorative dentisty, treatment after spontaneous tooth migrations, and treatment where there are disturbances of function. Then follows discussion of surgical-orthodontic treatment and retention.

19.2 General aspects of adult orthodontics

Psychological factors play an important part in treatment of adults. Oral hygiene and cooperation are often better than when treating children. Because the structure of bone and collagen changes with age, adults react to orthodontic treatment somewhat differently from children. The size and direction of appliance forces need to be adapted to adult conditions.

19.2.1 Psychological factors

With the growth of welfare services and the increased availability of orthodontic care, the demand for treating adults has also grown. In past decades a visibly abnormal

arrangement of the teeth was not much remarked upon. Currently the emphasis is on retaining one's natural teeth; the transition to a partial or full denture as the response to unesthetic teeth is no longer considered an appropriate mode of treatment.
Children generally accept wearing an orthodontic appliance. The increase in dental awareness has reduced the disinclination of adults to wear appliances. People are more and more willing to accept the inconvenience with the prospect of a significant improvement in their appearance and a better chance of keeping their own teeth.
Adult orthodontic treatment can give great satisfaction to the treating dentist, and the patients are usually very interested and thankful for the improvements.[56] In general, wearing of orthodontic appliances by those who have requested them creates no problem, certainly when the appliance is hardly visible. Even though the sensitivity of the oral structures is greater in adults than in children, this is seldom a source of difficulty.

19.2.2 Oral hygiene and cooperation

Adults are usually more aware than children of the importance of good oral hygiene. This applies particularly to those who seek orthodontic treatment. At the same time, the consequences for an adult of neglected oral hygiene are more serious than for children. Particularly when periodontal pockets are present and plaque is allowed to accumulate, pathologic processes can develop. With adults it is irresponsible to undertake orthodontic treatment if oral hygiene is not optimal. Moreover, under such circumstances the cooperation in other respects (e.g., good wearing of, manipulation of, and respect for appliances) often is insufficient.

19.2.3 Structure of bone and collagen

The most important difference between orthodontic treatment of adults and children is that with adults there is no prospect of using the possibility to change the relationships of individual facial bones, such as can be done in a growing child with facial orthopedic techniques. Purely orthodontic tooth movement is all that is possible, and there are also some limits compared with what is possible with children.
The bone of adults and especially of older people is different in structure and composition and reacts differently from that of children. The activity of osteoblasts and osteoclasts is reduced. The cortical bone is denser and after middle age it becomes thinner in cross section.[67] The quantity of bone formed no longer matches that broken down. The total amount of bone diminishes as a result.
In trabecular bone the number and thickness of the trabeculae reduce. The cortical bone not only becomes thinner but fenestration in the cortical plates appears.[136] Further, the turnover rate of collagen becomes smaller with age also. In addition, the space for the periodontal membrane becomes narrower.
The above changes that occur with age result in orthodontic treatment of adults that is slower than that of children. Specifically, it takes longer before the first tooth movements can be observed.
Moreover, it is essential with older patients to avoid major movements in a labial (buccal) or lingual direction. Otherwise, undesirable bone loss will occur. This is related to the reduced cell activity and denser structure of the cortical plate.[37] In

general one should aim to confine adult tooth movements to within the cortical plates, and to prevent root resorption as much as possible.[208]

19.2.4 Magnitude and direction of forces

Even more than with children it is important with adults that orthodontic forces be small and long-acting. The reduced cell activity, the thinner periodontal membrane, and the usually reduced area of attachment between root and alveolar bone demand very small forces.[37,56,129,209,237] Hyalinisation and necrosis must be avoided as much as possible.[167] The appliances used in adult orthodontics should be activated less often and less strongly than for children.
In applying forces, account should be taken of the intra-alveolar root length. The smaller the attached part of the root, the more the centre of resistance will move apically.[135]

19.3 Periodontal aspects

In treating adults it is important to secure and maintain as good a condition of the periodontal tissues as is possible. The appliances that will be used and the tooth movements that will be performed should be directed to this end. Furthermore, in some circumstances periodontal defects may be ameliorated by orthodontic treatment.

19.3.1 Preparatory treatment

Orthodontic treatment of periodontally vulnerable patients should only take place after optimal oral hygiene has been achieved, supragingival and subgingival plaque and calculus have been removed, any necessary root planing performed, and the accessible surfaces polished (initial therapy). There should be no sign of inflammation. The papillary bleeding test should be negative.

19.3.2 Periodontal therapy during and after orthodontic treatment

If there has been any pathologic process involving the periodontal tissues, it is necessary after the initial therapy to delay use of orthodontic appliances until an acceptable situation has been achieved. If the papillary bleeding test is still positive the initial therapy should be repeated and a flap operation contemplated.[40] However, it is more and more the rule to employ scaling, planing, and polishing rather than surgical intervention.
An inflamed periodontal pocket bleeds on probing. The reliability of this method of recognising inflammatory phenomena is related to the pocket depth. With 4 mm-deep pockets, blood from the pocket is easily visible. Blood from deeper pockets usually does not reach the gingival margin, hence lack of visible bleeding does not mean absence of inflammation in deep pockets. When a pocket is deeper than 4 mm a filter

paper point can be inserted and checked after 30 seconds for the presence of blood.[169] Because the use of orthodontic appliances in an inflamed area increases the danger of attachment loss, it is necessary to be extremely cautious when deep pockets are present. Pockets 6 to 8 mm deep can remain as they are if no further unfavourable influences appear, as long as the area is well cared for by the patient and professionally cleaned every 3 months.[51] Under these conditions it is reasonable to begin orthodontic treatment.

If plaque accumulation is avoided and care is taken not to move a tooth bearing plaque or calculus, then there will be no periodontal sequelae to orthodontic treatment. However, the risk of developing undesirable periodontal changes is increased. Pockets that have been trouble-free for some time can flare up. To prevent such occurrences as much as possible, monthly professional prophylaxes can be desirable.

Especially with deep pockets it is always possible during orthodontic treatment for unexpected inflammatory phenomena to occur (blood or pus from the pocket). If this does occur immediate action is called for. According to the circumstances it must be decided whether the orthodontic appliance should be kept in place or wholly or partly removed. In patients with unusually susceptible periodontal tissues it is advisable, in addition to monthly professional prophylaxes, to irrigate the site every 2 days with chlorhexidine. In doing this a syringe should be used to irrigate only the places in most danger.

On concluding the orthodontic treatment an acceptable periodontal situation must be maintained. This will be achieved if the patient keeps up a high standard of oral hygiene and has regular (3-month) professional prophylaxes. A recall system for this purpose is recommended.

19.3.3 Appliances that conserve periodontal structures

Plaque is the predominant factor in the development of periodontal disease. Its accumulation should be avoided by every means. As is well known, overhanging restoration margins are undesirable. Crown preparations should be finished some distance away from the gingival borders where possible.

Orthodontic bands seldom fit closely cervically, and even when they do there is still the obtrusive band thickness at the margin. Altogether there is an increased chance of plaque accumulation. Attachments bonded directly to the enamel have the advantage of only encroaching on a part of the buccal surface. Moreover, they can usually be placed some distance away from the gingival margin. Bonded brackets and tubes may therefore cause less loss of periodontal tissue and bone than bands.[1,244] In that respect, the use of small bonding bases and care taken to not leave excess composite resin on the tooth during the bonding process are important. Arches that are in structure and shape easy to keep clean will help the oral hygiene. In addition there are some toothbrushes that are well designed to cope with the difficulties of cleaning fixed appliances.

Despite the fact that there are few quantitative data available concerning the undesirable consequences of removable acrylic resin appliances, this is not an aspect that can be ignored. Almost all removable appliances cause irritation of the mucosa from mechanical factors, plaque accumulation, or both. When the proper measures have been taken regarding the plate and oral hygiene, a satisfactory result can be

obtained in retracting maxillary incisors and closing spaces without giving rise to demonstrable periodontal damage.[46] Such an appliance can administer physiologically acceptable forces (possibly using elastic bands) with support from the palatal tissues countering anchorage loss.
In general, for reasons to do with periodontal health, the use of well-fitted bonded fixed appliances is preferred to removable appliances. Treatment with fixed appliances takes less time than if removable appliances are used, and more tooth movements are possible. A short treatment time is certainly, for periodontal reasons, more important in adults than children.

19.3.4 Tooth movements that conserve periodontal structures

From experiments on Beagle dogs the conclusion has been drawn that with tipping movements of the teeth, supragingival plaque is displaced subgingivally and infrabony pockets are caused. This did not appear to happen when plaque-free teeth were tipped.[53] Parallel movement did not give rise to any gingival inflammation in teeth of which the periodontal support was reduced as long as they were initially free of inflammation.[52] Further, it appeared that the most important factor in the development, exacerbation, and relapse of periodontal disease was the presence of plaque in pockets.[50] When there was bodily movement in the presence of plaque, gingivitis did not change to a destructive and progressive periodontitis, such as that seen in tipping movements.[52]
The aforementioned findings have led to the conclusion that in orthodontic treatment of adults plaque must be avoided to the utmost and tipping movements prevented as much as possible also.[210] If teeth have to be intruded it is essential they be plaque-free.

19.3.5 Regeneration of periodontal tissues in orthodontic treatment

By uprighting teeth that had tilted but have a clean and flat root surface, a periodontal defect can correct itself. Mucogingival tissue from the sulcus fills the defect toward the cervical aspect as long as no inflammation is present. It takes some 6 months before osteoid converts to bone and the improvement is visible on a radiograph.[40,115,164,216] Regeneration of periodontal tissue can take place when a mesially tipped mandibular second permanent molar is uprighted (Fig. 19-1) and severely protruding mandibular incisors are retracted. Note that the prognosis for this is more favourable when bonded attachments are used rather than orthodontic bands. Increased height of the cervical bone margin by 1 to 2 mm has been described.[40,164]
The temporary splinting of teeth after orthodontic treatment can encourage the conversion of osteoid to bone, as long as the oral environment is kept spotlessly clean.

19.4 Late treatment of orthodontic anomalies

It happens more often that adults who would have been better treated as children seek orthodontic treatment when older. It is by no means uncommon for parent and

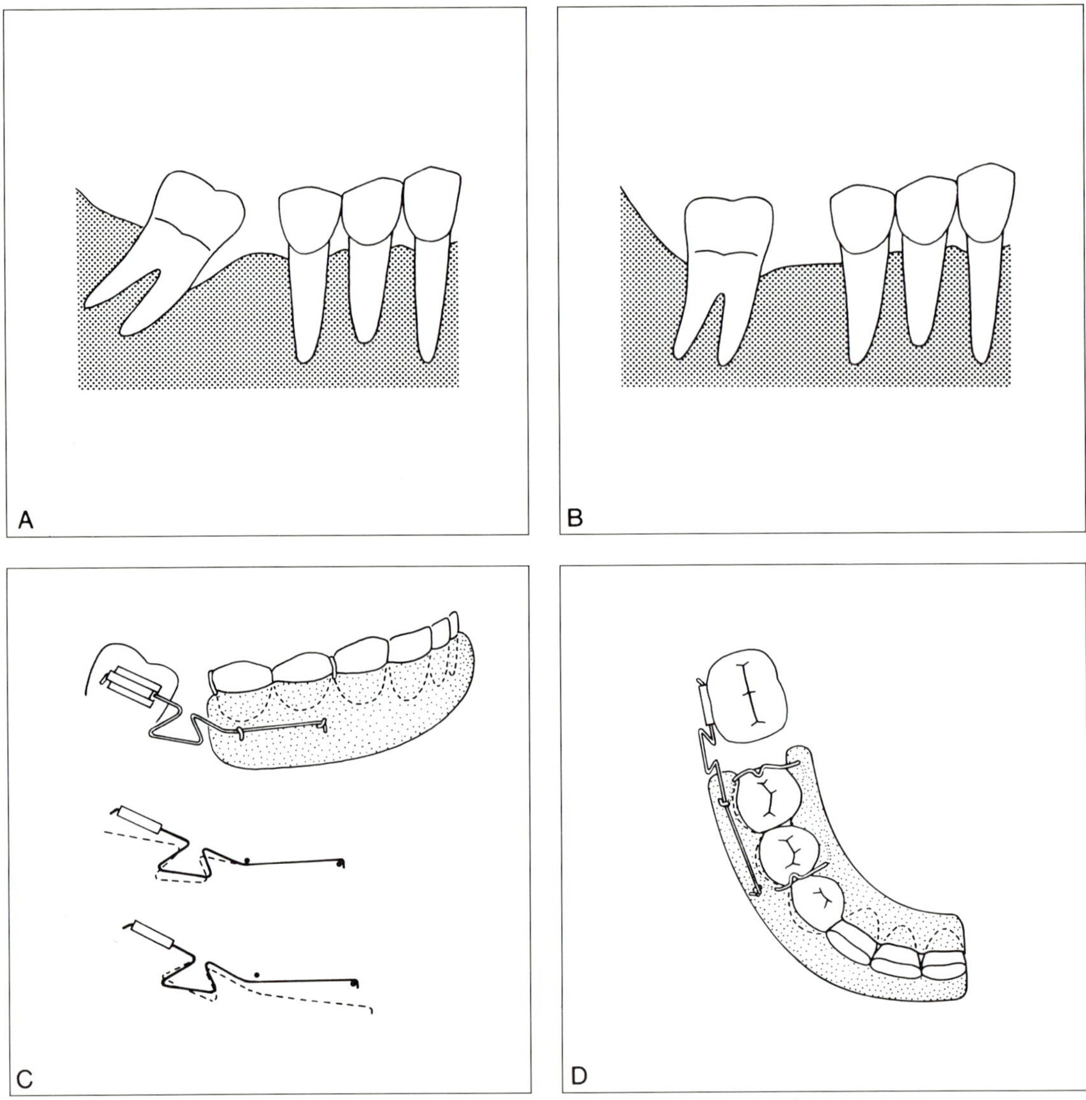

Fig. 19-1 Uprighting a mandibular second permanent molar that has drifted mesially and has tilted after extraction of the first permanent molar.

A *The second permanent molar has a periodontal pocket mesially, is in poor occlusion, and is unsatisfactory for use as an abutment for a bridge to replace the first molar.*

B *After uprighting the second permanent molar, regeneration of the bone can occur if the root surface is flat and clean and no inflammation is present.*

C *To upright the second permanent molar without driving it distally and extruding it demands a technique giving a combination of a force and a couple. With the approach illustrated here and in D (according to E.H.M. Dijkman) the molar can be uprighted and moved mesially as required. Extrusion of the molar is prevented by an intruding force generated by contact between the extension and the underside of the distal hook. The mesiolingual rotation and buccal translation need to be absorbed or corrected later. The wire segment fixed in the second molar tube (using a triangular loop for extra flexibility and ease of activation) is engaged under the distal hook and over the mesial one of the removable acrylic resin appliance. The dotted lines adjoining the sketches of the wire segment indicate the unactivated shape of the wire.*

D *The plate is in place with occlusal rests on the premolars. These rests need to be carefully fitted so that they do not cause occlusal interference. The sagittal position of the molar can be influenced by an elastic band placed between the distal hook on the plate and the distal end of the wire that protrudes from the molar tube.*[111]

child to receive orthodontic treatment simultaneously or at least shortly after one another.

As already has been pointed out, the possibilities for adults are more limited than for children, particularly because there is no scope for facial orthopedic changes in adults. Hence, in adults with pronounced deviations, extractions will be required more often than in similar instances in children.

It will also be more likely that combined surgical-orthodontic therapy will be considered appropriate (see 19.8).

19.5 Orthodontic aid in restorative dental treatment

This subject deals principally with uprighting and movement of teeth with the aim to improve the situation for provision of a prosthesis, and the vertical movement of teeth to facilitate better restoration.

19.5.1 Uprighting and relocation of teeth

The need to upright a tooth in most cases will concern a mandibular second permanent molar that has tipped mesially after the extraction of the adjacent first molar. When an absent tooth is to be replaced with a bridge, the required alignment of the abutment teeth is not determined just by the occlusion and articulation but also by the need to insert the casting.[38,110]

Uprighting a mandibular second molar involves a problem in avoiding extrusion, certainly when there is a wish to avoid distal movement.[111] Extrusion leads to occlusal disturbances, excessive mobility, and possible increase in lower face height, with a more distal occlusion of the teeth. A favourable consequence of uprighting of molars —the regeneration of a periodontal defect—has already been pointed out (Fig. 19-1, page 342).

Another movement sometimes desired is the uprighting and translation of the canines and central incisors in the maxilla in patients with agenesis of the lateral incisors. It can involve establishing a suitable space for a prosthesis either between the canine and central incisor or perhaps between the canine and first premolar (see 10.6).

Further, in a mandibular arch that is reduced in length, it can be desirable to move a mandibular second premolar distally and then provide a bridge between the two premolars to establish a better contact with the maxillary arch and enhance its stability.
A last example is that the need for a bridge to replace a lost mandibular first permanent molar can be eliminated if the second molar (without an antagonist) is moved mesially.

19.5.2 Forced eruption

Forced eruption covers the extrusion of teeth with the aid of orthodontic appliances, or by grinding the tooth out of occlusion (Fig. 19-2).
Subsequent to such treatment, a root that had lost much substance because of caries or trauma can still be used for restoration.[88] In such a case the orthodontic force can be applied to a pin fitted in the root canal, for example.
In certain cases an infrabony pocket can be eliminated by forced eruption. When a tooth is extruded actively the encircling bone builds up toward the occlusal surface and the bone defect decreases. The same result can usually be obtained with teeth that are in occlusion by grinding them out of occlusion in phases. If the bony defect is confined to one root surface, sometimes levelling the bone height around the other sides of the tooth by surgery is indicated.
A coincidental advantage gained by extruding teeth and reducing their clinical crowns is that the ratio between the clinical crown and root lengths becomes more favourable.[87]
With the aid of a removable plate with a bite plane it is possible to obtain forced eruption of the posterior teeth.[2] However, this carries with it the risk of increasing the lower face height, as mentioned above, with changes in the sagittal occlusion. If the plate covers the occlusal surfaces of the teeth that should not erupt, the remaining ones may extrude.
With the use of fixed appliances the height of the attachments can be adapted to the level of the bone. In the course of the treatment the attachments will be brought to a uniform level and as a result the topography of the bone will improve.[216] The associated vertical movements of the crowns will then need to be compensated for by occlusal adjustment by grinding or restorations.
In conclusion, it will be noted that when forced eruption is involved, the height of the attached gingiva increases because the mucogingival junction does not change its level.

19.6 Orthodontic treatment after spontaneous tooth migrations

Orthodontic problems with adults can be divided into two categories[134]: *(1)* those present from childhood on, which can be attributed to faulty development of the dentition and abnormal facial growth, and *(2)* those abnormalities that occur in adulthood or worsen as the result of loss of teeth, abnormal functional activity, or periodontal disease. Pathologic tooth movement related to age can involve single teeth or several teeth. Diastemata can develop, especially between the maxillary incisors. These often are associated with eversion and supraposition of the incisors.

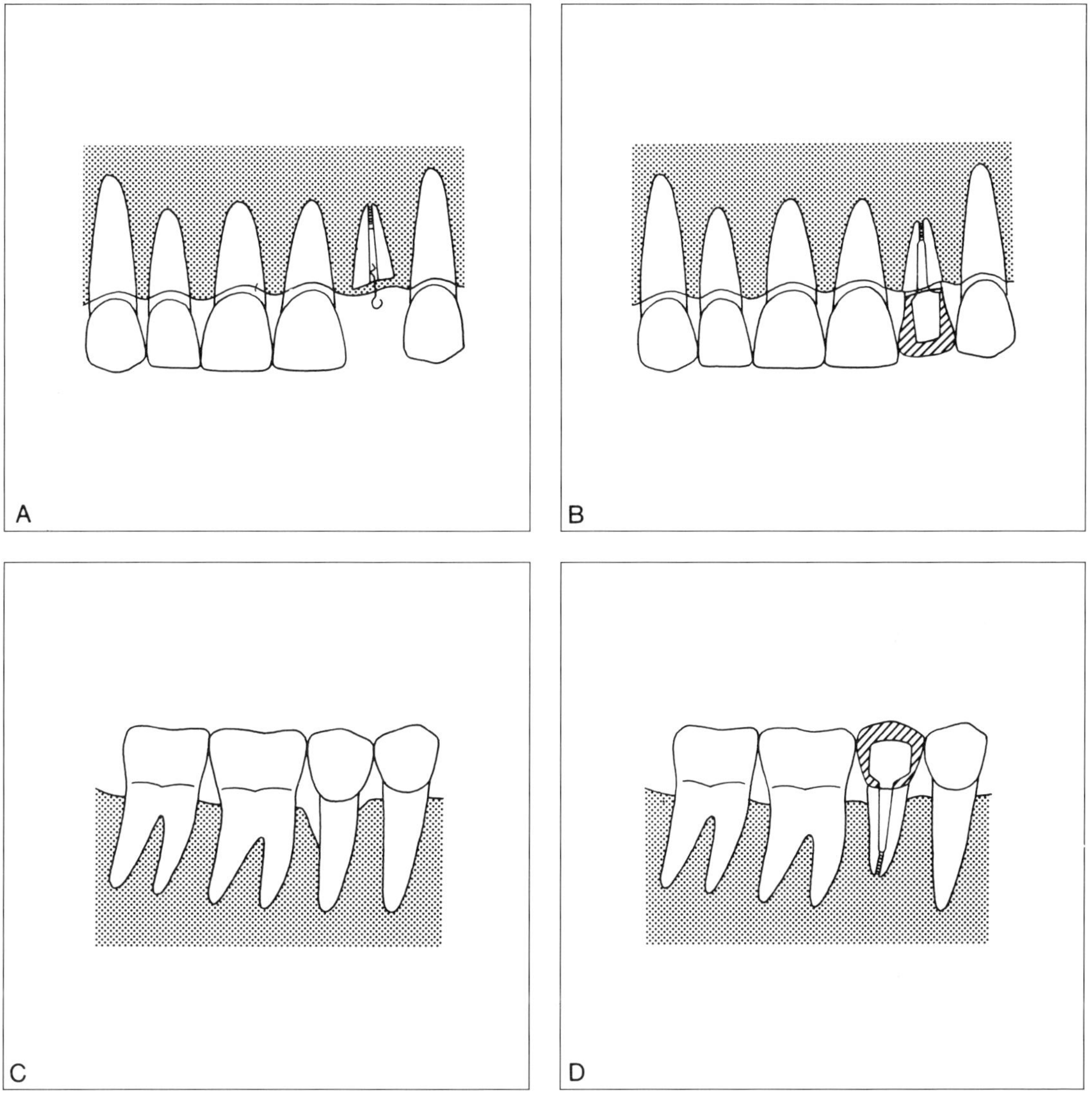

Fig. 19-2 Examples of forced eruption of teeth.

A The extrusion of a tooth that had broken off apically to the cervical margin, using an orthodontic appliance. After root treatment a hook can be fixed in the root canal and an elastic band can be used to provide an extruding force. A removable acrylic resin appliance with a guiding fork can be used to direct the elastic band and provide anchorage (Fig. 16-6, page 304).

B After extrusion, the remains of the root can be used to restore the tooth.[88]

C A normally functioning tooth erupts further after being ground clear of the occlusion. This phenomenom can be used to eliminate a periodontal defect such as the large distal pocket on a mandibular second premolar illustrated here.

D With the overeruption of the tooth, cervical bone is formed and a favourable periodontal situation has developed. Finally, the restoration can be made.

Premolars and molars can rotate and tip. The occlusion in the posterior regions can collapse with the result that sagittal and vertical overbites increase. These symptoms are often experienced by patients with severe periodontal disease. Such abnormalities cannot be treated satisfactorily without orthodontic therapy.[210]
In previous paragraphs specific aspects of orthodontic treatment of patients with vulnerable periodontal tissues have been discussed. Those matters will not be revisited. We will merely remark that plaque control is most important, that teeth with calculus or other irritating irregularities should never be moved, and that professional prophylaxis is of great significance.
When the necessary precautions are taken and good account is taken of the limiting conditions during treatment, almost every patient who asks for orthodontic treatment can be provided with it, regardless of susceptible periodontal tissues.[164]

19.7 Orthodontic treatment of functional disturbances

The most important functional disturbances in adults are abnormal lip posture, premature contacts and forced bites, serious occlusal interferences, and the mandibular dysfunction syndrome.

19.7.1 Abnormal lip posture

When the lips provide inadequate support against labial displacement of incisors undesired changes can occur with advancing age. As the periodontal support decreases, resistance to displacement also diminishes; forces exerted by the tongue or occlusion tending to procline the incisors may get the upper hand. The chance of undesirable tooth movement occurring is particularly great if lip seal is poor and/or the lower lip lies partly or wholly behind the maxillary incisors. Among other things, treatment must be directed at improving the relationship between the lips and incisors.

19.7.2 Premature contacts and forced bites

Premature contacts of themselves are no reason for instituting orthodontic therapy. They can be satisfactorily eliminated by restorations or occlusal grinding. However, if for some other reason orthodontic treatment is required, correction of premature contacts can usefully be done as a part of that treatment.
Forced bites of limited extent in adults require no treatment when the dentition shows no undesirable consequences, the periodontal tissues are healthy, and no complaints are felt concerning the masticatory muscles and temporomandibular joints.[164] When conditions are less satisfactory orthodontic treatment can secure a significant improvement. This applies especially to forced bites of an extensive character with excessively mobile teeth. This is seen particularly in protrusive forced bites with one or more incisors in reversed overbite. It is also possible for a protrusive forced bite to originate from incorrect restoration of posterior teeth so that the maxillary incisors are excessively loaded toward the labial aspect, with all the associated sequellae.

19.7.3 Serious occlusal interferences

There is only a limited number of conditions regarding tooth positions to which early loss of periodontal structures can be attributed. The presence of an orthodontic anomaly does not mean that a traumatic occlusion exists. Only in exceptional circumstances does an orthodontic anomaly predispose to traumatic occlusion.[164] Indeed, traumatic occlusion also does not necessarily lead to gingivitis or periodontitis, nor does gingivitis have to lead to periodontitis.[165,205] Whether or not occlusal trauma can affect deepening of a pocket, or significantly affect the level of attachment, is by no means cut and dried.[164] It usually is held that occlusal trauma does not cause periodontal pockets. However, if there are already abnormalities in the periodontal tissues, occlusal trauma may well exacerbate them.[169]
Damage to the palatal gingiva of the maxillary incisors and gingiva labial to the mandibular incisors, as occurs with some Class II/2 anomalies, can result in progressive destructive changes.[165] The same applies to a protrusive forced bite with the resultant movement up and down of the associated teeth in their sockets, and to severely mesially tipped molars.[113]
In the average orthodontic anomaly with normal lip posture and seal, no extra danger exists for the development of periodontal disease. Nevertheless, in certain extreme abnormalities orthodontic treatment can reduce the chance of developing such disorders.

19.7.4 Mandibular dysfunction syndrome

As suggested earlier, orthodontic treatment should be considered when complaints are expressed concerning the masticatory muscles and temporomandibular joints.[213] This is especially so when treatment is required for other reasons such as a reversed overbite and disturbing crossbites.[89] In most cases, however, the mandibular dysfunction syndrome would preferably be treated with other therapy.

19.8 Combined surgical-orthodontic therapy

In the beginning this field of treatment emphasized correcting pronounced facial deformities, without giving much thought to achieving a good dental situation. For that reason orthodontic support was often lacking, and this would have been justified in many cases by considerations of the poor quality of the dentition and the oral hygiene, making such appliance therapy unwise.
At present extreme orthodontic anomalies are treated with the help of surgery in adults in increasing numbers. To reach a satisfactory result there will usually be orthodontic treatment both before and after surgery. Good cooperation between orthodontist and oral surgeon, with knowledge of each other's potential, is essential for a successful outcome. Chapter 20 covers this subject, which is exclusively the terrain of specialists.

19.9 Retention

It is just as applicable to adult orthodontic treatment as it is to that of children that normalising the occlusion and articulation and bringing about a good lip position are essential for a stable result. Even so, in many patients permanent or semipermanent retention (removable acrylic resin appliances worn at night only) must be employed, unless there are clear reasons to assume that no relapse, or at worst one that would be acceptable, will occur.

With an acrylic resin plate, worn 24 hours a day for the first few months and subsequently nights only, the improvements achieved in the maxilla can be maintained. As long as the appliance is correctly made, oral hygiene remains optimal, and the plate is kept clean and intact, there should be no problems.

Retention can also be achieved with splints. This can be secured by using composite resin at the contact points of corrected incisors to hold their relationships. If the composite resin is limited in size and kept near the incisal surface, it is not difficult for an adult to have sufficient access to the interproximal areas to keep them well cleaned.

It is also possible to connect the incisors by bonding a thin twisted orthodontic wire (e.g., twist-o-flex) lingually. This is better esthetically and allows independent movement of the splinted teeth because the flexible wire is only fixed in the middle of the lingual surface.[241]

In general, semipermanent retention enables better oral hygiene to be achieved (via flossing, interdental brushing) than with permanent retention.[164]

If a bridge is made after orthodontic treatment it will of course act as permanent retention. If missing teeth are replaced using a partial denture (preferably skeletal) it will function as a semipermanent retainer. Consistent wear and care would be essential.

One can also attempt to prevent relapse of a deep bite in patients predisposed to this, by building up a ledge on the palatal surface of the maxillary incisors onto which the mandibular incisors can bite. In addition, retention of an increased intercanine width or correction of marked malalignment of the mandibular incisors can be secured by bonding a thin orthodontic wire lingually to the canines, closely adapted to the lingual surface of the incisors. Cleaning the lingual surface of the mandibular incisors is made quite difficult by this, and good oral hygiene in that region is seldom achieved. Consequently, the indications for a canine-to-canine bar should be considered with care and limited to special cases.

Splints probably have no significance for the health of the periodontal tissues but do affect the mental well-being of the patient. They prevent relapse of orthodontic anomalies and have a stabilising effect on excessively mobile teeth. Splints, however, can never be expected to give rise to improved periodontal conditions.[168]

In adults with susceptible periodontal tissues, severing the supra-alveolar fibres to improve the chance of avoiding relapse in not advised. When periodontal surgery nonetheless is considered necessary, it is best done after orthodontic treatment is completed, with the hope that after the tissues have healed their reorientation may assist in stabilising the result.[51,210]

19.10 Supplementary remarks

When orthodontic treatment is considered for esthetic reasons, other therapeutic possibilities should also be reviewed. Certainly since the introduction of acid etching for direct bonding of composite resins, especially using labial veneers, the possibilities for esthetic changes have broadened considerably.[11,182] The contour of individual teeth can be built up and improved, and bridges can also be provided (see 10.6).
Thanks to the incorporation of orthodontic therapy, certain patients with periodontal disease for whom no good remedy otherwise could be found are able to receive satisfactory treatment. Moreover, as has been pointed out, uprighting teeth and retracting canines and incisors from extreme labial or lingual situations into the arch may improve their condition, and periodontal structures lost earlier may at least partly be regenerated.
On the other hand, periodontal therapy can also contribute to the performance of orthodontic treatment, making the institution of orthodontic treatment a wise decision. In particular this has to do with surgical correction of gingival recession that may be esthetically disturbing, and the elimination of persistent frenula and muscle attachments at locations where attached gingiva are absent.
In the future, adults will probably continue to seek more orthodontic treatment. The complexity of this treatment makes it desirable that it be undertaken by orthodontists rather than general practitioners.
Simple orthodontic treatment of adults can nevertheless be performed by a general practitioner who has sufficient knowledge and skill in the field. It often would be wise to enlist the advice of an orthodontist. The treatment plan then should be devised in consultation with the specialist. This calls for close cooperation and interchange of ideas to ensure that all are working toward the same end. It concerns treatment in the field of restorative dentistry, treatment of periodontal disorders, or treatment of disturbances of function just as much as the isolated orthodontic problem.
A final remark concerns the recent techniques developed for use of attachments bonded not labially or buccally, but lingually on the teeth.[65,156] By this means orthodontic treatment can be performed with an appliance that cannot be seen. The extraordinary complexity of this technique makes it unlikely, certainly in the short term, that this approach will have wide application.

Chapter 20

Combined Surgical-Orthodontic Therapy

20.1 Introduction

Facial deformities can be so great that normal orthodontic treatment cannot provide a satisfactory remedy, even when incorporating facial orthopedic techniques for patients who are young enough. In such situations it is only by using surgical treatment that the form of the facial skeleton can be so changed that a more acceptable condition will result. Usually the surgery is combined with orthodontic treatment.

Surgical-orthodontic therapy requires the consideration of several specific matters. These include indications, psychological aspects, diagnosis and treatment planning, preferred patient age at operation, treatment procedures, operative corrections, retention and relapse, and risks of operation.

20.2 Indications

Orthodontic anomalies often disturb facial harmony. Most are best treated conservatively. Sometimes, however, the deformity is so great that without surgical reconstruction of the facial skeleton it will not be possible to secure a good result.

Disproportion in the craniofacial skeleton can be present from the beginning of morphogenesis (i.e., be congenital). It can also occur as the result of trauma (e.g., condyle fracture), early ankylosis of the temporomandibular joint, tumours, sequelae to radiotherapy, and also from growth disorders that distort an originally normal face. Extreme growth of the mandible giving rise to a disturbing degree of mandibular prognathism is a good example of the latter.

In serious deformities of the craniofacial skeleton the dentoalveolar compensatory mechanism fails and a severely deviant occlusion with abnormal positions of the teeth, particularly the anterior teeth, will result.

Most patients for whom surgical-orthodontic treatment is considered will in the first place have asked their dentist or family physician about the possibilities for treatment. They would usually then have been referred to an orthodontist or oral surgeon. The initiative for combined surgical-orthodontic treatment generally does not come from the patient, though in the case of people seeking cosmetic improvements (plastic surgery) that certainly is not so.[166]

Surgical-orthodontic therapy should also be contemplated when it is possible to achieve good occlusion with normal orthodontic procedures but an acceptable appearance cannot be attained. On the one hand this applies to situations in which facial esthetics would in fact be made worse as a consequence of securing a good occlusion. For example, in retracting maxillary and mandibular incisors over a considerable distance the lips may fall inwards excessively particularly in patients with a marked chin, or the nasolabial angle might become unacceptably great. On the other hand, there are patients who after orthodontic treatment, still need surgical correction outside the immediate dentomaxillary area. Examples of this are the provision of paranasal onlays where the canine fossae are excessively hollow, and correction of the form and position of the bony chin.
Functional disturbances such as inadequate lip seal, indistinct speech, and poor mastication can indeed influence a decision to institute surgical-orthodontic treatment for severe facial deformities. The most important influence, however, is of psychological origin.
Indeed, the patient's desire to improve his or her appearance is the essential deciding factor. Those who are satisfied with the condition of their teeth and facial appearance and do not suffer from social or psychological disadvantage connected with those factors do not need surgical-orthodontic treatment. Such treatment is only appropriate when the patient, after being made fully aware of all the treatment difficulties, still emphatically wishes to go ahead.

20.3 Psychological aspects

Improvement of appearance brings with it increased self-confidence and inner well-being.[74] This is particularly so for patients for whom a serious deformity has been corrected.
The social climate in which we live sets great store by physical attractiveness; the face is the focus of this attention. The form of the face has a great influence on the feeling of self-esteem and on establishing and maintaining interpersonal contacts.[91]
A patient with a serious facial deformity, to whom the possibilities of surgical-orthodontic treatment have been explained, will build up an image of how he or she will fit into society once the handicap has been corrected. Of course this sometimes exceeds the limits of reality. However, the majority of patients who have experienced such an improvement are indeed very satisfied with the result. They are delighted by the improvement in their appearance, feel better accepted by other people, make friends more easily, and have a more positive outlook on their own potential. As a result they have a tendency to quickly forget the seriousness of their former deformity.[91,148]
Children with a severe facial deformity also suffer psychologically and socially. The significance increases sharply once they leave their own sheltered environment in order to attend school. The psychological pressure can be so great that an operation at an early age can be justified even if that leads to a less satisfactory physical result than would be achieved at a later age. There may also be a need for further surgery later, but the immediate benefits counter any such disadvantages.

The improvements that can be achieved with surgical-orthodontic treatment are often so pronounced that the patient subsequently encounters many obvious reactions from other people. The patient must learn to live with a new appearance; this demands a certain ability to adapt, not only from the patient but from his or her family and friends also. Not every patient who undergoes substantial physical changes is able to manage it without emotional problems. Therefore it is essential to assess the patient beforehand and take all the steps necessary to inform and prepare him or her for what is involved. To undertake surgical-orthodontic treatment without giving full consideration to the psychological consequences is irresponsible. The patient must be strongly motivated but not desperate. Most importantly, the patient's feet should be firmly on the ground.

20.4 Diagnosis and treatment planning

The orthodontist and oral surgeon should jointly establish a diagnosis and choose the treatment for patients who are potential candidates for surgical-orthodontic therapy. In doing so, consideration has to be given not only to psychological aspects and facial esthetics, but also to occlusion and function.[235]

For diagnosis, comprehensive records are necessary in addition to the history and detailed clinical examination of the patient. The latter should involve dynamic and static features. The records should include well-extended plaster models of the teeth and surrounding structures, radiographs of the skull and teeth such as might be needed to give unambiguous information, and standardised facial photographs. For treatment planning, montages of facial photographs (preferably life-size) and cephalometric and soft tissue tracings are essential aids.[58] In patients where displacement of jaws or segments thereof is being considered, a "trial operation" using plaster models properly mounted on a fully adjustable articulator is indispensable in order to properly simulate the changes being sought.

Over 100 different approaches have been presented for surgical correction of major facial deformities.[15,49] Which approach is most appropriate and which methods of operation are most suitable for the situation can only be determined after careful diagnosis and deliberation. Moreover, different teams have diverse viewpoints on these matters.[121] Fortunately there usually is more than one approach that will reach a satisfactory result.

In theory, dentofacial deformities can be divided into sagittal, vertical, and transverse components. Where there is no asymmetry the deformity usually is restricted to the sagittal and, to a lesser degree, vertical components. Besides, transverse elements are difficult to quantify.

The practical situation, however, is that although patients usually see their faces from the front in a mirror, their judgement of their deformity generally places the anteroposterior aspects of the profile at the top of the list of undesirable characteristics.[123]

In planning the surgery, the size of the jaws and their relation are foremost in consideration; the conditions within the dental arches are less important.

Naturally, the patient must be involved in the discussion over what is wrong and what can be done about it. Good cooperation between surgeon and orthodontist is not enough. The patient must be well instructed regarding the pros and cons of different approaches, their possible results, including the chance of relapse, the risks involved, and the physical and mental burdens that will accompany the procedures. These are not minor interventions and the survival rate is not 100%. For the patient this is not just a matter of statistics.

20.5 Patient age at operation

Two aspects are in opposition when choosing the best time for surgical intervention: *(1)* the needs and wishes of the patient and *(2)* long-term results.
Individual differences in the magnitude of the deformity and the psychological makeup of the patient are important. In exceptional circumstances, the latter consideration will justify early action (without, or with only limited orthodontic therapy) even if it means that usually a compromise result must be accepted and that the possibility that later surgery may be essential must be allowed for.
Most facial deformities first become disturbing during adolescence. It is far better to wait until facial growth is complete before using surgery. This applies especially to Class III anomalies and asymmetries and less to Class II anomalies where somewhat earlier intervention can be accepted.
In patients where further mandibular growth will have an important effect on the eventual result, surgery should be delayed until facial growth is totally, or almost totally, complete. As a rule of thumb it can be taken that girls should be at least 17 years old and boys 18.[63] However, there are great differences regarding the intensity and duration of growth of the face. In particular, boys can still show remarkable growth after age 17.[63] With the aid of lateral cephalographs taken at intervals of 6 to 12 months, the progress of the patient's growth can be estimated and the time for surgery chosen on a more individual, hence wiser, basis.

20.6 Treatment procedures

From the jointly devised treatment plan, the order in which the various steps should be taken and the phases during which certain aims should have been achieved will come to light. In general the choice will go to secure first an overall alignment of the dental arches, then the operation, followed by the continuation of the orthodontic treatment for detailed finishing.
Usually, both arches require orthodontic treatment and will have to match well to each other after surgery. Dentoalveolar compensations that have occurred from the deformity must be eliminated. This covers alteration of form of the arches, positions and inclinations of the teeth, and the correction of infra- and suprapositions. It is often necessary to use fixed appliances. This has the consequent advantage that the jaws or parts thereof can be splinted easily and well, after the operation, using those same appliances.

After the above orthodontic corrections have been obtained they must be checked to see that the result corresponds with what was planned in the set-up that was provided as a trial operation on the articulator. Then the orthodontist can place a closely fitting, strong splinting arch wire in the tubes and brackets. This arch wire is provided with extensions for attachment of elastic bands or steel ligatures with which the dental arches of the maxilla and the mandible can be firmly tied together. The patient is now orthodontically ready for surgery and the necessary preoperative documentation should be sent with the patient to the oral surgeon to ensure that the next phase in the treatment plan will proceed smoothly.

The operation is the most far-reaching and critical part of the treatment. Before operation it has been accurately outlined where and how, and how much, to alter the dentofacial skeleton, including possible use of bone grafts. When the desired changes have been achieved the separate sections are fixed together. Where segmental osteotomies have been performed the individual parts are given intramaxillary fixation using a strong, well-fitting arch wire in the attachments already used in the earlier orthodontic treatment. If preferred, the orthodontic appliance can be removed entirely just before the operation, and a surgical splint fabricated on the trial setup can be cemented in place after the operation. More complex surgery is stabilised using both jaws, fixed to each other via the teeth after interposing an acrylic resin interocclusal splint that was made before the operation. For this intermaxillary fixation, elastic bands are usually used for the first 24 to 48 hours; thereafter steel ligatures are inserted.

After the period of fixation (normally 6 weeks) the new situation is consolidated if healing has been uneventful. Subsequently it is necessary to wait some time, because among other things the patient cannot open his or her mouth sufficiently. Then the remaining tooth movements should be carried out. These will generally have to do with uprighting of teeth alongside saw cuts, and the improvement of the buccolingual occlusion of individual teeth.

20.7 Operative corrections

As pointed out earlier, there is a great number of techiques for correcting dentofacial deformities by means of surgery. In this sphere we shall only illustrate and describe summarily a few of the most commonly used approaches for correcting Class II/1 (Figs. 20-1 to 20-3) and Class III anomalies (Figs. 20-4 and 20-5), and for correcting the area of the chin (Fig. 20-6).

Depending on the situation, the operation will be restricted to one jaw only, though both could be involved. Sometimes it is only possible to reach a good result by combining two or more techniques. That applies especially to open bites, the surgical correction of which is complex. Often this requires the choice of segmental osteotomy in the maxilla with a total displacement of the mandible.

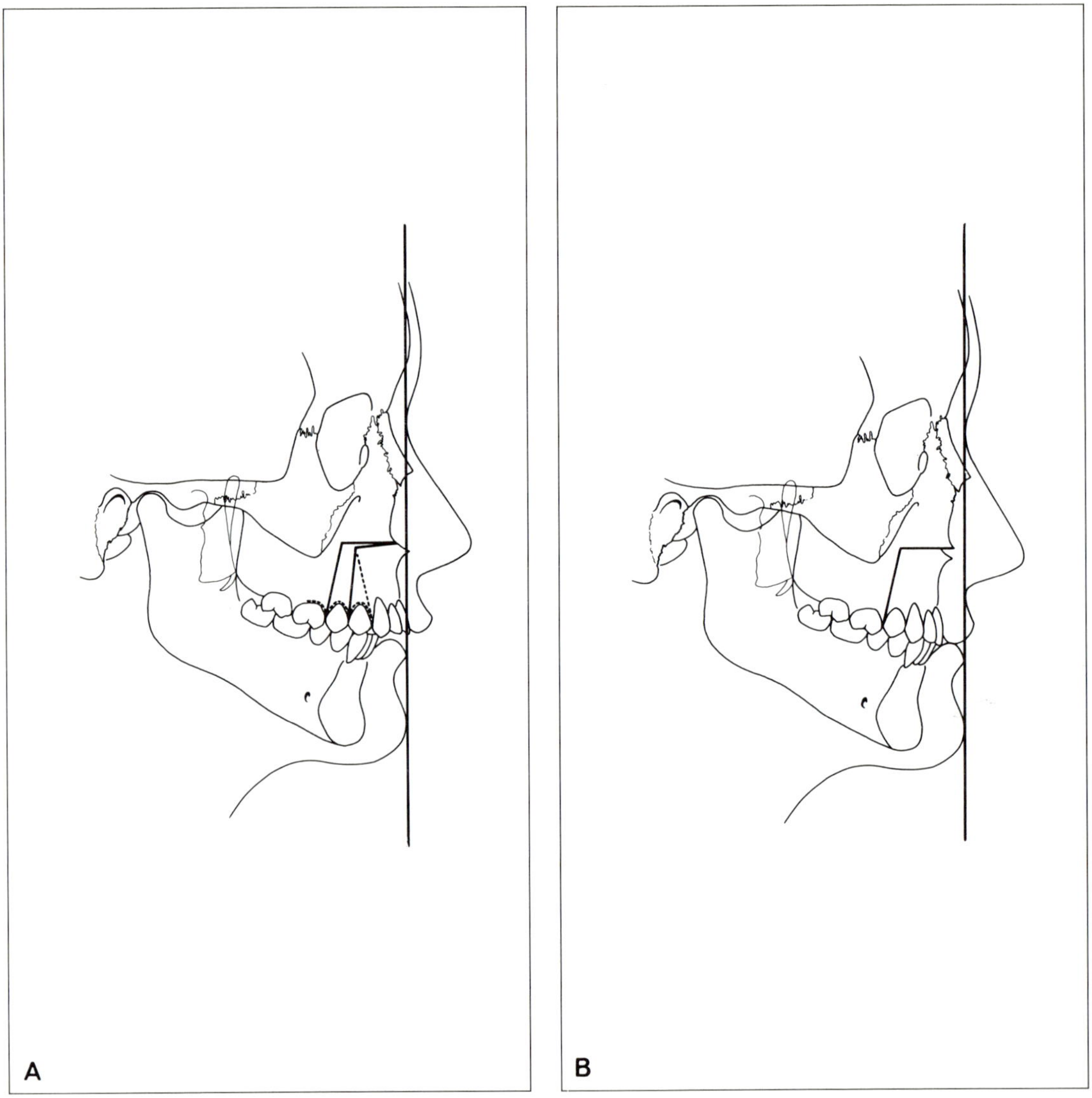

Fig. 20-1 Osteotomy of the anterior part of the maxilla according to Wassmund/Wunderer, for a Class II/1 anomaly with maxillary prognathism and an anterior open bite. (From Van der Zwan and Boering.[230])

A After extraction (usually of teeth 15 and 25) and bone removal, the anterior section is displaced dorsally. The midline is split if necessary to secure the required increase in width distally in the premolar-canine region. The course of the incision is indicated in this illustration and the following one by a dotted line.

B After displacing and repositioning the anterior segment, intramaxillary fixation is sufficient.

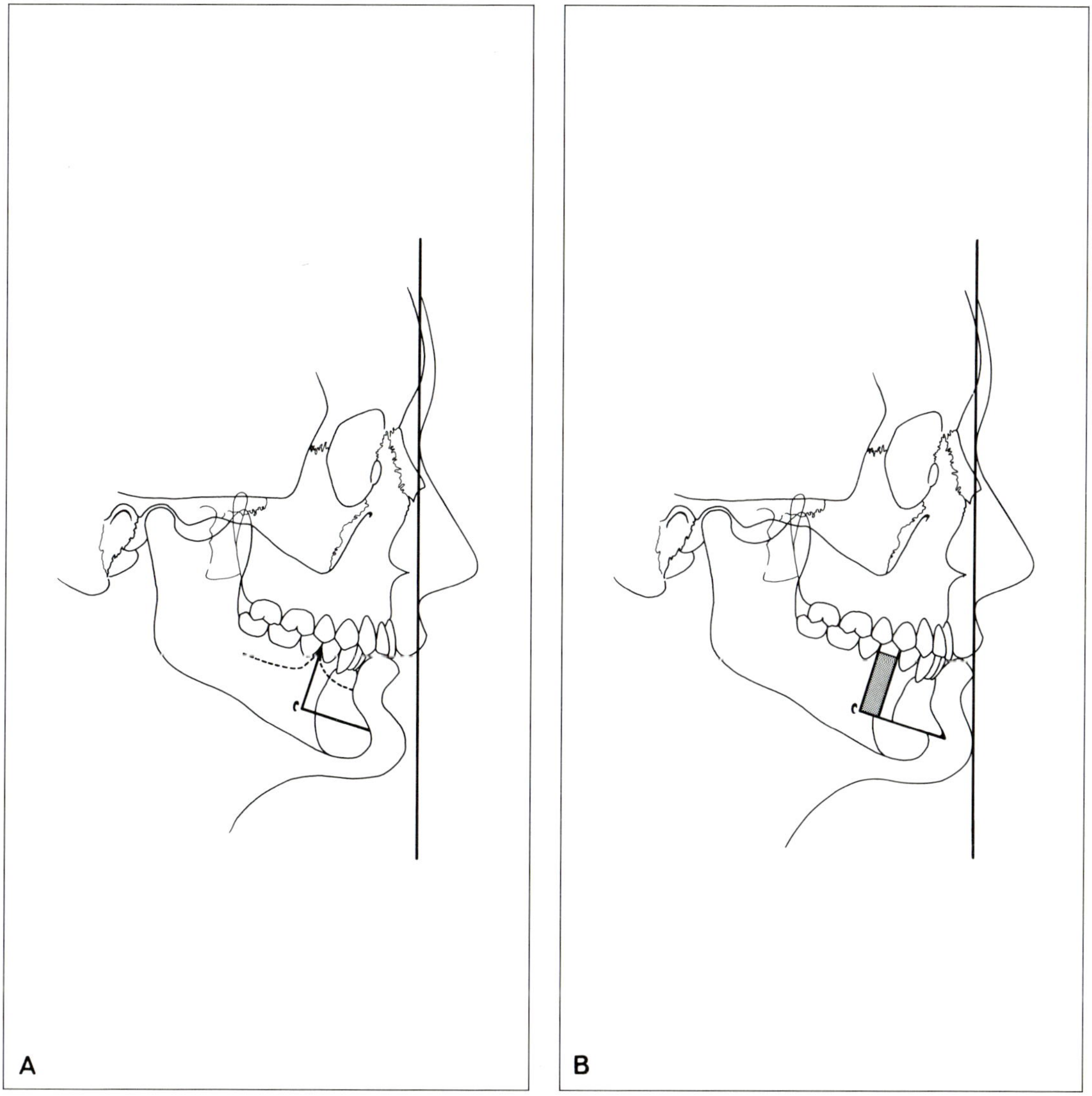

Fig. 20-2 Osteotomy of the anterior part of the mandible according to Hofer, for a Class II/1 anomaly with prominent chin and deep plica mentalis. (From Van der Zwan and Boering.[230])

A The anterior segment is cut free. The vertical cut usually lies between first and second premolars.

B The free segment is moved ventrally. The projecting bone margin is rounded and the opened up space is filled with bone. Intramaxillary fixation is sufficient.

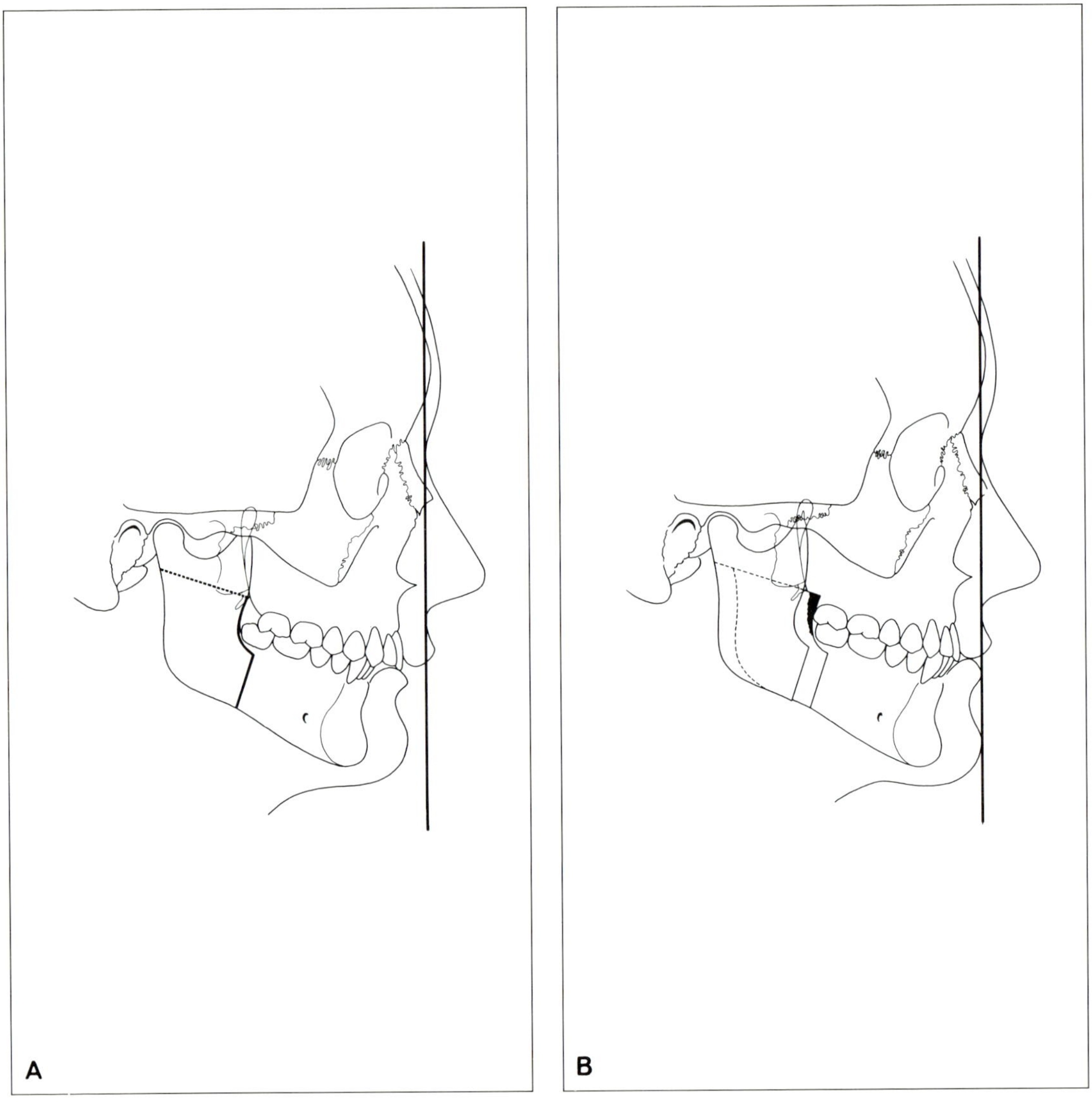

Fig. 20-3 Osteotomy of the mandible according to Obwegeser-Dal Pont for a Class II/1 anomaly with mandibular retrognathy (sagittal split osteotomy). (From Van der Zwan and Boering.[230])

A The cortical bone of the lingual surface of the ramus is sawn through caudal to the condyle and the coronoid process. The cortical bone of the buccal surface of the corpus is sawn through ventral to the jaw angle. Then the inner and outer plates of the part of the jaw between the two cuts are split apart sagittally.

B Next the corpus of the mandible is displaced ventrally and fixed to the lateral section of the ramus with steel ligatures. The sharp point formed by the anterior border of the lingual part of the ramus is rounded off. Intermaxillary fixation is essential.

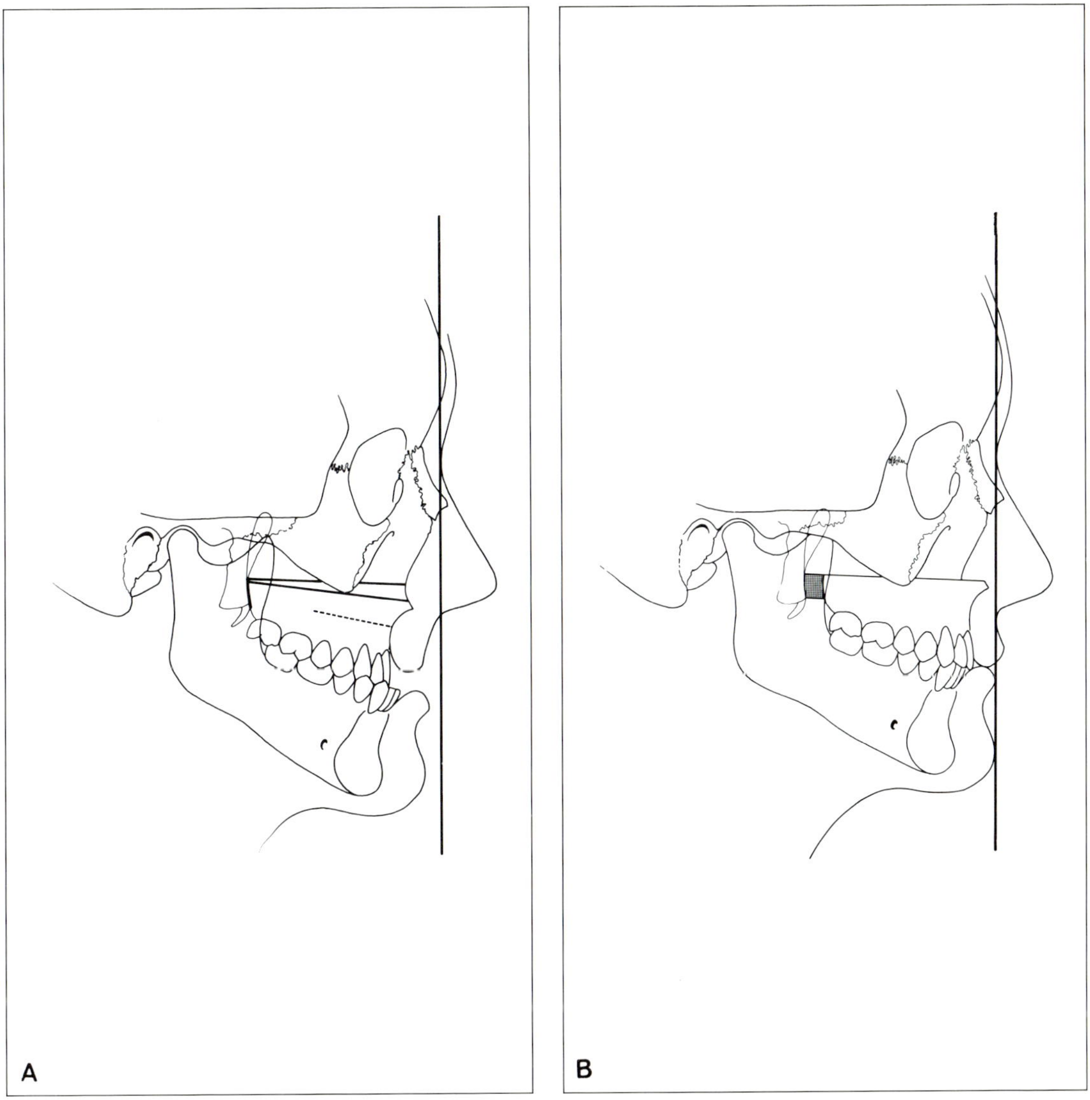

Fig. 20-4 Osteotomy of the maxilla analogous to a Le Fort I fracture for a Class III anomaly with maxillary retrognathy. (From Van der Zwan and Boering.[230])

A The entire maxilla is cut through slightly cranial to the nasal floor and freed from the surrounding bony structures.

B The free part of the maxilla is displaced ventrally and fixed to the bone cranially with steel ligatures. If the displacement is more than 5 mm ventrally, a bone implant between maxilla and pterygoid process is indicated. Intermaxillary fixation is required in addition to the steel ligatures suspending the maxilla.

This example shows, in addition, both the reduction of the height of the lower third of the face due to performing an osteotomy and the effective ventral movement of the labial surface of the mandible as the result of the mandible rotating forward (autorotation). This feature is particularly favourable for Class II/1 anomalies with a long lower face. For these conditions the Le Fort I osteotomy ventrally and cranially is most appropriate.

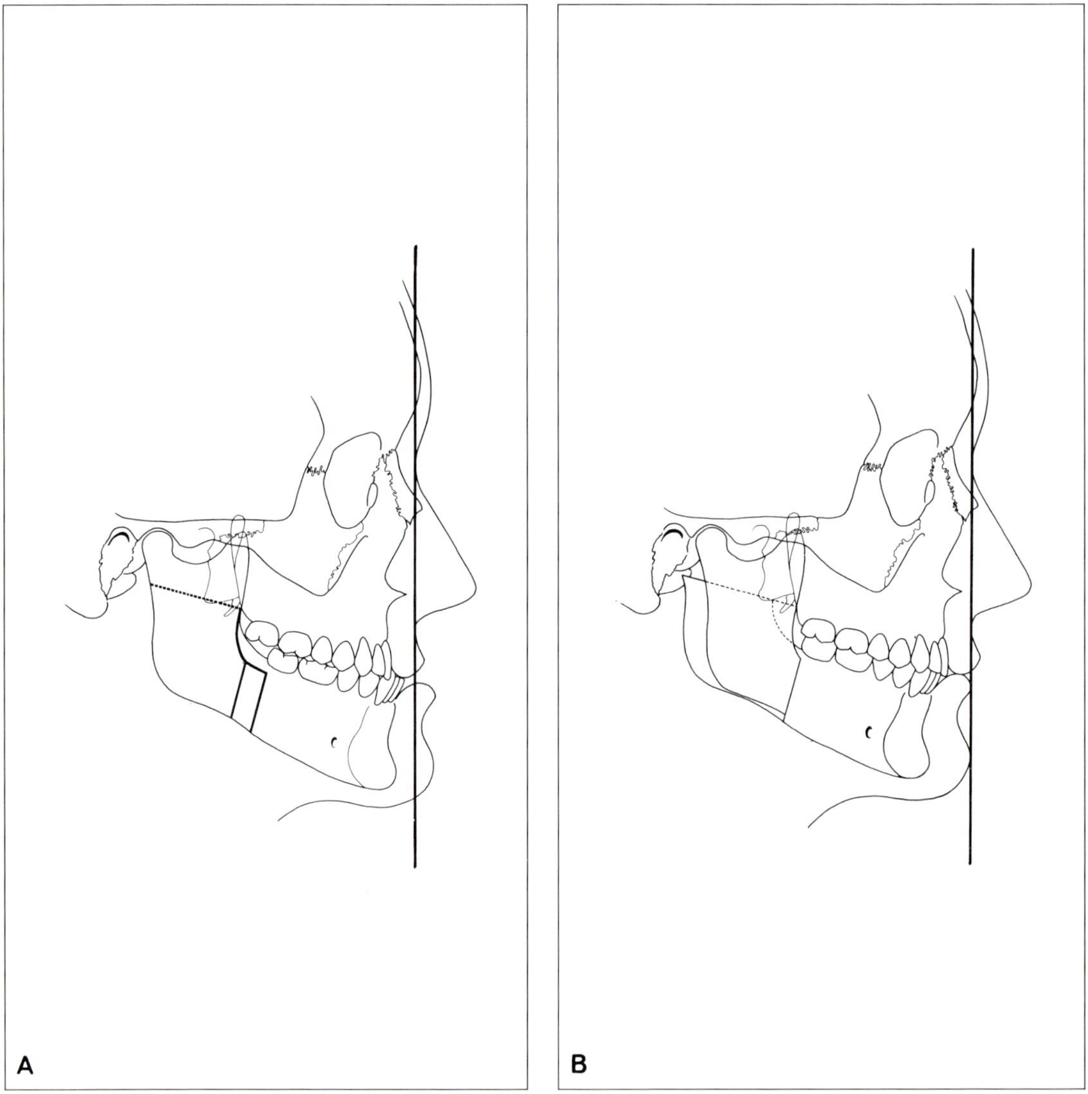

Fig. 20-5 Osteotomy of the mandible according to Obwegeser-Dal Pont for a Class III anomaly with mandibular prognathism. (From Van der Zwan and Boering.[230])

A The ramus needs to be reduced in width ventrally by removing a strip of bone buccally. This is followed by a sagittal split.

B After displacement and fixation, the lingual plate of the ascending ramus projects dorsally. This will resorb naturally. Intermaxillary fixation is essential.

Using this approach the corpus of the mandible can be tilted and rotated if required.

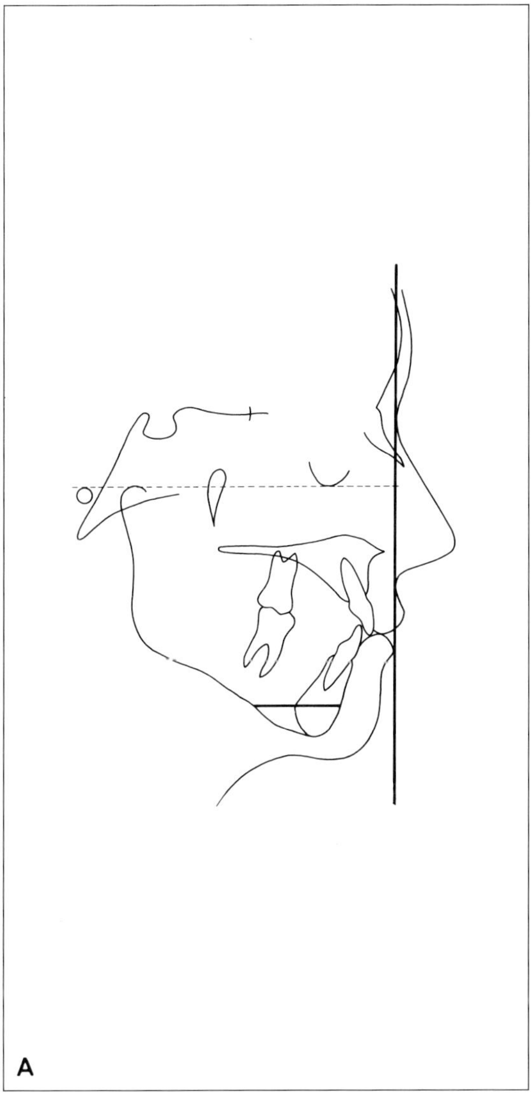

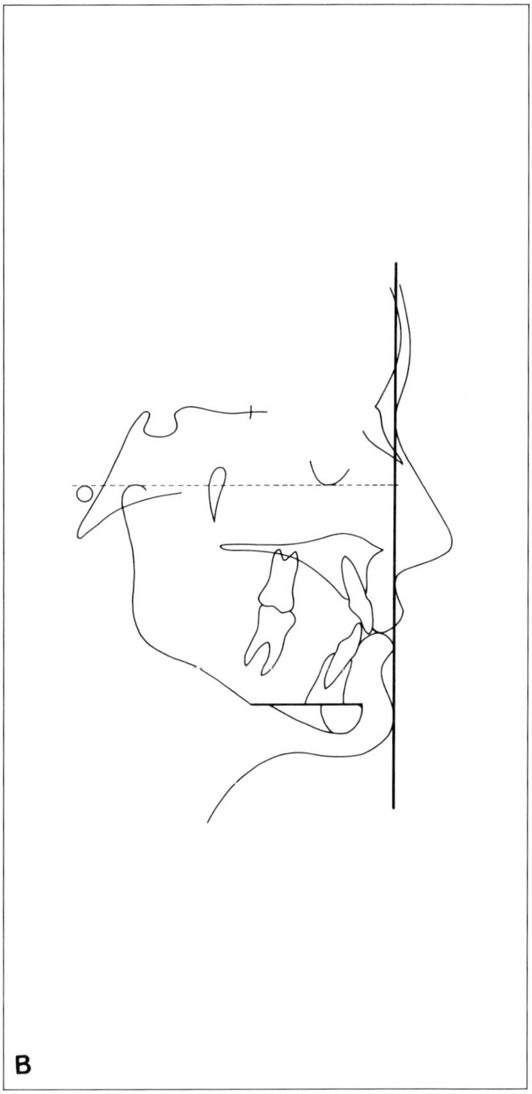

Fig. 20-6 Osteotomy through the chin and mandible for a receding chin. (From Van der Zwan and Boering.[230])

A In patients with an increased lower face height, a simultaneous height reduction and increase in chin prominence can be obtained.
B The segment that is either free or only attached to muscles is moved ventrally. This provides a good chin prominence, a definite plica mentalis, and a much improved profile. Fixation is with steel ligatures.

By modifying the above approach the chin can be moved in all three dimensions.

20.8 Retention and relapse

The results achieved with operative corrections can later regress somewhat, particularly when it concerns mandibular prognathism.[45] In these patients postoperative growth plays a more important part than does relapse. Corrections done before the age of 16 will, for that reason, give worse ultimate results than those that were delayed until a later age.[62]
The only procedures of this nature that can be performed without risk before growth is complete are ventral displacement of the anterior aspect of the body of the mandible and dorsal displacement of the anterior section of the maxilla. After other operative procedures, the situation deteriorates if the mandible still grows.[62]
With surgical corrections of Class II/1 anomalies where the mandible is sectioned, a danger exists that the condyles will not remain in their fossae but will be drawn forward. Should that occur and bone union follow with the condyles drawn forward, the condyles will return distally once fixation has been removed and the mandible will have returned to its original distorelation.[48,240]
Open bites also have a great tendency to regress partially after surgery, particularly when the operation has been done on the mandible. Anomalies that have a functional origin (tongue interposition, disturbed nasal respiration) remain unstable after surgical correction if the functional disturbance has not also been eliminated.[221]
Results achieved with surgical corrections of the maxilla and the midface are generally permanent.[62,63] These are probably stable because few if any muscles are involved, in contrast to those involving the mandible. Research results in monkeys justify the proposal that sectioning and then rejoining muscles in particular situations increases the chance of securing a better functional and skeletal balance and thus less relapse.[132] Of course, good interdigitation provides stability.[230]
Retention of surgical correction is used where necessary (as advised previously) through immobilisation by fixation of the dental arches and by using steel ligatures through the bone to fix bone segments and to suspend the maxillomandibular complex from stable cranial bone structures. After healing and consolidation of the newly formed bone at the created bone junctions, the immobilisation of the mandible and the fixation of the dental arches can be discontinued. The steel ligatures in the bone are not removed; they cause no problems over time.
For avoiding relapse of corrected tooth positions the same rules apply as for orthodontic treatment without surgery. Mostly a wire is fixed lingually to the mandibular incisors using composite resin on the canines; in the maxilla a removable acrylic resin retainer is provided.

20.9 Risks of operation

Apart from the dangers possible with any operation and the chance of relapse, there are specific risks involved with surgical-orthodontic intervention. They depend largely on the nature of the operation.
Threatening situations during or shortly after surgery occur in 0.1% to 0.3% of

operations. In the same order of magnitude is the risk of necrosis in the bone segments.
Damage to or loss of teeth (1%) occurs more often, particularly adjacent to the cuts in segmental osteotomies. Periodontal damage and loss of vitality occur slightly more often (2% to 3%), while the chance of loss of sensory nerve supply to teeth is higher (5% in the maxilla, 30% in the mandible).
Although especially disagreeable, permanent disturbance of the nerve supply to the lower lip and chin (partial loss of sensibility: 10% to 40%, total loss of sensibility: 2%) is of varying significance to different patients. The risk of permanent nerve damage in maxillary surgery is considerably less.
If there is insufficient aftercare, the degree of opening of the mouth can remain restricted (i.e., less than 40 mm), and in approximately 10% of patients temporomandibular joint problems occur, though usually only temporarily.
The risk for eyes and/or tear ducts in connection with a high facial osteotomy is less than 1%.
The figures given above vary from author to author and are only intended as an overall indication. It certainly can be gathered that surgery in the maxilla shows clearly less chance of relapse and undesirable aftereffects than operations on the mandible.[64]

20.10 Supplementary remarks

Surgical-orthodontic therapy has some other favourable effects besides the functional and esthetic improvements mentioned. The chance of long-term retention of one's own dentition is enhanced if all goes well. Even if teeth are eventually lost, the conditions for providing a satisfactory prosthesis are better.
It is a misconception to think that surgical-orthodontic therapy takes less time than conventional orthodontic treatment. That really applies only to treatment requiring no pre- or postoperative orthodontic treatment.
Purely surgical treatment is indicated principally when the dental arches happen to match each other without further attention postoperatively, and where there is no other reason for orthodontic treatment. It also can be indicated where the general condition of the teeth is so bad that no orthodontic treatment could be undertaken.
Finally, the possibility should be mentioned of using alveolotomy to move an ankylotic maxillary incisor to its correct position after facial growth is complete. The life span of such a tooth is, however, limited.

References

1. Alstad, S., Zachrisson, B.U. Longitudinal study of periodontal treatment in adolescents.
Am. J. Orthod. 76: 277-286, 1979.
2. Amsterdam, M., Corn, H. Graduate Seminar Series, University of Pennsylvania, School of Dental Medicine, 1969-1972.
3. Andreasen, J.O. The influence of traumatic intrusion of primary teeth on their permanent successors. A radiographic and histologic study in monkeys.
Int. J. Oral Surg. 5: 207-219, 1976.
4. Andreasen, J.O. *Traumatic injuries of the teeth.* 2nd ed.
Munksgaard, Copenhagen, 1981.
5. Andreasen, J.O. Challenges in clinical dental traumatology.
Endodont. Dent. Traumatol. 1: 45-55, 1985.
6. Andreasen, J.O., Hjørting-Hansen, E. Replantation of teeth. I. Radiographic and clinical study of 110 human teeth replanted after accidental loss.
Acta Odontol. Scand. 24: 263-286, 1966.
7. Andreasen, J.O., Sundström, B., Ravn, J.J. The effect of traumatic injuries to primary teeth in their permanent successors. I. A clinical and histological study of 117 injured permanent teeth.
Scand. J. Dent. Res. 79: 219-283, 1971.
8. Arya, B.S., Savara, B.S., Thomas, D.R. Prediction of first molar occlusion.
Am. J. Orthod. 63: 610-621, 1973.
9. Atkinson, C.D. The case against early extraction of mandibular primary canines.
J. Am. Dent. Assoc. 104: 302-304, 1982.
10. Bachmann, H. Die Häufigkeit von Nichtanlagen bleibender Zähne (ausgenom men der Weisheitszähne). Ergebnis der Auswertung von 8694 Orthopantomo grammen 9-10 jähriger Schulkinder aus Zürich.
Med. Diss. Zürich, 1974.
11. Banker, C.A., Berlocher, W.C., Mueller, B.H. Alternative methods for the management of persistent maxillary central diastema.
Gen. Dent. 30: 136-139, 1982.
12. Baume, L.J. Auswirkung des Extraktion von Zähnen auf das deforme Gebiss. Erster Teil.
Schweiz. Monatschr. Zahnheilkd. 49: 295-337, 1939.
13. Baume, L.J. Physiological tooth migration and its significance for the development of occlusion. I, II, III and IV.
J. Dent. Res. 29: 123-132, 331-337, 338-348, 440-447, 1950.
14. Behrents, R.G. Growth in the aging craniofacial skeleton. Monograph No. 17. Craniofacial Growth Series.
Center for Human Growth and Development. The University of Michigan, Ann Arbor, Mich., 1985.
15. Bell, W.H., Proffit, W.R., White, R.P. Surgical correction of dentofacial deformities.
W.B. Saunders Co., Philadelphia, 1980.
16. Bergström, K., Jensen, R., Martensson, B. The effect of superior labial frenectomy in cases with midline diastema.
Am. J. Orthod. 63: 633-638, 1973.
17. Bjerklin, K., Kurol, J. Prevalence of ectopic eruption of the maxillary first permanent molar.
Swed. Dent. J. 5: 29-34, 1981.
18. Bjerklin, K., Kurol, J. Ectopic eruption of the maxillary first permanent molar: etiologic factors.
Am. J. Orthod. 84: 147-155, 1983.
19. Björk, A., Jensen, E., Palling, M. Mandibular growth and third molar impaction.
Acta Odontol. Scand. 14: 231-272, 1956.
20. Björk, A., Skieller, V. Facial development and tooth eruption. An implant study at the age of puberty.
Am. J. Orthod. 62: 339-383, 1972.
21. Bodin, I., Julin, P., Thomsson, M. Hyperodontia.
Dentomax.-Fac. Radiol. 10: 35-42, 1981.
22. Boersma, H. Het centraal diasteem in de bovenkaak.
Ned. Tijdschr. Tandheelk. 82: 410-414, 1975.
23. Boese, L.R. Increased stability of orthodontically rotated teeth following gingivectomy in *Macaca nemestrina.*
Am. J. Orthod. 56: 273-290, 1969.

24. Booy, C. Personal communication, 1958.
25. Brandt, S.K., Shapiro, S.D., Kittle, P.E. Immature primary molar in the newborn. *Pediatr. Dent.* 5: 210-213, 1983.
26. Brauer, J.E. A report of 113 early or premature extractions of primary molars and the incidence of closure of space. *J. Dent. Child.* 8: 222-224, 1941.
27. Breakspear, E.K. Further observations on early loss of deciduous molars. *Dent. Pract. (Bristol)* 11: 233-252, 1961.
28. Brown, I.D. Some further observations on submerging deciduous molars. *Br. J. Orthod.* 8: 99-107, 1981.
29. Brown, L.H., Berkman, S., Cohen, D., Kaplan, A.L., Rosenberg, M. A radiological study of the frequency and distribution of impacted teeth. *J. Dent. Assoc. South Afr.* 37: 627-630, 1982.
30. Burgersdijk, R.C.W. Personal communication, 1986.
31. Chipman, M.R. Second and third molars: their role in orthodontic therapy. *Am. J. Orthod.* 47: 498-520, 1961.
32. Chow, M.H. Natal and neonatal teeth. *J. Am. Dent. Assoc.* 100: 215-216, 1980.
33. Clinch, L.M. A longitudinal study of the results of premature loss of deciduous teeth between 3-4 and 13-14 years of age. *Dent. Pract. Dent. Rec. (Bristol)* 9: 109-128, 1959.
34. Davey, K.W. Effect of premature loss of deciduous molars on the anteroposterior position of maxillary first permanent molars and other maxillary teeth. *J. Can. Dent. Assoc.* 32: 406-416, 1966.
35. De Smit, A. Gelaatsprofielen. Academisch Proefschrift, Gent, 1985.
36. Diamond, M. Posterior growth of maxilla. *Am. J. Orthod. Oral Surg.* 32: 359-364, 1966.
37. Diedrich, P. Kieferorthopädische Aspekte bei parodontal erkrankten Patienten. *ZWR* 91: 26-35, 1982.
38. Diedrich, P. Die Aufrichtung gekippter Molaren als präprothetische und parodontitisprophylaktische Massnahme. *Dtsch. Zahnärztl. Z.* 2: 159-164, 1986.
39. Dorenbos, J. Algemeen tandheelkundige en orthodontische aspecten bij traumata van fronttanden. *Ned. Tijdschr. Tandheelk.* 79: 398-405, 1972.
40. Dragoo, M.R. Periodontics and orthodontics. In: *Orthodontics and periodontics.* Pg. 33-51, Eds. E. Hösl, B.U. Zachrisson, A. Baldauf. Quintessence Publ. Co., Chicago, 1985.
41. Duterloo, H.S. Knochenstruktur und Zahnbewegung. *Fortschr. Kieferorthop.* 41: 177-185, 1980.
42. Edwards, J.G. A surgical procedure to eliminate rotational relapse. *Am. J. Orthod.* 57: 35-46, 1970.
43. Edwards, J.G. The diastema, the frenum, the frenectomy: a clinical study. *Am. J. Orthod.* 71: 489-508, 1977.
44. Efstratiadis, S.S., Kent, R.L., Lebret, L.M.L., Moorrees, C.F.A. Spatial position of mandibular third molars in monozygotic twins. *Angle Orthod.* 54: 271-282, 1984.
45. Egyedi, P. Evaluation of operations for mandibular protrusion. *Oral Surg. Oral Med. Oral Pathol.* 19: 451-458, 1965.
46. Eliasson, L.A., Hugoson, A., Kurol, J., Siwe, H. The effects of orthodontic treatment on periodontal tissues in patients with reduced periodontal support. *Eur. J. Orthod.* 4: 1-9, 1982.
47. Engström, C., Engström, H., Sagne, S. Lower third molar development in relation to skeletal maturity and chronological age. *Angle Orthod.* 53: 97-106, 1983.
48. Epker, B.N., Wessberg, G.A. Mechanisms of early skeletal relapse following surgical advancement of the mandible. *Br. J. Oral Surg.* 20: 175-182, 1982.
49. Epker, B.N., Wolford, L.M. *Dentofacial deformities: surgical-orthodontic correction.* The C.V. Mosby Co., St. Louis, 1985.
49a. Ericson, S., Kurol, J. Early treatment of palatally erupting maxillary canines by extraction of the primary canines. *Eur. J. Orthod.* 10: 283-295, 1988.
49b. Ericson, S., Kurol, J. Resorption of maxillary lateral incisors due to ectopic eruption of the canines. A clinical and radiographic analysis of predisposing factors. *Am. J. Orthod.* 94: 503-513, 1988.
50. Ericsson, I., Thilander, B. Orthodontic forces and recurrence of periodontal disease. An experimental study in the dog. *Am. J. Orthod.* 74: 41-50, 1978.
51. Ericsson, I., Thilander, B. Orthodontic relapse in dentitions with reduced periodontal support: an experimental study in dogs. *Eur. J. Orthod.* 2: 51-57, 1980.
52. Ericsson, I., Thilander, B., Lindhe, J. Periodontal conditions after orthodontic tooth movements in the dog. *Angle Orthod.* 48: 210-218, 1978.

53. Ericsson, I., Thilander, B., Lindhe, J., Okamoto, H. The effect of orthodontic tilting movements on the periodontal tissues of infected and noninfected dentitions in dogs. *J. Clin. Periodontol.* 4: 278-293, 1977.
54. Fanning, E.A. Effect of extraction of deciduous molars on the formation and eruption of their successors. *Angle Orthod.* 32: 44-53, 1962.
55. Fanning, E.A. Third molar emergence in Bostonians. *Am. J. Phys. Anthrop.* 20: 339-346, 1962.
56. Fastlight, G. Adult orthodontics. *J. Clin. Orthod.* 16: 606-618, 1982.
57. Ferguson, F.S. Prevalence of labial-lingual and vertical malocclusion in the primary dentition. *J. Pedodont.* 4: 187-191, 1980.
58. Fish, L.C., Epker, B.N. Surgical-orthodontic cephalometric prediction tracing. *J. Clin. Orthod.* 14: 36-52, 1980.
59. Fränkel, R. Lip seal training in the treatment of skeletal open bite. *Eur. J. Orthod.* 2: 219-228, 1980.
60. Fränkel, R., Falck, F. Zahndurchbruch und Vererbung beim Deckbiss. *Fortschr. Kieferorthop.* 28: 175-182, 1967.
61. Freihofer, H.P.M. Results after midface osteotomies. *J. Maxillofac. Surg.* 1: 30-36, 1973.
62. Freihofer, H.P.M. Results of osteotomies of the facial skeleton in adolescence. *J. Maxillofac. Surg.* 5: 267-297, 1977.
63. Freihofer, H.P.M. The timing of facial osteotomies in children and adolescents. *Clin. Plast. Surg.* 9: 445-456, 1982.
64. Freihofer, H.P.M. Personal communication, 1986.
65. Fujita, K. New orthodontic treatment with lingual bracket mushroom arch wire appliance. *Am. J. Orthod.* 76: 657-675, 1979.
66. Gardiner, J.H. Erupted teeth in the newborn. *Proc. R. Soc. Med.* 54: 504-506, 1961.
67. Garn, S.M. *The earlier gain and the later loss of cortical bone.* Charles C Thomas Publ., Springfield, Ill., 1970.
68. Garn, S.M., Lewis, A.B., Bonne, B. Third molar formation and its development course. *Angle Orthod.* 32: 270-279, 1962.
69. Garn, S.M., Lewis, A.B., Kerewsky, R.S. Third molar agenesis and variation in size of the remaining teeth. *Nature* 201: 839, 1964.
70. Garn, S.M., Lewis, A.B., Vicinus, J.H. Third molar polymorphism and its significance to dental genetics. *J. Dent. Res.* 42: 1344-1363, 1963.
71. Garn, S.M., Lewis, A.B., Walenga, A.J. Maximum-confidence values for the human mesiodistal crown dimension of human teeth. *Arch. Oral Biol.* 18: 841, 1968.
72. Gellin, M.E., Haley, J.V. Managing cases of overretention of mandibular primary incisors where their permanent successors erupt lingually. *J. Dent. Child.* 49: 118-122, 1982.
72a. Goldstein, R.E., *Change Your Smile.* 2nd ed. Quintessence Publ. Co., Chicago, 1988.
73. Gorlin, R.J., Goldman, H.M. (eds.) *Thoma's oral pathology.* Vol. I and II. 6th ed. The C.V. Mosby Co., St. Louis, 1970.
74. Graber, L.W. Psychiological considerations of orthodontic treatment. In: *Psychological aspects of facial form.* Monograph No. 11. Craniofacial Growth Series. Pg. 81-117, Eds. G.W. Lucker, K.A. Ribbens, J.A. McNamara Jr. Center for Human Growth and Development. The University of Michigan, Ann Arbor, Mich., 1980.
75. Graber, T.M. *Orthodontics.* 3rd ed. W.B. Saunders Co., Philadelphia, 1972.
76. Graber, T.M., Kaineg, T.F. The mandibular third molar — its predictive status and role in incisor crowding. *Proc. Finn. Dent. Soc.* 77: 37-44, 1981.
77. Grahnen, H. Hypodontia in the permanent dentition. A clinical and genetical investigation. *Odontol. Revy* Suppl. 3: 76, 1956.
78. Gravely, J.F. A radiographic survey of third molar development. *Br. Dent. J.* 119: 397-401, 1965.
79. Groper, J.N. A simplified treatment for correcting an ectopically erupting maxillary first permanent molar. *J. Dent. Child.* 52: 374-376, 1985.
80. Haaviko, K., Altonen, M., Mattila, K. Predicting angular development and eruption of the lower third molar. *Angle Orthod.* 48: 39-48, 1978.
81. Hallett, G.E.M., Burke, P.H. Symmetrical extraction of first permanent molars. Factors controlling results in the lower arch. *Trans. Eur. Orthod. Soc.* 37: 238-255, 1961.
82. Hargreaves, J.A., Graig, J.W. *The management of traumatised anterior teeth of children.* 2nd ed. Livingstone, London, 1981.

83. Helm, S., Siersbaek-Nielsen, S. Crowding in the permanent dentition after early loss of deciduous molars or canines.
Trans. Eur. Orthod. Soc. 49: 137-149, 1973.

84. Hoffding, J., Kisling, E. Premature loss of primary teeth. II. The specific effects on occlusion and space in the permanent dentition.
J. Dent. Child. 45: 284-287, 1978.

85. Holm, U. Problems of compensative extraction in cases with loss of first permanent molars.
Trans. Eur. Orthod. Soc. 46: 409-427, 1970.

86. Holm, U. 25 Jahre Erfahrungen mit der Sechsjahrmolarenextraktion in der Kieferorthopädie. In: Studieweek 1980, Pg. 99-112.
Ned. Ver. Orthod. Studie, 1980.

87. Ingber, J.S. Forced eruption: Part I. A method of treating isolated one and two wall infrabony osseous defects — rational and case report.
J. Periodontol. 45: 199-206, 1974.

88. Ingber, J.S. Forced eruption: Part II. A method of treating nonrestorable teeth — periodontal and restorative considerations.
J. Periodontol. 47: 203-216, 1976.

89. Ingervall, B. Orthodontic treatment in adults with temporomandibular dysfunction symptoms.
Am. J. Orthod. 73: 551-559, 1978.

90. Ingervall, B., Eliasson, G.B. Effect of lip training in children with short upper lip.
Angle Orthod. 52: 222-233, 1982.

91. Jacobson, A. Psychological aspects of dentofacial esthetics and orthognathic surgery.
Angle Orthod. 54: 18-35, 1984.

92. Jakobsson, S.O. Diastema medial en longitudinell undersökning.
Odont. Tidschr. 73: 127-148, 1965.

93. Johnson, D.B. Supernumerary lateral incisor teeth.
Br. J. Orthod. 1: 149-157, 1974.

94. Joho, J.P., Marechaux, S.C. Trauma in the primary dentition: a clinical presentation.
J. Dent. Child. 47: 167-174, 1980.

95. Joondeph, D.R., McNeill, R.N. Congenitally absent second premolars: an interceptive approach.
Am. J. Orthod. 59: 50-66, 1971.

96. Judd, W.V. Concensus development conference.
Ind. Health Serv. Dent. Newsl. 18: 63-80, 1980.

97. Kaplan, R.G. Mandibular third molars and postretention crowding.
Am. J. Orthod. 66: 411-430, 1974.

98. Kates, G.A., Needleman, H.L., Holmes, L.B. Natal and neonatal teeth: a clinical study.
J. Am. Dent. Assoc. 109: 441-443, 1984.

99. Kim, Y.H., Fogels, H.R., Shiere, F.R. Factors of tooth rotation and axial inclination of lower premolars.
J. Dent. Res. 39: 673, 1960.

100. Kohnstamm, G.A. *Duimzuigen bij kleine en grote kinderen.*
Van Loghum Slaterus, Deventer, 1981.

101. Korf, S.R. The eruption of permanent central incisors follows premature loss of their antecedents.
J. Dent. Child. 32: 39-44, 1965.

102. Krakowiak, F.J. Ankylosed primary molars.
J. Dent. Child. 45: 288-292, 1978.

103. Kristerson, L. Autotransplantation of human premolars.
Int. J. Oral Surg. 14: 200-213, 1985.

104. Kristerson, L., Andreasen, J.O. Autotransplantation and replantation of tooth germs in monkeys.
Int. J. Oral Surg. 13: 324-333, 1984.

105. Kristerson, L., Lagerström, L. Influence of orthodontic treatment upon root development of autotransplanted bicuspids.
Am. J. Orthod., in press.

106. Kurol, J. Infraocclusion of primary molars: an epidemiologic and familial study.
Community Dent. Oral Epidemiol. 9: 94-102, 1981.

107. Kurol, J., Koch, G. The effect of extraction of infraoccluded deciduous molars: a longitudinal study.
Am. J. Orthod. 87: 46-55, 1985.

108. Kurol, J., Thilander, B. Infraocclusion of primary molars and the effect on occlusal development. A longitudinal study.
Eur. J. Orthod. 6: 277-293, 1984.

109. Kurol, J., Thilander, B. Infraocclusion of primary molars with aplasia of the permanent successor: a longitudinal study.
Angle Orthod. 54: 283-294, 1984.

110. Kuijpers-Jagtman, A.M. Aspecten van preprothetische orthodontische therapie. In: *Het tandheelkundig jaar.* Pg. 50-58, Eds. W.A.M. van der Kwast, C.L. Davidson, M.A.J. Eykman, A.F. Käyser, J. van der Waal. Bohn, Scheltema & Holkema, Utrecht, 1983.

111. Kuijpers-Jagtman, A.M., Dijkman, E.H.M. Vroegtijdig verlies van ondermolaren en preprothetische orthodontische mogelijkheden. In: *Het tandheelkundig jaar.* Pg. 93-103, Eds. W.A.M. van der Kwast, C.L. Davidson, M.A.J. Eykman, A.F. Käyser, J. van der Waal. Bohn, Scheltema & Holkema, Utrecht, 1984.

112. Lagerström, L. Personal communication, 1985.

113. Lang, N.P. Das präprothetische Aufrichten von gekippten unteren Molaren im Hinblick auf den parodontalen Zustand.
Schweiz. Mschr. Zahnheilk. 87: 560-569, 1977.

114. Lang, R. Uprighting partially impacted molars.
J. Clin. Orthod. 9: 646-650, 1985.

115. Lange, D.E. Indications and procedures for mucogingival surgery. In: *Orthodontics and periodontics.* Pg. 79-103, Eds. E. Hösl, B.U. Zachrisson, A. Baldauf.
Quintessence Publ. Co., Chicago, 1985.

116. Larsson, E. Dummy- and finger-sucking habits in 4-year-olds.
Swed. Dent. J. 68: 219-224, 1975.

117. Levine, N. Injury to the primary dentition.
Dent. Clin. North Am. 26: 461-480, 1982.

118. Lewis, T.E. Incidence of fractured anterior teeth as related to their protrusion.
Angle Orthod. 29: 128-131, 1959.

119. Linder-Aronson, S. The effect of premature loss of deciduous teeth. A biometric study in 14- and 15-year-olds.
Acta Odontol. Scand. 18: 101-122, 1960.

120. Lindqvist, B., Thilander, B. Extraction of third molars in cases of anticipated crowding in the lower jaw.
Am. J. Orthod. 81: 130-139, 1982.

121. Litt, R.A. Surgical orthodontics — science or art.
Pacific Coast Soc. Orthod. Bull. 51: 55-59, 1979.

122. Lo, R.T., Moyers, R.E. Studies in the etiology and prevention of malocclusion. I. The sequence of the permanent dentition.
Am. J. Orthod. 39: 460-467, 1953.

123. Lucker, G.W. Esthetics and a quantitative analysis of facial treatment. In: *Psychological aspects of facial form.* Monograph No. 11. Craniofacial Growth Series. Pg. 49-79, Eds. G.W. Lucker, K.A. Ribbens, J.A. McNamara Jr.
Center for Human Growth and Development. The University of Michigan, Ann Arbor, Mich., 1980.

124. Lundström, A. The significance of early loss of deciduous teeth in the etiology of malocclusion.
Am. J. Orthod. 41: 819-826, 1955.

125. Lysell, G., Lysell, L. Persistence of deciduous teeth to advanced age.
Trans. R. Schools Dent. Stockholm and Umea 5: 55-59, 1960.

126. Magnusson, T.E. The effect of premature loss of deciduous teeth on the spacing of the permanent dentition.
Eur. J. Orthod. 1: 243-249, 1979.

127. Magnusson, B.O., Persliden, B. Development and its aberrations. In: *Pedodontics.* Pg. 79-128, Ed. B.O. Magnusson.
Munksgaard, Copenhagen, 1981.

128. Mamandras, A.H. Growth of lips in two dimensions: a serial cephalometric study.
Am. J. Orthod. 86: 61-66, 1984.

129. Marks, M.H., Corn, H. The role of tooth movement in periodontal therapy.
Dent. Clin. North Am. 13: 229, 1969.

130. Massler, M., Savara, B.S. Natal and neonatal teeth. A review of twenty four cases reported in the literature.
J. Pediatr. 36: 349-359, 1950.

131. McEwen, J.D., McHugh, W.D. An epidemiological investigation into the effects of the loss of first permanent molars.
Trans. Eur. Orthod. Soc. 46: 337-348, 1970.

132. McNamara Jr., J.A., Carlson, D.S., Yellich, G.M., Hendricksen, R.P. Muskuloskelettale Adaptation nach kieferchirurgischen Eingriffen. In: *Kieferorthopädie: Konzepte & Perspektiven.* Pg. 193-214, Ed. E. Hösl, R. Diernberger, P. Grosse.
Verlag Zahnärztlich-Medizinisches Schriftum, München, 1980.

133. McNeil, R.W., Joondeph, D.R. Congenitally absent maxillary lateral incisors: treatment planning considerations.
Angle Orthod. 43: 24-29, 1973.

134. Melsen, B. Preprosthetic movement of anterior teeth.
Belg. Tijdschr. Tandheelk. 37: 111-114, 1982.

135. Melsen, B. Behandlungsprobleme bei Erwachsene Patienten.
Fortschr. Kieferorthop. 34: 112-127, 1983.

136. Melsen, F., Melsen, B., Mosekilde, L., Bergman, S. Histomorphometric analysis of normal bone from the iliac crest.
Acta Pathol. Microbiol. Immunol. Scand. [A] 86: 70-81, 1978.

137. Messer, L.B., Cline, J.T. Ankylosed primary molars: results and treatment recommendations from an eight-year longitudinal study.
Pediatr. Dent. 2: 37-47, 1980.

138. Meyer, W. Der verbogene obere mittlere Schneidezahn.
Zahnärztl. Welt 10: 406-407, 1955.

139. Modeer, T., Odenrick, L. Post-treatment periodontal status of labially erupted maxillary canines.
Acta Odontol. Scand. 38: 253-256, 1980.

140. Moore, A.W. The mechanism of adjustment to wear and accident in the dentition and periodontium.
Angle Orthod. 26: 50-58, 1956.

141. Moorrees, C.F.A. *The dentition of the growing child. A longitudinal study of dental development between 3 and 18 years of age.* Harvard University Press, Cambridge, Mass., 1959.

142. Moorrees, C.F.A., Chadha, J.M. Crown diameters of corresponding tooth groups in the deciduous and permanent dentition. *J. Dent. Res.* 41: 466-470, 1962.

143. Moorrees, C.F.A., Chadha, J.M. Available space for the incisors during dental development. A growth study based on physiologic age. *Angle Orthod.* 35: 12-22, 1965.

144. Moorrees, C.F.A., Reed, R.B. Correlation among crown diameters of human teeth. *Arch. Oral Biol.* 9: 685-697, 1964.

145. Moorrees, C.F.A., Reed, R.B. Changes in dental arch dimensions expressed on the basis of tooth eruption as a measure of biologic age. *J. Dent. Res.* 44: 129-141, 1965.

146. Moyers, R.E. *Handbook of orthodontics.* 3rd ed. Year Book Medical Publ., Chicago, 1973.

147. Mueller, B.H., L'Homme, P.R., Schoenbrodt, F.A., Ayer, W.A. The effect of primary-canine extraction on the IMPA. *J. Dent. Child.* 45: 461-464, 1978.

148. Munro, I.R. The psychological effects of surgical treatment of facial deformity. In: *Psychological aspects of facial form.* Monograph No. 11. Craniofacial Growth Series. Pg. 171-199, Eds. G.W. Lucker, K.A. Ribbens, J.A. McNamara Jr. Center for Human Growth and Development. The University of Michigan, Ann Arbor, Mich., 1980.

149. Nicholas, N.K. Dental injuries in primary and intermediate school children. *N. Z. Dent. J.* 76: 8-11, 1980.

150. Nordquist, G.G., McNeil, R.W. Orthodontic vs. restorative treatment of the congenitally absent lateral incisor. Longterm periodontal and occlusal evaluation. *J. Periodontol.* 46: 139-143, 1975.

151. Northway, W.M. Anteroposterior arch dimension changes in French-Canadian children: a study of the effects of dental caries and premature extractions. M.Sc. Thesis, Montreal, 1977.

152. Northway, W.M. Transplantation of teeth and tooth germs. *Int. Dent. J.* 31: 240-249, 1981.

153. Northway, W.M., Wainright, F.L., Demirjian, A. Effects of premature loss of deciduous molars. *Angle Orthod.* 54: 295-329, 1984.

154. Olive, R.J., Basford, K.E. Transverse dentoskeletal relationships and third molar impaction. *Angle Orthod.* 51: 41-47, 1981.

155. Owen, D. The incidence and nature of space closure following the premature extraction of deciduous teeth. A literature survey. *Am. J. Orthod.* 59: 37-49, 1971.

156. Paige, S.F. A lingual light-wire technique. *J. Clin. Orthod.* 16: 534-544, 1982.

157. Peck, H., Peck, S. An index for assessing tooth shape deviations as applied to mandibular incisors. *Am. J. Orthod.* 61: 384-401, 1972.

158. Pfyffer, A. Über die Spätfolgen der Sechsjahrmolar-Extraktion. *Schweiz. Monatschr. Zahnheilk.* 61: 565-590, 1951.

159. Plint, D.A. The effect on the occlusion of the loss of one or more permanent molars. *Trans. Eur. Orthod. Soc.* 46: 239-336, 1970.

160. Popovich, F., Thompson, G.W., Main, P.A. The maxillary interincisal diastema and its relationship to the superior labial frenulum and intermaxillary suture. *Angle Orthod.* 47: 265-271, 1977.

161. Prahl-Andersen, B., Berendsen, W.J.H. Enige gevolgen van vroegtijdig verlies van tweede melkmolaren in de onderkaak. *Ned. Tijdschr. Tandheelk.* 86: 89-92, 1979.

162. Prahl-Andersen, B., Kowalski, C.J., Heydendael, P.H.J. (Eds.) *A mixed longitudinal, interdisciplinary study of growth and development.* Academic Press, New York, 1979.

163. Pulver, F., Croft, W. A simple method for treating ectopic eruption of the first permanent molar. *Pediatr. Dent.* 5: 140-141, 1983.

164. Ramfjord, S.P. Orthodontics and periodontal prophylaxis. In: *Orthodontics and periodontics.* Pg. 113-125, Eds. E. Hösl, B.U. Zachrisson, A. Baldauf. Quintessence Publ. Co., Chicago, 1985.

165. Ramfjord, S.P., Ash Jr., M.M. *Occlusion.* 3rd ed. W.B. Saunders Co., Philadelphia, 1983.

166. Redmond, A.C., Donner, L., Tilghman, D. Psychological evaluation of facial change following orthognathic surgery. In: *Psychological aspects of facial form.* Monograph No. 11. Craniofacial Growth Series. Pg. 119-141, Eds. G.W. Lucker, K.A. Ribbens, J.A. McNamara Jr. Center for Human Growth and Development. The University of Michigan, Ann Arbor, Mich., 1980.

167. Reitan, V.K. Anfängliches Gewebsverhalten während der Wurzelspitzenre sorption. *Inf. Orthod. Kieferorthop.* 6: 194-211, 1974.

168. Renggli, H.H. Indicaties en contra-indicaties van vaste en afneembare parodontaalspalken. *Belg. Tijdschr. Tandheelk.* 37: 90-93, 1982.

169. Renggli, H.H. Personal communication, 1983.

170. Reychler, A. De derde molaren. *Acta Stomatol. Belg.* 80: 51-58, 1983.

171. Richardson, E.R., Malhotra, S.K., Semenya, K. Longitudinal study of three views of mandibular third molar eruption in males. *Am. J. Orthod.* 86: 119-129, 1984.

172. Richardson, M.E. The relationship between the relative amount of space present in the deciduous dental arch and the rate and degree of space closure subsequent to extraction of a deciduous molar. *Dent. Pract.* (Bristol) 16: 111-118, 1965.

173. Richardson, M.E. The early developmental position of the lower third molar relative to certain jaw dimensions. *Angle Orthod.* 40: 226-230, 1970.

174. Richardson, M.E. Development of the lower third molar from 10 to 15 years. *Angle Orthod.* 43: 191-193, 1973.

175. Richardson, M.E. The development of third molar impaction. *Br. J. Orthod.* 2: 231-234, 1975.

176. Richardson, M.E. Late lower arch crowding in relation to primary crowding. *Angle Orthod.* 52: 300-312, 1982.

177. Richardson, M.E. Lower molar crowding in the early permanent dentition. *Angle Orthod.* 55: 51-57, 1985.

178. Ricketts, R.M. Perspectives in the clinical application of cephalometrics. *Angle Orthod.* 51: 115-150, 1981.

179. Ricketts, R.M. A principle of arcial growth of the mandible. *Angle Orthod.* 42: 368-386, 1972.

180. Ricketts, R.M., Turley, P., Chaconas, S., Schulhof, R.J. Third molar enucleation: diagnosis and technique. *J. Calif. Dent. Assoc.* 4: 52-57, 1976.

181. Riedel, R.A. Post-pubertal occlusal changes. In: *The biology of occlusal development.* Monograph No. 7. Craniofacial Growth Series. Pg. 113-140, Ed. J.A. McNamara Jr. Center for Human Growth and Development. The University of Michigan, Ann Arbor, Mich., 1977.

182. Roeters, J.F.M. Toepassing en verwerking van voorgevormde kunstharsvensters ter verbetering van esthetiek van frontelementen. *Ned. Tijdschr. Tandheelk.* 88: 131-135, 1981.

183. Roeters, J.J.M., Van der Linden, F.P.G.M. Problems after trauma of maxillary central permanent incisors: lessons from a case report. *Quintessence Int.* 9: 639-647, 1985.

183a. Roeters, J.J.M., De Kloet. Kosmetische Zahnheilkunde mit Komposit. Quintessenz Verlag GmbH, Berlin, 1990.

184. Rönnerman, A. Early extraction of deciduous molars and canines. *Trans. Eur. Orthod. Soc.* 41: 153-168, 1965.

185. Rönnerman, A. The effect of early loss of primary molars on tooth eruption and space conditions. A longitudinal study. *Acta Odontol. Scand.* 35: 229-239, 1977.

186. Salzmann, J.A. A study of orthodontic and facial changes and effects on dentition attending the loss of first molars in five hundred adolescents. *J. Am. Dent. Assoc.* 25: 892-905, 1938.

187. Sampson, W.J., Richards, L.C., Leighton, B.C. Third molar eruption patterns and mandibular dental arch crowding. *Aust. Orthod. J.* 8: 10-20, 1983.

188. Schiller, W. Positional changes in mesioangular impacted mandibular third molars during a year. *J. Am. Dent. Assoc.* 99: 460-464, 1979.

189. Schröder, U., Granath, L. A new interceptive treatment of cases with missing maxillary lateral incisors. *Swed. Dent. J.* 5: 155-158, 1981.

190. Schulhof, R.J. Third molars and orthodontic diagnosis. *J. Clin. Orthod.* 10: 272-281, 1976.

191. Schulze, C. Über Retention und Reinklusion (Depression) erster und zwei ter Molaren. *Zeitschr. Zahn-, Mund- und Kieferheilkd.* 37: 338-375, 1962.

192. Schwarz, A.M. *Lehrgang der Gebissreglung.* Band II. Urban & Schwarzenberg, Wien, 1953.

193. Schwarz, D. Die Problematik des Sechsjahrmolaren in der Kinderstomatolo gische Betreuung. *Stomatol. DDR* 30: 423-433, 1980.

194. Schwarze, C.W. The influence of third molar germectomy — a comparative long-term study. Trans. Third Intern. Orthod. Congr. 551-562. The C.V. Mosby Co., St. Louis, 1975.

195. Eipel, C.M. Prevention of malocclusion. *Trans. Eur. Orthod. Soc.* 24: 203-213, 1948.
196. Selliseth, N.E. The significance of traumatised primary incisors on the development and eruption of permanent teeth. *Trans. Eur. Orthod. Soc.* 46: 443-459, 1970.
197. Shapiro, P.A. Mandibular arch form and dimension. *Am. J. Orthod.* 66: 58-70, 1974.
198. Shiere, F.R., Frankl, S.N. The effect of deciduous tooth infections on permanent teeth. *Dent. Progress* 2: 59-68, 1961.
199. Slagsvold, O., Bjercke, B. Indications for autotransplantation in cases of missing premolars. *Am. J. Orthod.* 74: 241-257, 1978.
200. Slagsvold, O., Bjercke, B. Applicability of autotransplantation in cases of missing upper anterior teeth. *Am. J. Orthod.* 74: 410-421, 1978.
201. Spalding, P.M., Fields, H.W., Torney, D., Cobb, H.B. The changing role of endodontics and orthodontics in the management of traumatically intruded permanent incisors. *Pediatr. Dent.* 7: 104-110, 1985.
202. Spouge, J.D., Feasby, W.H. Erupted teeth in the newborn. *Oral Surg. Oral Med. Oral Pathol.* 22: 198-208, 1966.
203. Steigman, S., Koyoumdjisky-Kaye, E., Matrai, Y. Submerged deciduous molars in preschool children: an epidemiologic survey. *J. Dent. Res.* 52: 322-326, 1973.
204. Steigman, S., Koyoumdjisky-Kaye, E., Matrai, Y. Submerged deciduous molars and congenital absence of premolars. *J. Dent. Res.* 52: 842, 1973.
205. Svanberg, G. Influence of trauma from occlusion on the periodontium of dogs with normal or inflamed gingiva. *Odontol. Revy* 25: 165-178, 1974.
206. Svendsen, H., Malmskov, O., Björk, A. Prediction of lower third molar impaction from the frontal cephalometric projection. *Eur. J. Orthod.* 7: 1-16, 1985.
207. Tait, R.V. Mesial migration and lower third molar tilt. *Br. J. Orthod.* 9: 41-47, 1982.
208. Ten Hoeve, A., Mulie, R.M. The effect of antero-postero incisor repositioning on the palatal cortex as studied with laminagraphy. *J. Clin. Orthod.* 10: 804-822.
209. Thilander, B. Indication for orthodontic treatment in adults. *Eur. J. Orthod.* 1: 227-241, 1979.
210. Thilander, B. Orthodontic treatment in dentitions with reduced periodontal support. *Belg. Tijdschr. Tandheelk.* 37: 119-125, 1982.
211. Thilander, B., Skagius, S. Orthodontic sequelae of extraction of permanent first molars. A longitudinal study. *Trans. Eur. Orthod. Soc.* 46: 429-442, 1970.
212. Thunhold, K. Early loss of the first molars 25 years after. *Trans. Eur. Orthod. Soc.* 46: 349-365, 1970.
213. Tränkmann, J. Kieferorthopädische Behandlungsmassnahmen vor der prothetische Versorgung Erwachsener. 1. Teil. *ZWR* 88: 309-311, 1979.
214. Tuverson, D. Orthodontic treatment using canines in place of missing lateral incisors. *Am. J. Orthod.* 58: 109-127, 1970.
215. Ungar, A.L. Incidence and effects of premature loss of deciduous teeth. *Int. J. Orthod.* 24: 613-621, 1938.
216. Vanarsdall, R. Correction of periodontal problems through orthodontic treatment. In: *Orthodontics and periodontics.* Pg. 127-167, Eds. E. Hösl, B.U. Zachrisson, A. Baldauf. Quintessence Publ. Co., Chicago, 1985.
217. Van Beers, W.J.D.M., Van der Linden, F.P.G.M. Retentie van blijvende ondermolaren. In preparation.
218. Van der Linden, F.P.G.M. Theoretical and practical aspects of crowding in the human dentition. *J. Am. Dent. Assoc.* 89: 139-153, 1974.
219. Van der Linden, F.P.G.M. Zwei Varianten der Klasse II/1. *Fortschr. Kieferorthop.* 36: 51-72, 1975.
220. Van der Linden, F.P.G.M. Models in the development of the human dentition. In: *The biology of occlusal development.* Monograph No. 7. Craniofacial Growth Series. Pg. 43-60, Ed. J.A. McNamara Jr. Center for Human Growth and Development. The University of Michigan, Ann Arbor, Mich., 1977.
221. Van der Linden, F.P.G.M. Stabilität Kieferorthopädisch chirurgischer Korrekturen. *Inf. Orthod. Kieferorthop.* 10: 461-471, 1978.
222. Van der Linden, F.P.G.M. Changes in the position of posterior teeth in relation to ruga points. *Am. J. Orthod.* 74: 142-161, 1978.
223. Van der Linden, F.P.G.M. *Development of the dentition.* Quintessence Publ. Co., Chicago, 1983.

224. Van der Linden, F.P.G.M. *Facial growth and facial orthopedics.* Quintessence Publ. Co., Chicago, 1986.
225. Van der Linden, F.P.G.M. (ed.) *Transition of the human dentition.* Monograph No. 13. Craniofacial Growth Series. Center for Human Growth and Development. The University of Michigan, Ann Arbor, Mich., 1982.
226. Van der Linden, F.P.G.M., Boersma, H. *Diagnosis and treatment planning in dentofacial orthopedics.* Quintessence Publ. Co., Chicago, 1987.
227. Van der Linden, F.P.G.M., Duterloo, H.S. *The development of the human dentition. An atlas.* Harper & Row, New York, 1976.
228. Van der Veen, J.A. *Frenulum labii superioris.* Academisch Proefschrift, Groningen, 1971.
229. Van der Veen-Le Grand, C.E. De spoon-prothese. *Ned. Tijdschr. Tandheelk.* 89: 437-442, 1982.
230. Van der Zwan, J., Boering, G. *Operatieve kaakorthopedie.* Stafleu & Tholen, Alphen aan den Rijn, 1981.
231. Van Dijk, L., Bosker, H. Autotransplantatie van gebitselementen. *Ned. Tijdschr. Tandheelk.* 88: 242-246, 1981.
232. Venn, R.J. Ectopic eruption of permanent first molars: a clinical technique. *J. Pedodont.* 10: 81-88, 1985.
233. Vermeeren, J.I.J.F. De chirurgische behandeling van mesiodentes. *Ned. Tijdschr. Tandheelk.* 82: 415-416, 1975.
234. Vig, P.S., Cohen, A.M. Vertical growth of the lips: a serial cephalometric study. *Am. J. Orthod.* 75: 405-415, 1979.
235. West, R.A., McNeill, R.W. Diagnosis and treatment planning: a coordinated effort between oral and maxillofacial surgery and orthodontics. *J. Oral Surg.* 39: 809-816, 1981.
236. Williams, R., Hosila, F.J. The effect of different extraction sites upon incisor retraction. *Am. J. Orthod.* 69: 388-410, 1976.
237. Williams, S., Melsen, B., Agerbaek, N., Asboe, V. The orthodontic treatment of malocclusion in patients with previous periodontal disease. *Br. J. Orthod.* 9: 178-184, 1982.
238. Willis, T.A. The impacted mandibular molar. *Angle Orthod.* 36: 165-168, 1966.
239. Wilson, H.E. Long term observation on the extraction of second permanent molars. *Eur. Orthod. Soc.* 50: 215-221, 1974.
240. Worms, F.W., Speidel, T.M., Bevis, R.R., Waite, D.E. Posttreatment stability and esthetics of orthognatic surgery. *Angle Orthod.* 50: 251-273, 1980.
241. Zachrisson, B. Clinical implications of recent ortho-perio research findings. In: *Orthodontics and periodontics.* Pg. 169-186, Eds. E. Hösl, B.U. Zachrisson, A. Baldauf. Quintessence Publ. Co., Chicago, 1985.
242. Zachrisson, B., Thilander, B. Treatment of dento-alveolar anomalies. In: *Introduction to orthodontics.* Pg. 135-184, Eds. B. Thilander, O. Rönning. Tandläkarförlaget, Stockholm, 1985.
243. Zachrisson, B.U. Improving orthodontic results in cases with maxillary incisors missing. *Am. J. Orthod.* 73: 274-289, 1978.
244. Zachrisson, B.U., Alnaes, L. Periodontal condition in orthodontically treated and untreated individuals. II. Loss of attachment, gingival pocket depth and clinical crown height. *Angle Orthod.* 43: 402-411, 1973.

Index

* Numbers in italics refer to figures

U

V